Thieme

Pocket Atlas of Sectional Anatomy

Computed Tomography and Magnetic Resonance Imaging

Volume III
Spine, Extremities, Joints

Torsten B. Moeller, MD
Department of Radiology
Marienhaus Klinikum
Saarlouis/Dillingen, Germany

Emil Reif, MD
Department of Teleradiology
reif & moeller diagnostic-network
Dillingen, Germany

Second Edition
725 illustrations

Thieme
Stuttgart · New York · Delhi · Rio de Janeiro

Library of Congress Cataloging-in-Publication Data is available from the publisher.

Original translation of 1st edition by Barbara Herzberger, MD, Munich, Germany

Illustrator: Barbara Gay, Stuttgart, Germany

1st French edition 2008
1st Greek edition 2014
1st Hungarian edition 2010
1st Italian edition 2007
1st Japanese edition 2008
1st Korean edition 2010
1st Polish edition 2007
1st Portuguese edition 2009
1st Russian edition 2010
1st Spanish edition 2007
1st Turkish edition 2007

Thieme Publishers Stuttgart
Rüdigerstrasse 14, 70469 Stuttgart, Germany
+49 [0]711 8931 421,
customerservice@thieme.de

Thieme Publishers New York
333 Seventh Avenue, New York, NY 10001, USA
+1-800-782-3488,
customerservice@thieme.com

Thieme Publishers Delhi
A-12, Second Floor, Sector-2, Noida-201301
Uttar Pradesh, India
+91 120 45 566 00,
customerservice@thieme.in

Thieme Publishers Rio,
Thieme Publicações Ltda.
Edifício Rodolpho de Paoli, 25° andar
Av. Nilo Peçanha, 50 – Sala 2508
Rio de Janeiro 20020-906 Brasil
+55 21 3172 2297 / +55 21 3172 1896

Cover design: Thieme Publishing Group

Typesetting by primustype Robert Hurler GmbH, Notzingen, Germany

Printed in Italy by L.E.G.O., Vicenza

5 4 3 2 1

ISBN 978-3-13-143172-1

Also available as an e-book:
eISBN 978-3-13-201962-1

For my American relatives

Bernie and Arlene, Bryan and Nancy, Rick, Krista, and Ella Rose, Bill, Kayla, Abby and Liviana, Shirley, Mike, Austin and Amanda, Michael and Kendall, Audrey, Mike and Kristen, Katelyn and Matt, Claudia and Larry, Bryan and Stacy, Jamie and Shawn, Meghan and Jason

Contents

Preface

We have been greatly gratified and much encouraged by the very positive responses to our volume III of the *Pocket Atlas of Sectional Anatomy*, the "Musculoskeletal Atlas," and by its wide distribution and the many foreign-language editions. This success was a spur to further improvements. Accordingly, to the existing images of the first edition, which focus on the regions in the proximity of the joints, we have added new images and illustrations of the complete upper and lower arm and thigh and lower leg in two planes. With these we bridge and fill the previous gap regarding bone or soft tissue lesions of the diaphysis such as those caused by inflammation or tumors. The regular structure of the book has been preserved: the uniform color schemes for the different muscles, vessels, nerves, and other anatomical structures; and the comparison of high-quality (3-tesla) magnetic resonance images with the drawings. We thus hope to achieve precision and clarity and to facilitate locating and identifying the relevant anatomical structures.

As with the other volumes, the work would not have been possible without the invaluable support of so many dedicated assistants. We express our cordial thanks to all of them.

Special thanks go to Carina Engler for her consistent commitment to obtaining optimal images and to our entire MRI team, as well as to Nicole Bigga for making the 3-tesla images.

We wish the readers of this book once again as much pleasure and joy in using it as we had in making the images and the illustrations.

Torsten B. Moeller, MD
Emil Reif, MD

- Arteries
- Nerves
- Veins
- Bones
- Fatty tissue
- Cartilage
- Tendon
- Disk, labrum etc.
- Fluid

Muscles of Trunk:
Serratus anterior
Omohyoid
Trapezius
Subclavius
Intercostal

Muscles of Shoulder:
Deltoid
Infraspinatus
Pectoralis major and pectoralis minor
Subscapularis
Coracobrachialis
Latissimus dorsi
Dorsal Muscles of Lower Arm:
Supinator
Extensor pollicis longus and brevis
Extensor indicis
Muscles of Hand:
Dorsal and palmar interosseous
Lumbrical

Volar Muscles of Upper Arm:
Biceps brachii
Brachialis

Dorsal Muscles of Upper Arm:
Triceps brachii
Anconeus

Dorsal Muscles of Lower Arm (superficial layer):
Extensor digitorum
Extensor digiti minimi
Extensor carpi ulnaris

Radial Muscles of Lower Arm:
Brachioradialis
Extensor carpi radialis longus
and Extensor carpi radialis brevis

Volar Muscles of Lower Arm (superficial layer):
Pronator teres
Flexor digitorum superficialis
Flexor carpi radialis and flexor carpi ulnaris
Palmaris longus and palmaris brevis

Volar Muscles of Lower Arm (deep layer):
Flexor digitorum profundus
Flexor pollicis longus
Pronator quadratus

Muscles of Little (Fifth) Finger:
Abductor digiti minimi brevis
Flexor digiti minimi brevis
Opponens digiti minimi

Muscles of Thumb:
Abductor pollicis longus
and abductor pollicis brevis
Opponens pollicis
Flexor pollicis brevis
Adductor pollicis

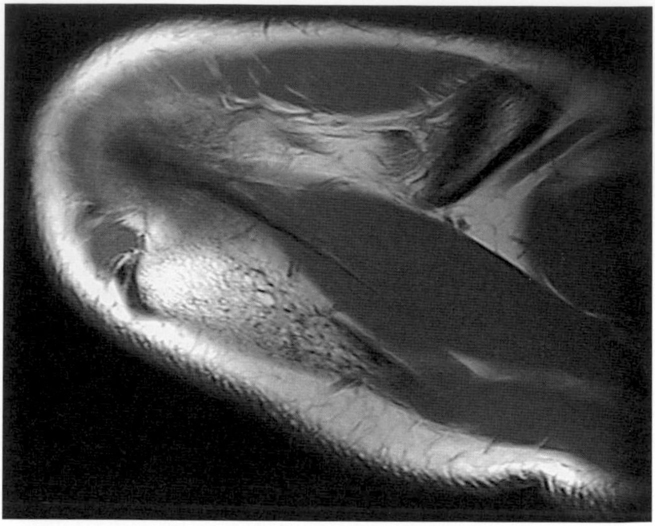

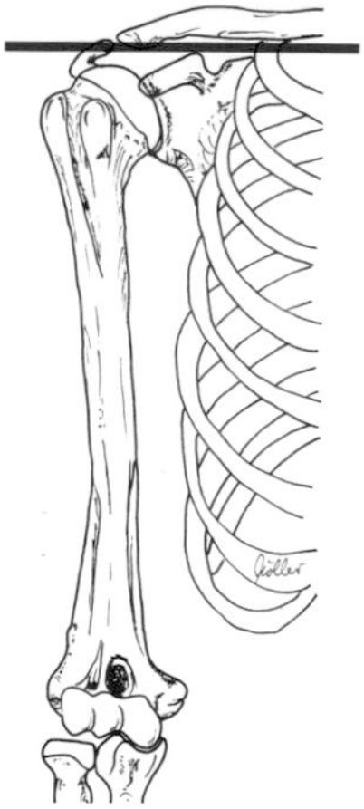

Ventral

Lateral ☐ Medial

Dorsal

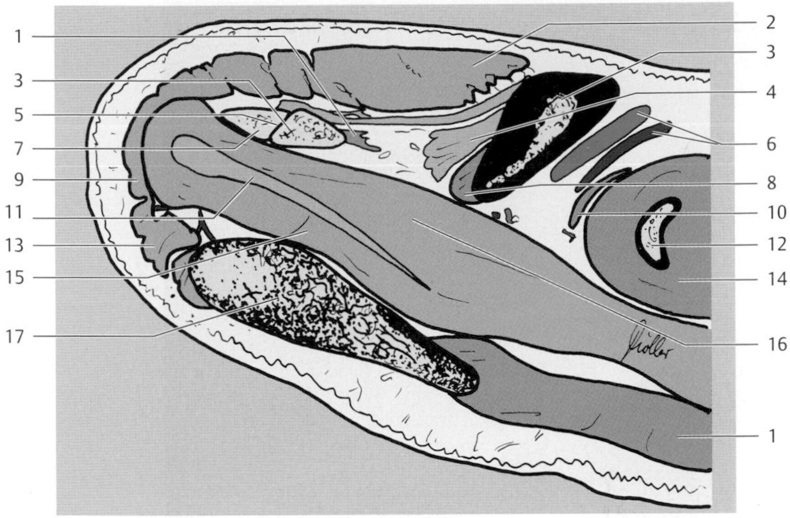

1 Trapezius muscle
2 Deltoid muscle (clavicular part)
3 Clavicle
4 Coracoclavicular ligament
5 Acromioclavicular joint
6 Suprascapular artery and vein
7 Acromion
8 Subclavius muscle
9 Deltoid muscle (acromial part)
10 Omohyoid muscle
11 Supraspinatus muscle (central tendon)
12 Rib
13 Deltoid muscle (spinal part)
14 Serratus anterior muscle
15 Supraspinatus muscle (dorsal ligament)
16 Supraspinatus muscle (ventral ligament)
17 Spine of scapula

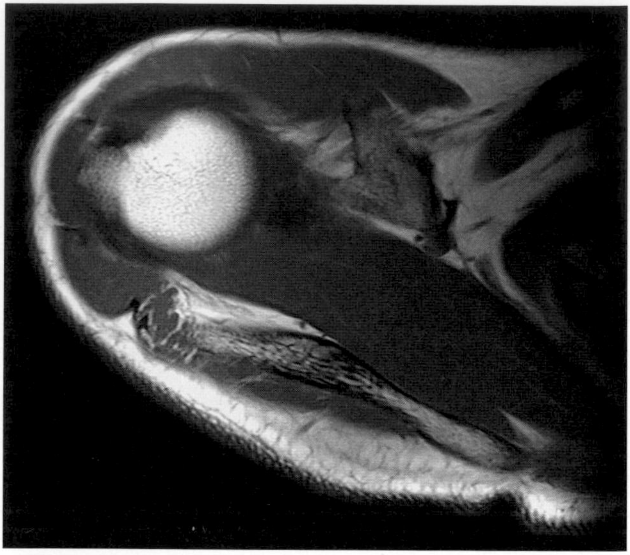

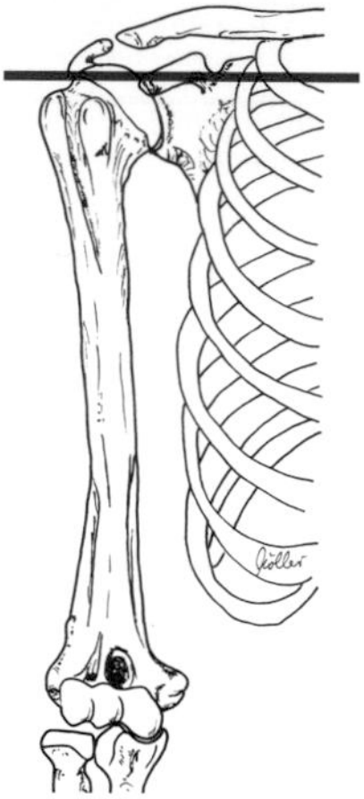

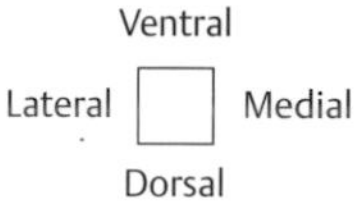
Ventral
Lateral
Medial
Dorsal

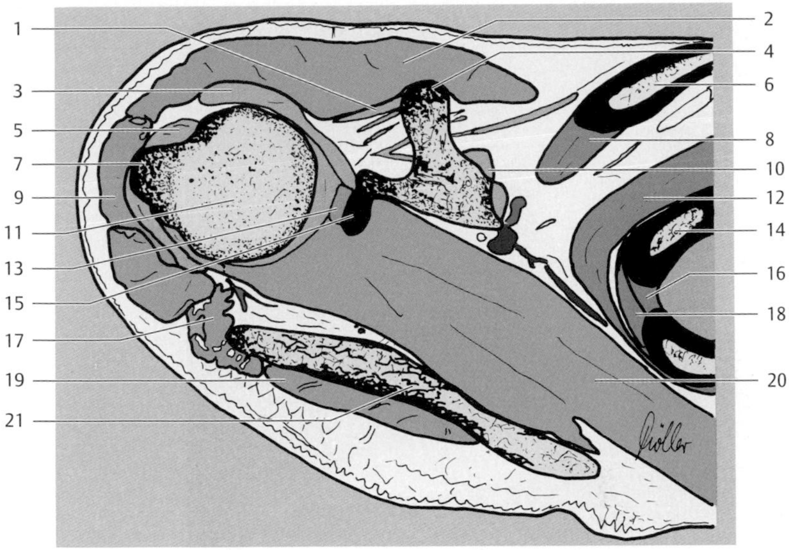

1 Coracohumeral ligament
2 Deltoid muscle (clavicular part)
3 Middle glenohumeral ligament
4 Coracoid process
5 Supraspinatus muscle (tendon)
6 Clavicle
7 Humerus (greater tubercle)
8 Subclavius muscle
9 Deltoid muscle (acromial part)
10 Coracoclavicular ligament
11 Head of humerus
12 Serratus anterior muscle
13 Superior glenoid labrum
14 Rib
15 Glenoid
16 Internal intercostal muscle
17 Deltoid muscle (spinal part)
18 External intercostal muscle
19 Infraspinatus muscle
20 Supraspinatus muscle
21 Spine of scapula

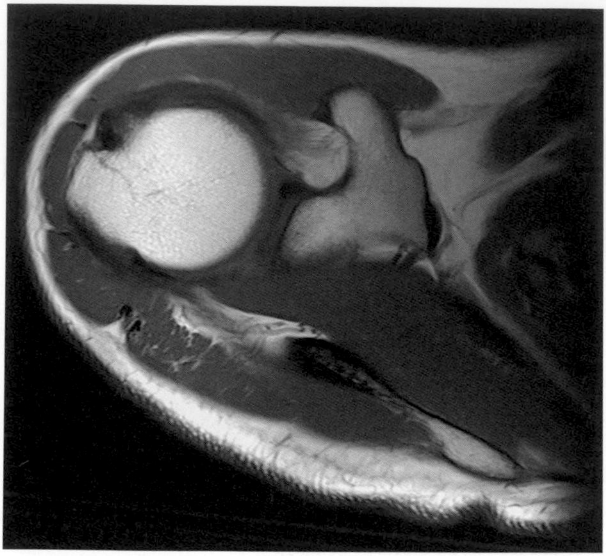

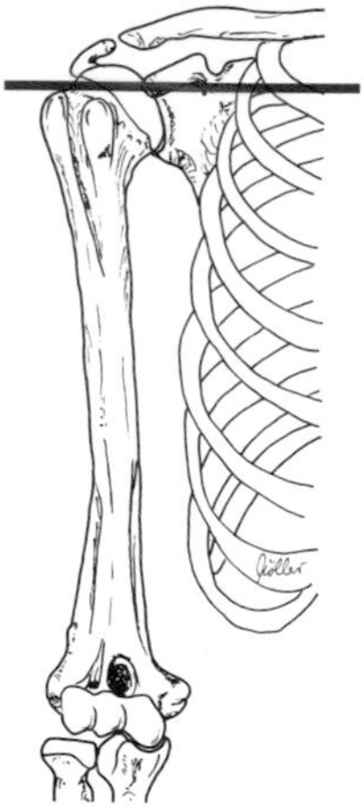

Ventral

Lateral Medial

Dorsal

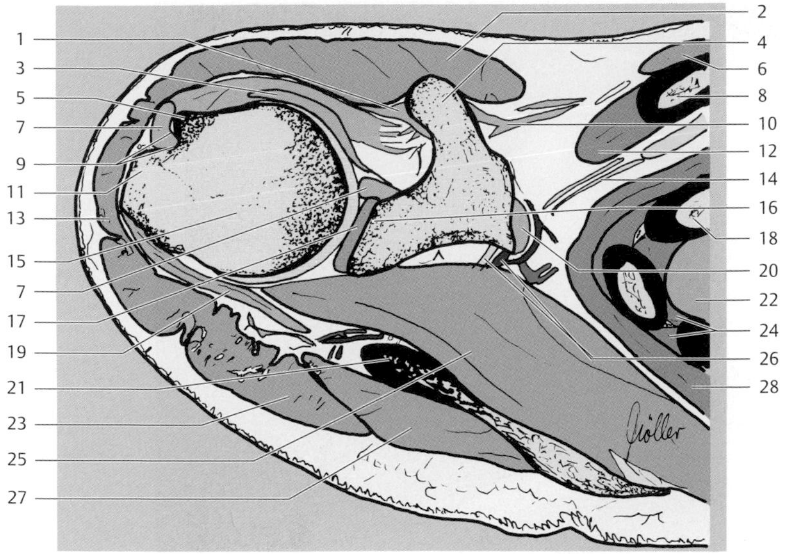

1 Coracohumeral ligament
2 Deltoid muscle (clavicular part)
3 Middle glenohumeral ligament
4 Coracoid process
5 Humerus (lesser tubercle)
6 Pectoralis major muscle
7 Biceps brachii muscle (long head, tendon)
8 Clavicle
9 Intertubercular sulcus (bicipital groove)
10 Pectoralis minor muscle (tendon)
11 Humerus (greater tubercle)
12 Subclavius muscle
13 Deltoid muscle (acromial part)
14 Brachial plexus
15 Head of humerus
16 Glenoid
17 Superior glenoid labrum
18 Rib
19 Infraspinatus muscle (tendon attachment)
20 Coracoclavicular ligament
21 Spine of scapula
22 Lung
23 Deltoid muscle (spinal part)
24 Internal and external intercostal muscles
25 Supraspinatus muscle
26 Suprascapular artery, vein and nerve
27 Infraspinatus muscle
28 Serratus anterior muscle

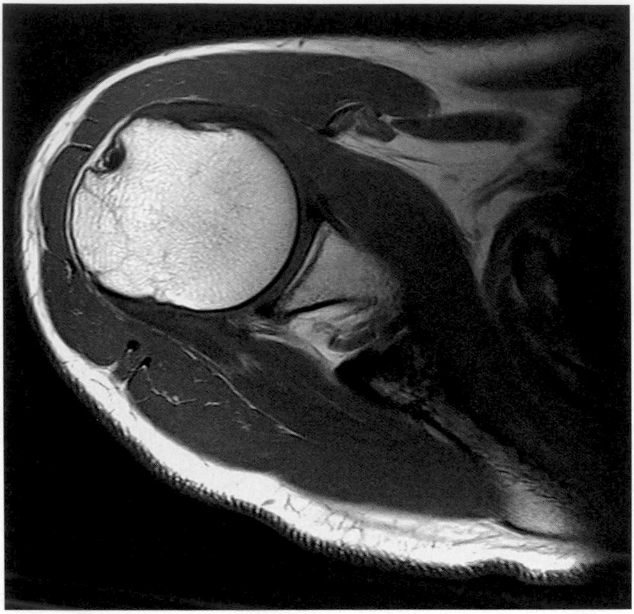

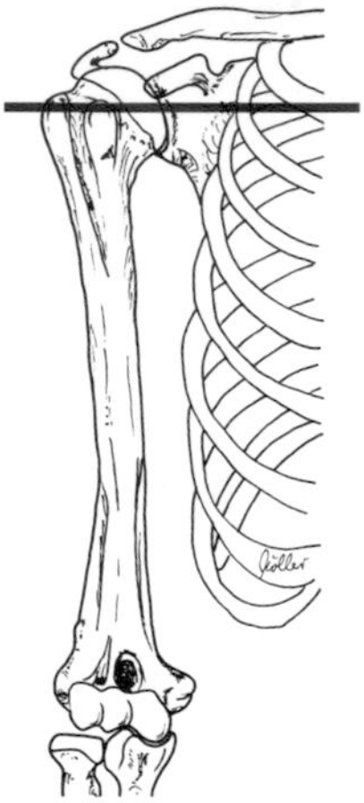

Ventral

Lateral ☐ Medial

Dorsal

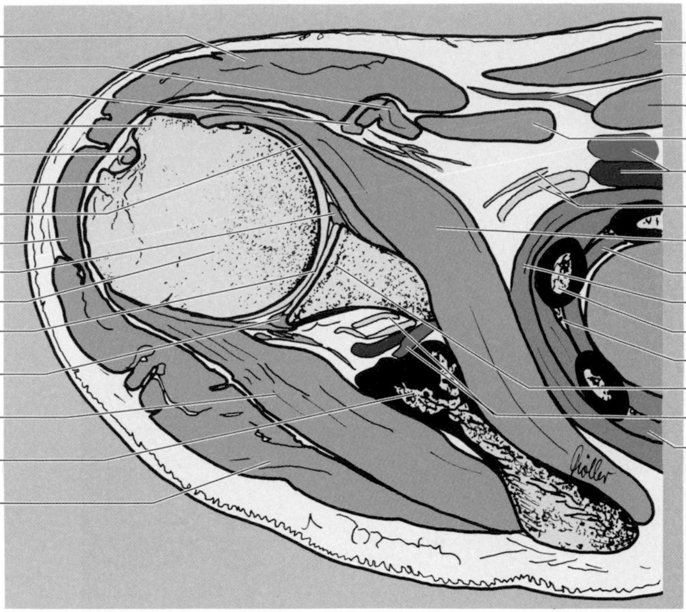

1 Deltoid muscle (clavicular part)
2 Pectoralis major muscle
3 Coracobrachialis muscle (+ tendon)
4 Cephalic vein
5 Biceps brachii muscle (short head, tendon)
6 Subclavius muscle
7 Humerus (lesser tubercle)
8 Pectoralis minor muscle
9 Biceps brachii muscle (long head, tendon)
10 Axillary artery and vein
11 Humerus (greater tubercle)
12 Brachial plexus and subscapular nerve
13 Middle glenohumeral ligament
14 Subscapularis muscle
15 Deltoid muscle (acromial part)
16 Internal intercostal muscle
17 Anterior glenoid labrum
18 Serratus anterior muscle
19 Head of humerus
20 Rib
21 Humeroscapular joint
22 Intercostal artery, vein, and nerve
23 Posterior glenoid labrum
24 Glenoid
25 Infraspinatus muscle
26 Suprascapular artery, vein, and nerve
27 Scapula
28 External intercostal muscle
29 Deltoid muscle (spinal part)

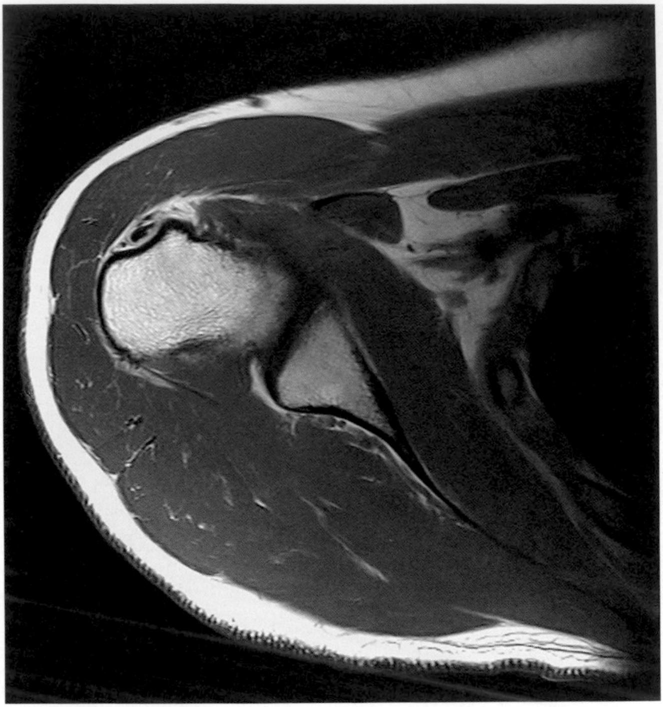

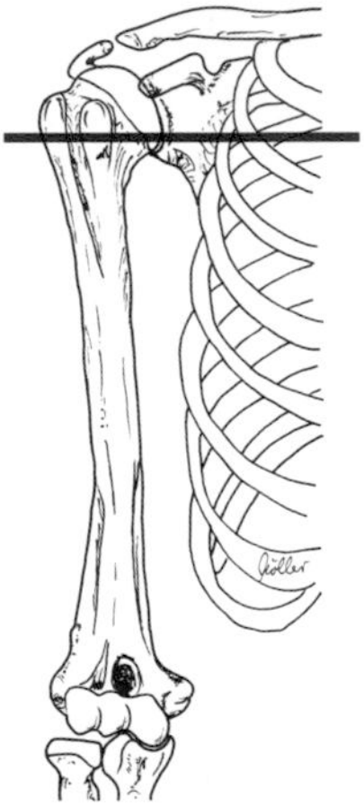

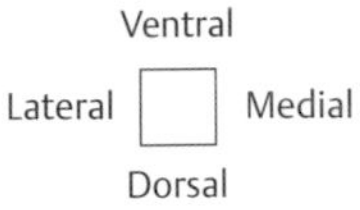
Ventral
Lateral
Medial
Dorsal

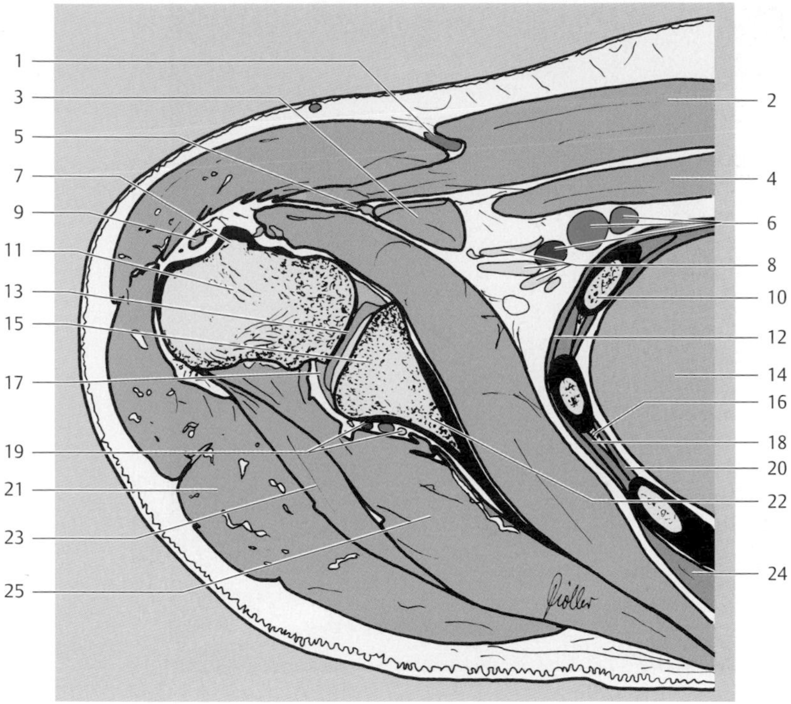

1 Cephalic vein
2 Pectoralis major muscle
3 Coracobrachialis muscle (+ tendon)
4 Pectoralis minor muscle
5 Biceps brachii muscle (short head, tendon)
6 Axillary artery and vein
7 Humerus (lesser tubercle)
8 Brachial plexus
9 Biceps brachii muscle (long head, tendon)
10 Rib
11 Humerus
12 Serratus anterior muscle
13 Inferior glenoid labrum
14 Lung
15 Glenoid
16 Intercostal artery, vein, and nerve
17 Joint capsule
18 External intercostal muscle
19 Suprascapular artery, vein, and nerve
20 Internal intercostal muscle
21 Deltoid muscle
22 Scapula
23 Teres minor muscle
24 Serratus posterior muscle
25 Infraspinatus muscle

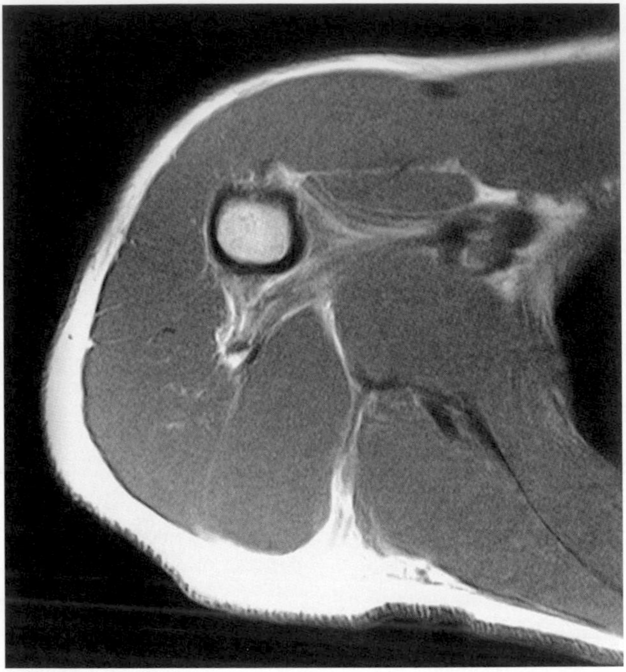

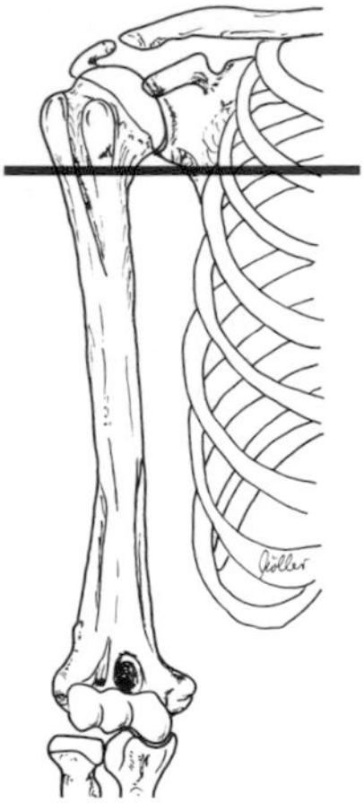

Ventral

Lateral Medial

Dorsal

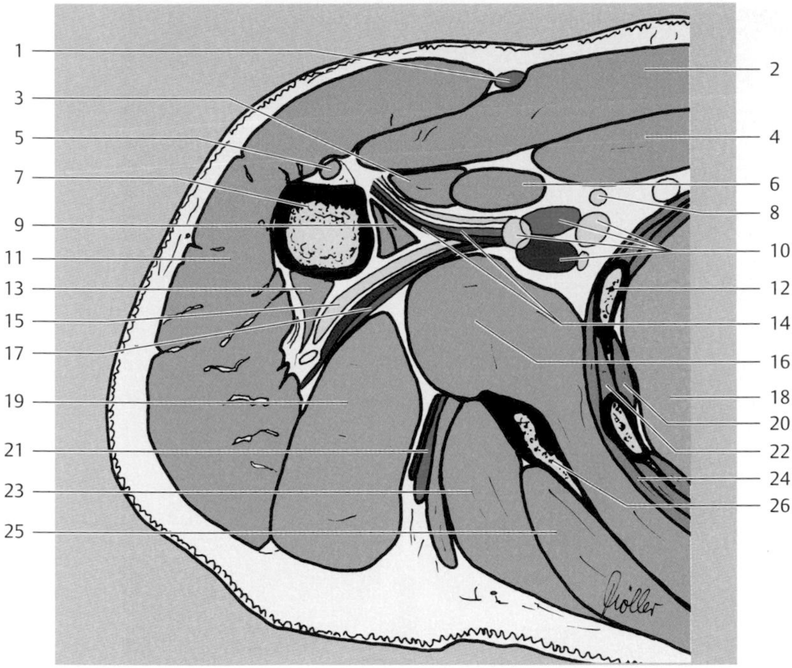

1 Cephalic vein
2 Pectoralis major muscle
3 Biceps brachii muscle (short head, tendon)
4 Pectoralis minor muscle
5 Biceps brachii muscle (long head, tendon)
6 Coracobrachialis muscle
7 Humerus
8 Long thoracic nerve
9 Latissimus dorsi muscle and teres major muscle
10 Axillary artery and vein and brachial plexus
11 Deltoid muscle
12 Rib
13 Triceps brachii muscle (lateral head)
14 Anterior circumflex humeral artery and vein
15 Axillary nerve
16 Subscapularis muscle
17 Posterior circumflex humeral artery and vein
18 Lung
19 Triceps brachii muscle (long head)
20 Internal intercostal muscle and innermost intercostal muscle
21 Circumflex scapular artery and vein
22 External intercostal muscle
23 Teres minor muscle
24 Serratus anterior muscle
25 Infraspinatus muscle
26 Scapula

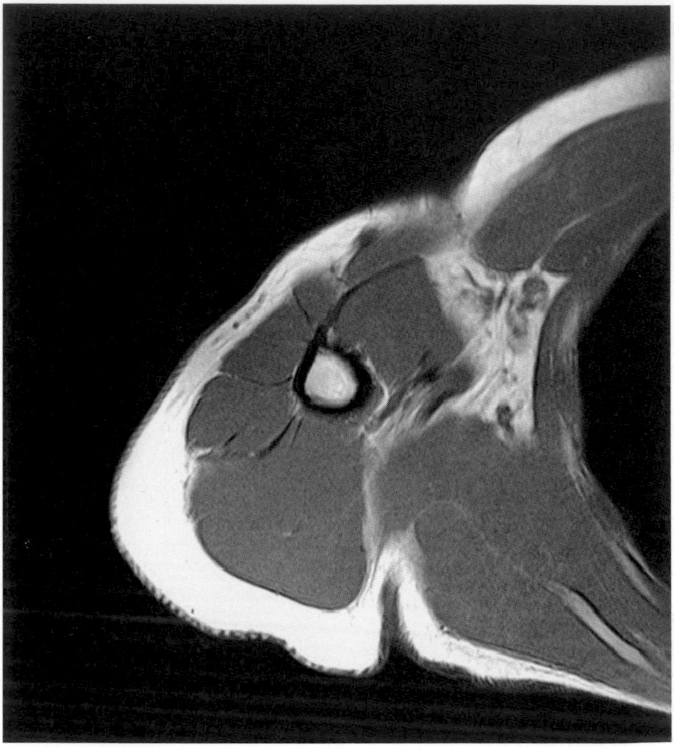

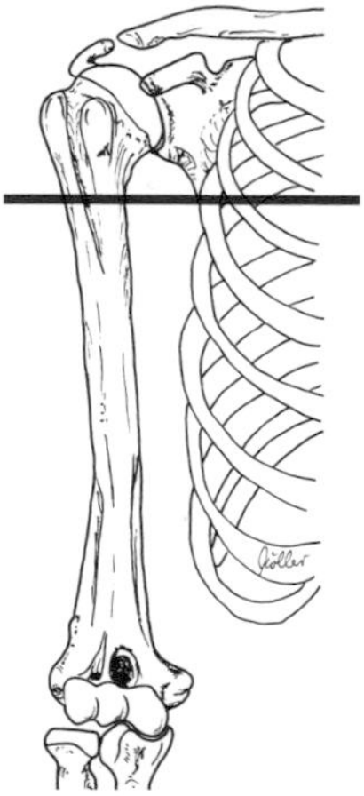

Ventral

Lateral ☐ Medial

Dorsal

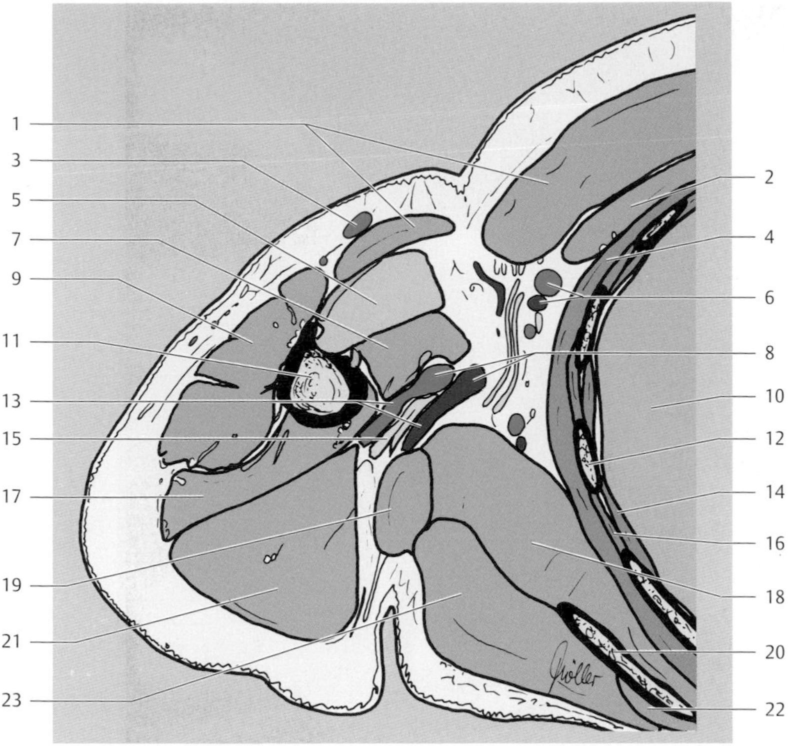

1 Pectoralis major muscle
2 Pectoralis minor muscle
3 Cephalic vein
4 Serratus anterior muscle
5 Biceps brachii muscle
6 Lateral thoracic artery and vein
7 Coracobrachialis muscle
8 Axillary artery and vein
9 Deltoid muscle
10 Lung
11 Humerus
12 Rib
13 Deep artery and vein of arm
14 Internal and innermost intercostal muscles
15 Radial nerve
16 External intercostal muscle
17 Triceps brachii muscle (lateral head)
18 Subscapularis muscle
19 Teres major muscle
20 Scapula
21 Triceps brachii muscle (long head)
22 Infraspinatus muscle
23 Teres major muscle and latissimus dorsi muscle

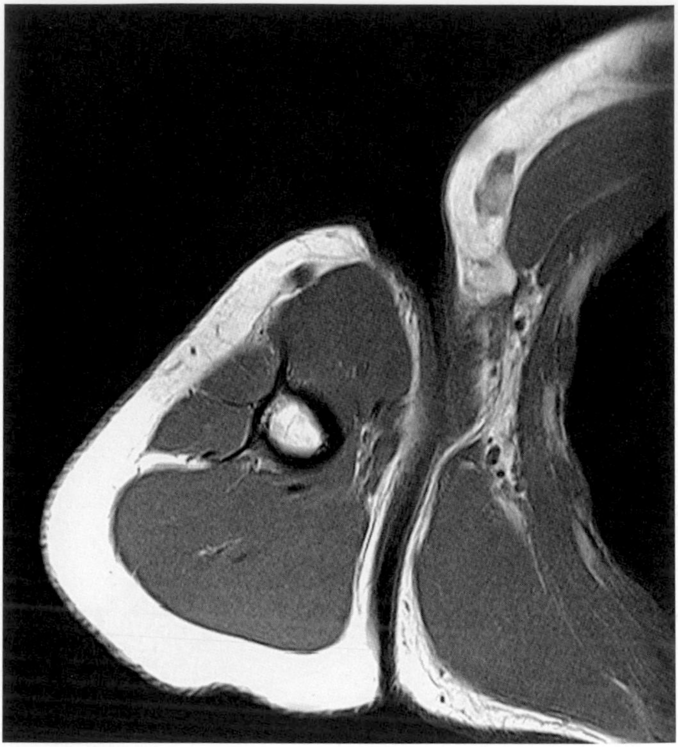

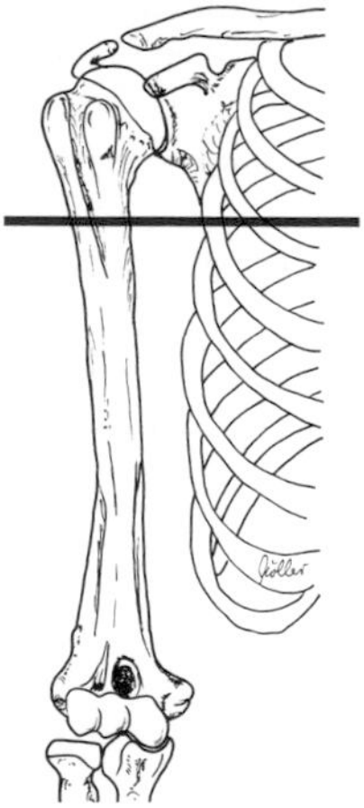

Ventral

Lateral ☐ Medial

Dorsal

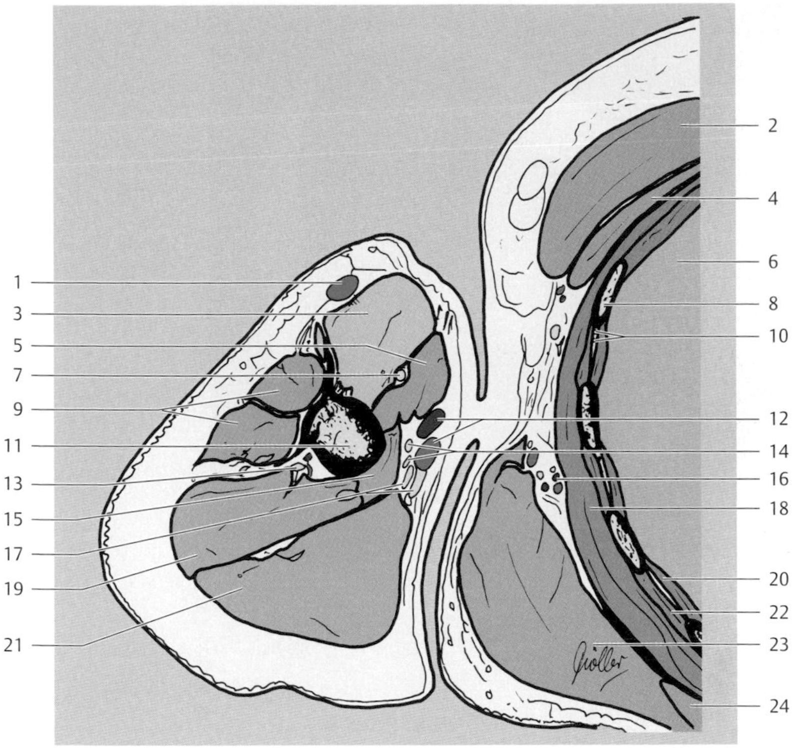

1 Cephalic vein
2 Pectoralis major muscle
3 Biceps brachii muscle
4 Pectoralis minor muscle
5 Coracobrachialis muscle
6 Lung
7 Musculocutaneous nerve
8 Rib
9 Deltoid muscle
10 Intercostal artery, vein, and nerve
11 Humerus (shaft)
12 Brachial artery and vein
13 Radial nerve
14 Median nerve
15 Triceps brachii muscle (medial head)
16 Thoracodorsal artery, vein and nerve
17 Ulnar nerve
18 Serratus anterior muscle
19 Triceps brachii muscle (lateral head)
20 Internal and innermost intercostal muscles
21 Triceps brachii muscle (lateral head)
22 External intercostal muscle
23 Teres major muscle and latissimus dorsi muscle
24 Infraspinatus muscle

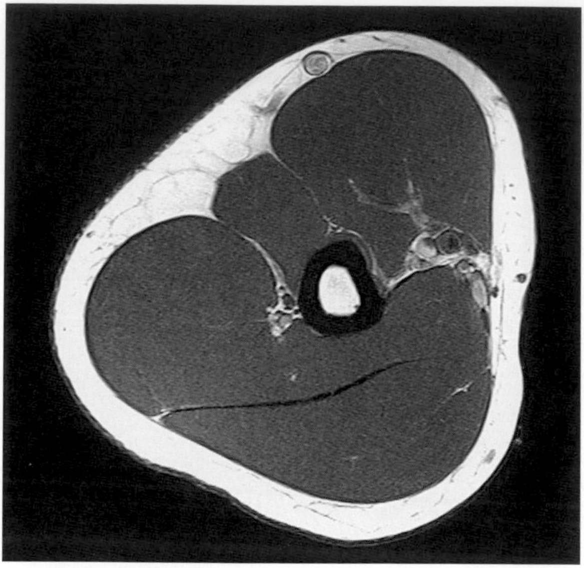

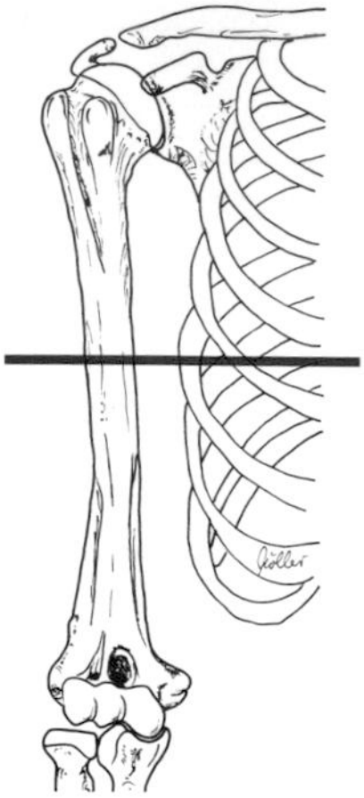
Röller

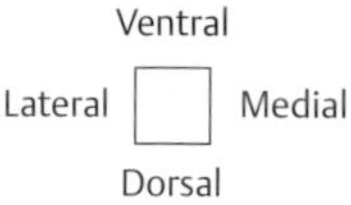
Ventral
Lateral
Medial
Dorsal

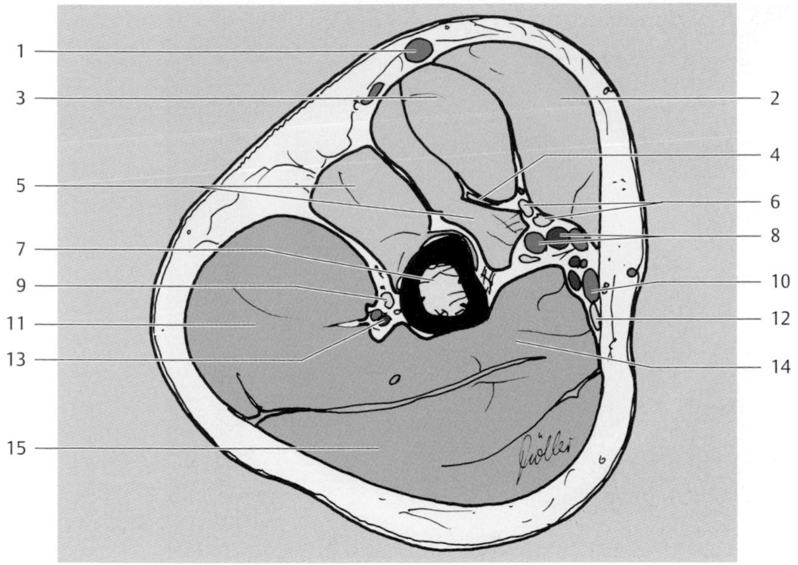

1 Cephalic vein
2 Biceps brachii muscle (short head)
3 Biceps brachii muscle (long head)
4 Musculocutaneous nerve
5 Brachial muscle
6 Median nerve
7 Humerus (shaft)
8 Brachial artery and vein
9 Radial nerve
10 Basilic vein
11 Triceps brachii muscle (lateral head)
12 Ulnar nerve
13 Deep brachial artery and vein
14 Triceps brachii muscle (medial head)
15 Triceps brachii muscle (long head)

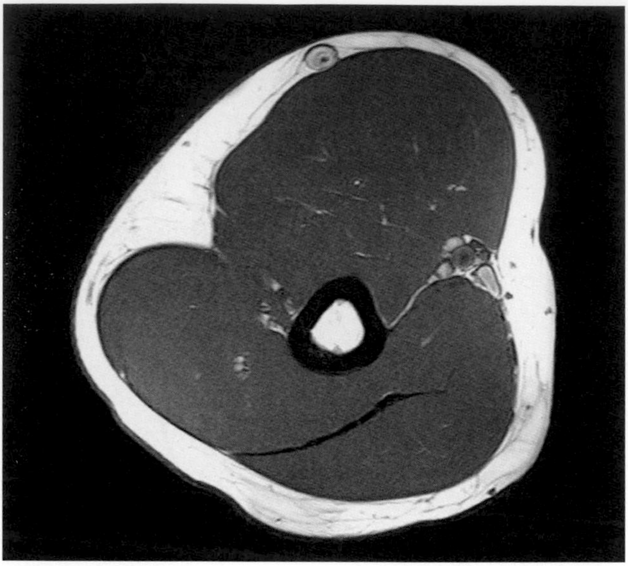

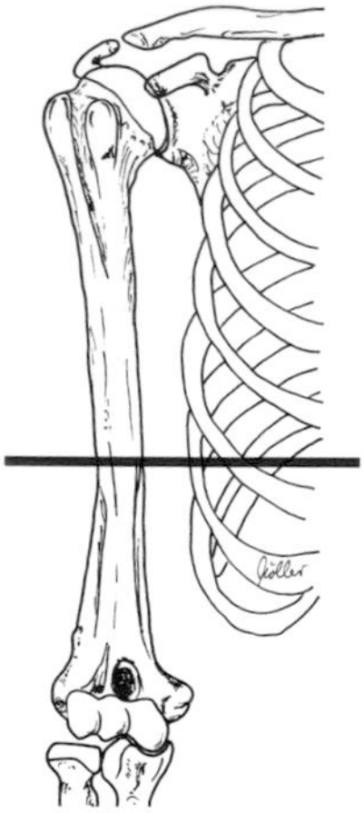

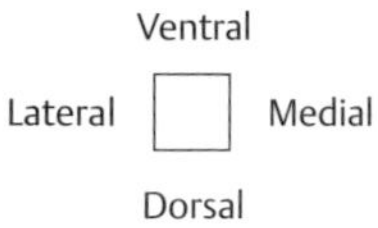
Ventral
Lateral
Medial
Dorsal

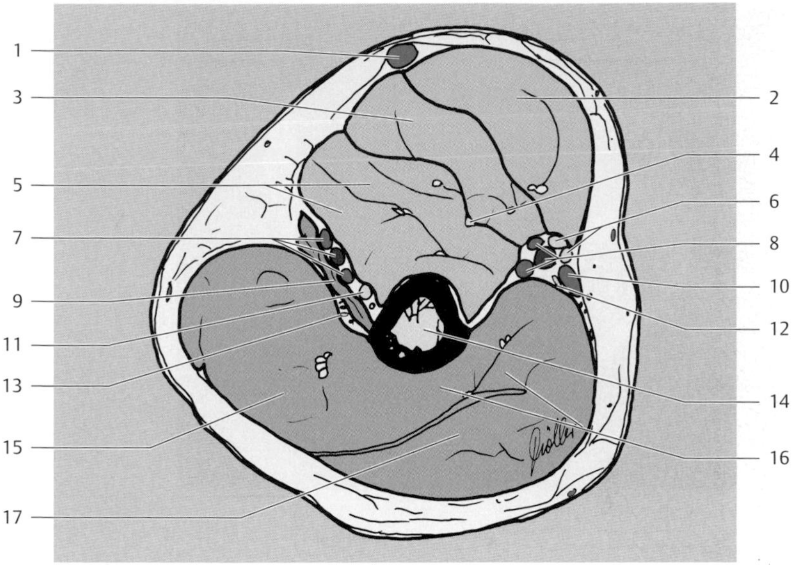

1 Cephalic vein
2 Biceps brachii muscle (short head)
3 Biceps brachii muscle (long head)
4 Musculocutaneous nerve
5 Brachialis muscle
6 Median nerve
7 Deep artery and vein of the arm
8 Brachial artery and vein
9 Brachioradialis muscle
10 Basilic vein
11 Radial nerve
12 Ulnar nerve
13 Posterior cutaneous nerve of arm (branch)
14 Humerus (shaft)
15 Triceps brachii muscle (lateral head)
16 Triceps brachii muscle (medial head)
17 Triceps brachii muscle (long head)

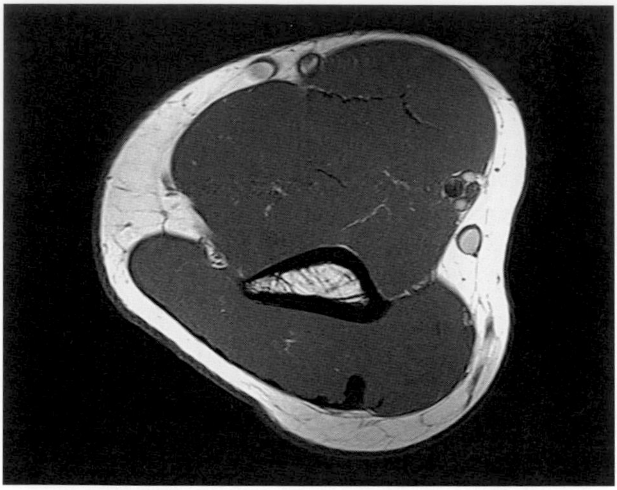

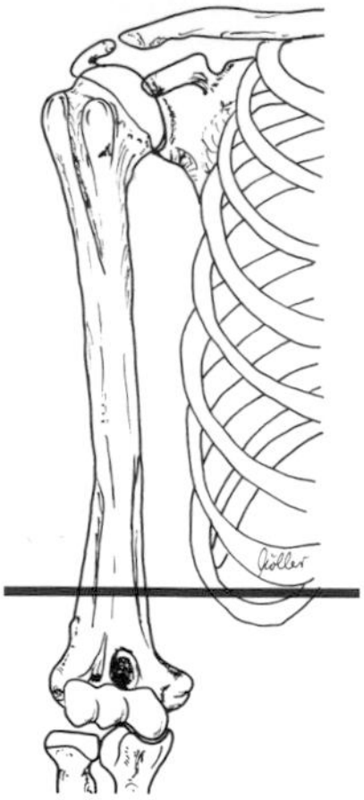

Ventral

Lateral ☐ Medial

Dorsal

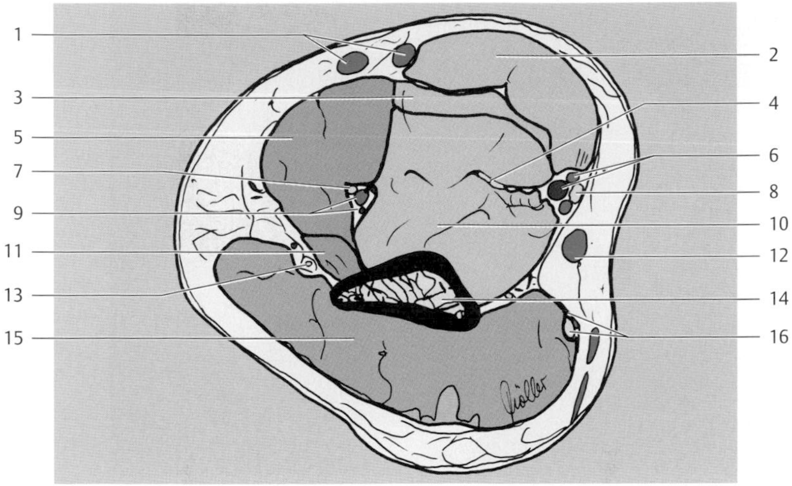

1	Cephalic vein	9	Deep brachial artery and vein
2	Biceps brachii muscle (short head)	10	Brachialis muscle
3	Biceps brachii muscle (long head)	11	Extensor carpi radialis longus muscle
4	Musculocutaneous nerve	12	Basilic vein
5	Brachioradialis muscle	13	Posterior cutaneous nerve of forearm
6	Brachial artery and vein	14	Humerus (shaft)
7	Radial nerve	15	Triceps brachii muscle
8	Median nerve	16	Ulnar nerve, artery, and vein

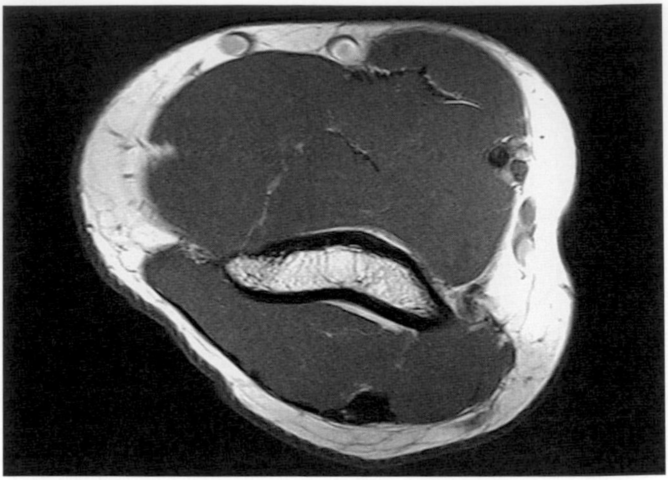

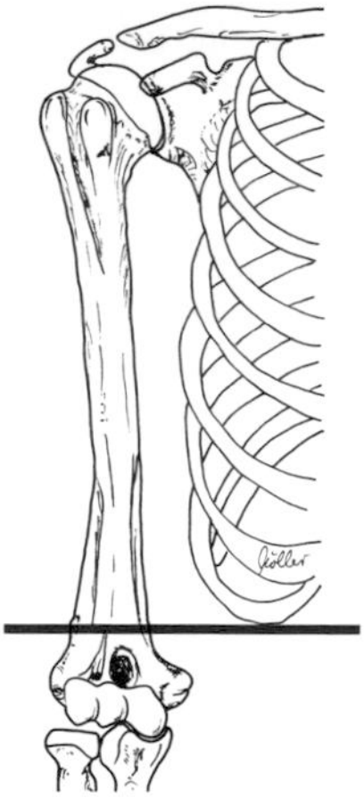
Göller

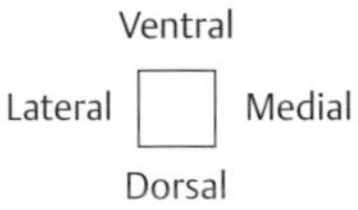
Ventral
Lateral
Medial
Dorsal

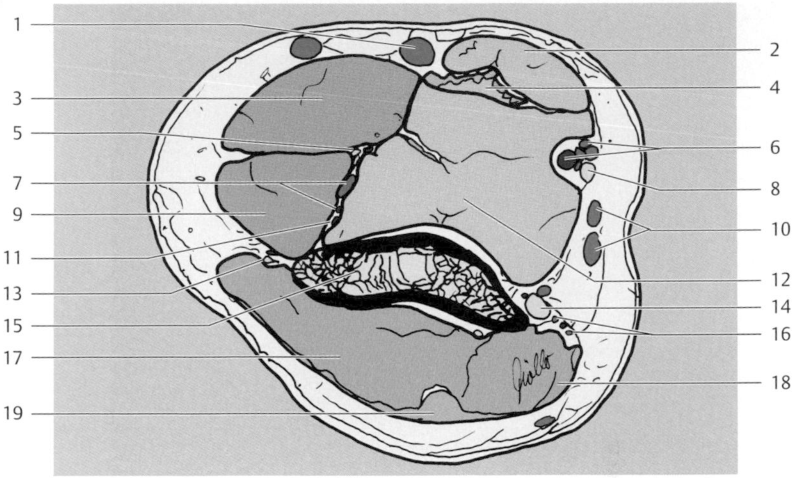

1 Cephalic vein
2 Biceps brachii muscle (short head)
3 Brachioradialis muscle
4 Biceps brachii muscle (long head and tendon)
5 Radial nerve
6 Brachial artery and vein
7 Deep brachial artery and vein
8 Median nerve
9 Extensor carpi radialis longus muscle
10 Basilic vein
11 Medial collateral artery
12 Brachialis muscle
13 Posterior cutaneous nerve of forearm
14 Ulnar nerve
15 Humerus (shaft)
16 Ulnar artery and vein
17 Triceps brachii muscle (lateral head)
18 Triceps brachii muscle (medial head)
19 Triceps brachii muscle (tendon)

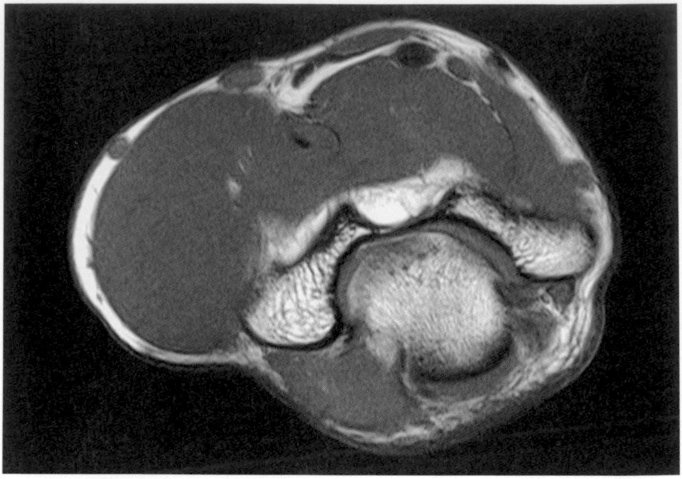

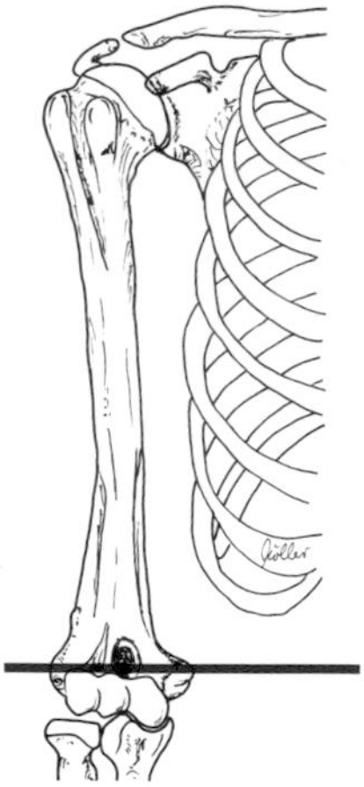
Göller

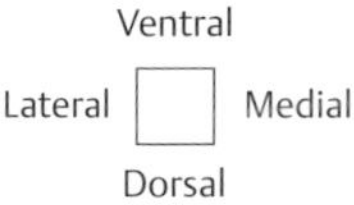
Ventral
Lateral
Medial
Dorsal

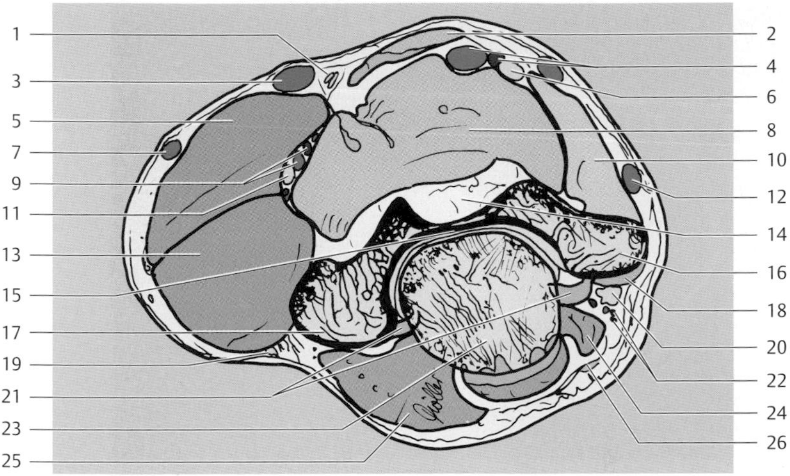

1 Cutaneous nerve of forearm
2 Biceps brachii muscle (+ tendon)
3 Median cubital vein
4 Brachial artery and vein
5 Brachioradialis muscle
6 Median nerve
7 Cephalic vein
8 Brachialis muscle
9 Collateral radial artery and vein
10 Pronator teres muscle
11 Radial nerve
12 Basilic vein
13 Extensor carpi radialis longus muscle
14 Olecranon fossa
15 Humero-ulnar joint
16 Medial epicondyle of humerus
17 Lateral epicondyle of humerus
18 Tendon attachment of ventral superficial muscles of forearm and collateral ligaments
19 Posterior cutaneous nerve of forearm (radial nerve)
20 Ulnar nerve
21 Joint capsule
22 Superior collateral ulnar artery and nerve
23 Olecranon
24 Triceps brachii muscle (+ tendon)
25 Anconeus muscle
26 Subcutaneous olecranon bursa

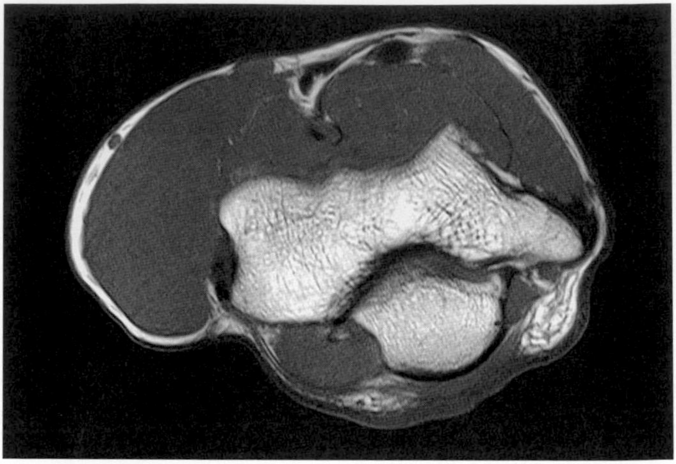

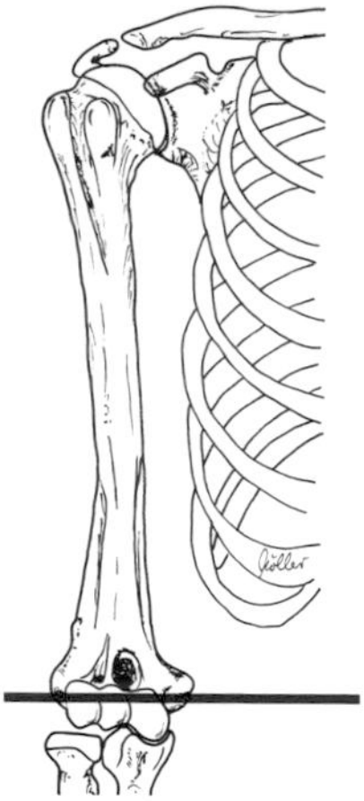

Ventral

Lateral Medial

Dorsal

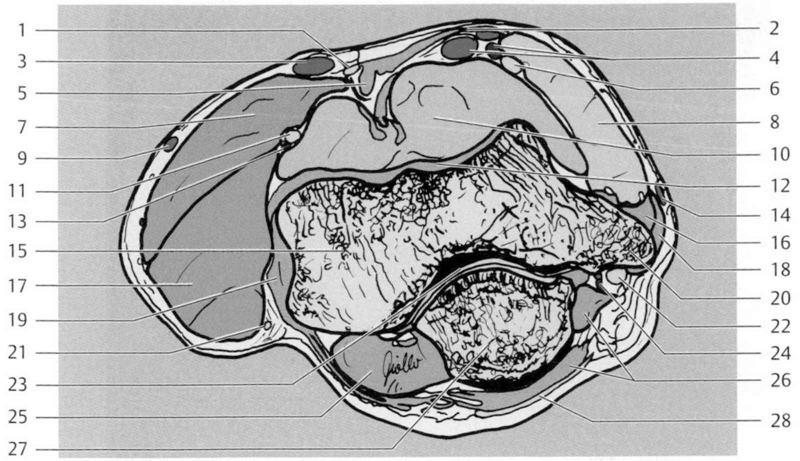

1 Cutaneous nerve of forearm
2 Bicipital aponeurosis
3 Median cubital vein
4 Brachial artery and vein
5 Biceps brachii muscle (tendon)
6 Median nerve
7 Brachioradialis muscle
8 Pronator teres muscle
9 Cephalic vein
10 Brachialis muscle (+ tendon)
11 Radial nerve
12 Articular capsule of elbow
13 Radial collateral artery and vein
14 Basilic vein
15 Humerus (capitulum)
16 Flexor carpi radialis muscle (tendon attachment)
17 Extensor carpi radialis longus muscle
18 Palmaris longus muscle (tendon attachment)
19 Lateral collateral ligament
20 Medial epicondyle of humerus
21 Posterior cutaneous nerve of forearm (radial nerve)
22 Ulnar nerve
23 Humero-ulnar joint
24 Superior collateral ulnar artery and vein
25 Anconeus muscle
26 Triceps brachii muscle (+ tendon)
27 Olecranon
28 Subcutaneous olecranon bursa

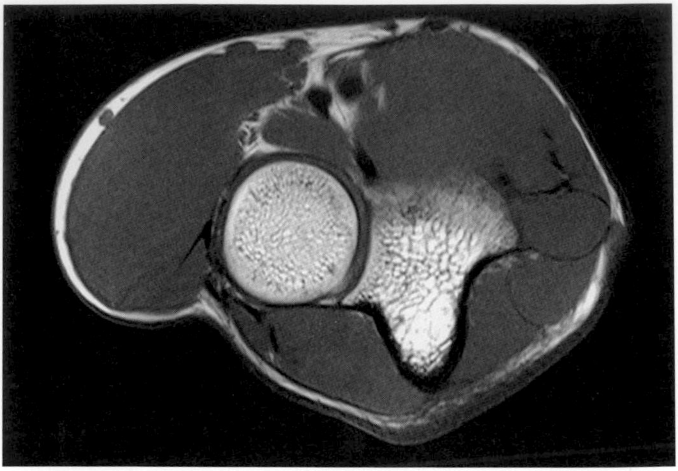

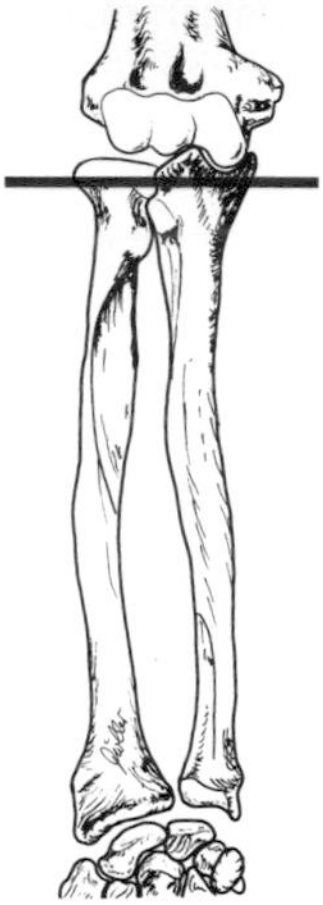

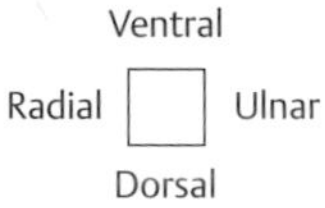
Ventral
Radial
Ulnar
Dorsal

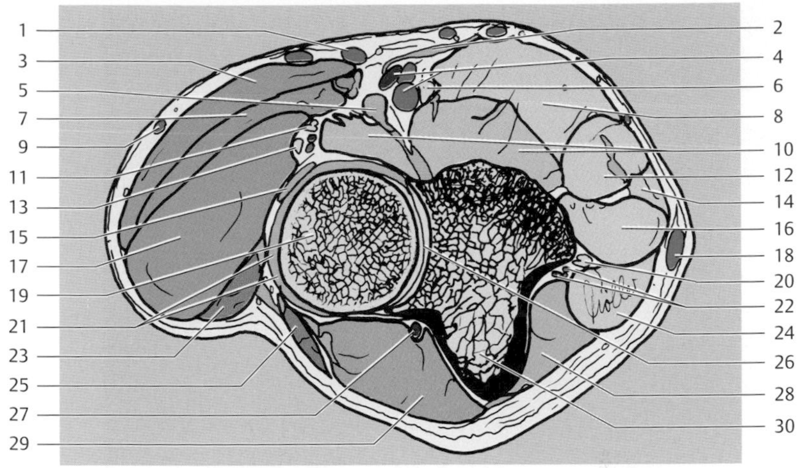

1 Median cubital vein
2 Bicipital aponeurosis
3 Brachioradialis muscle
4 Brachial artery and vein
5 Biceps brachii muscle (tendon)
6 Median nerve
7 Extensor carpi radialis longus muscle
8 Pronator teres muscle
9 Cephalic vein
10 Brachial muscle (+ tendon)
11 Radial nerve (superficial branch)
12 Flexor carpi radialis muscle
13 Radial nerve (deep branch)
14 Palmaris longus muscle
15 Supinator muscle (tendon)
16 Flexor digitorum superficialis muscle
17 Extensor carpi radialis longus muscle
18 Basilic vein
19 Head of radius
20 Ulnar nerve
21 Anular ligament
22 Superior ulnar collateral artery and vein
23 Extensor digitorum muscle
24 Flexor carpi ulnaris muscle
25 Extensor carpi ulnaris muscle
26 Proximal radioulnar joint
27 Recurrent interosseous artery
28 Flexor digitorum profundus muscle
29 Anconeus muscle
30 Ulna

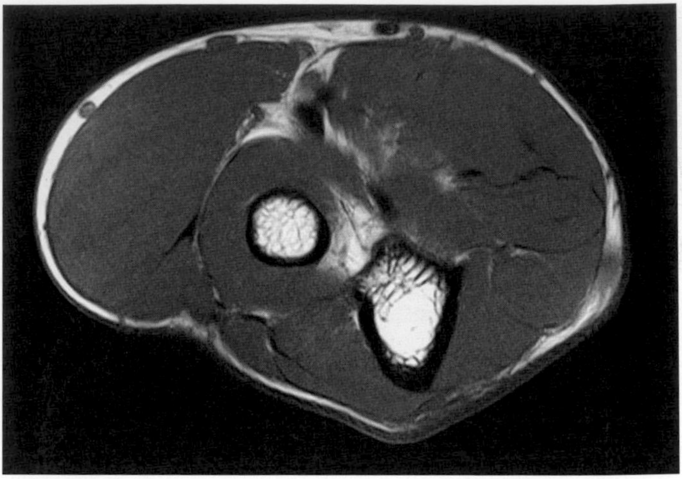

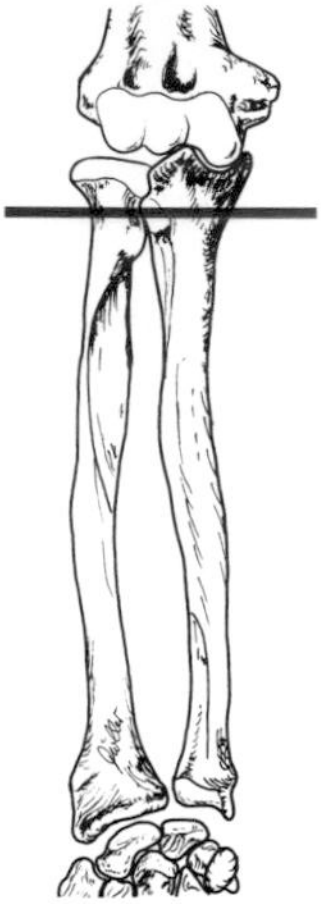

Ventral

Radial ☐ Ulnar

Dorsal

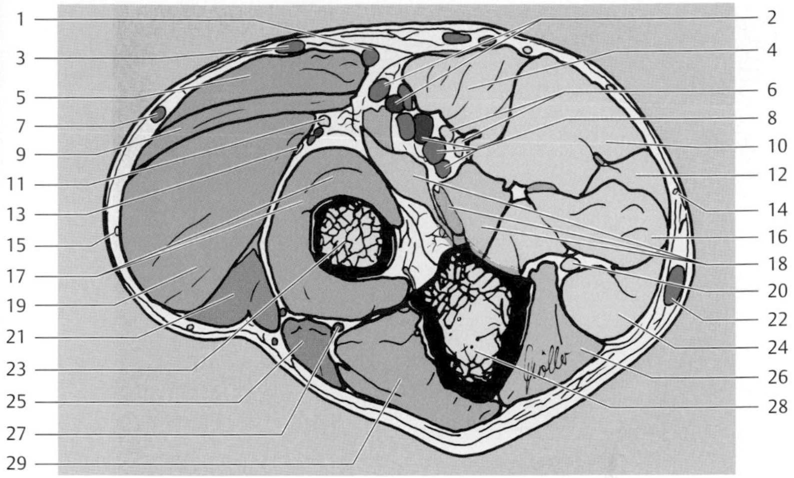

1 Deep median cubital vein
2 Radial artery and vein
3 Accessory cephalic vein
4 Pronator teres muscle
5 Brachioradialis muscle
6 Median nerve
7 Cephalic vein
8 Ulnar artery and vein
9 Extensor carpi radialis longus muscle
10 Flexor carpi radialis muscle
11 Radial nerve (superficial branch)
12 Palmaris longus muscle
13 Radial nerve (deep branch)
14 Medial cutaneous nerve of forearm
15 Posterior cutaneous nerve of forearm
16 Flexor digitorum superficialis muscle
17 Supinator muscle
18 Brachialis muscle (+ tendon attachment)
19 Extensor carpi radialis brevis muscle
20 Ulnar nerve
21 Extensor digitorum muscle
22 Basilic vein
23 Radius
24 Flexor carpi ulnaris muscle
25 Extensor carpi ulnaris muscle
26 Flexor digitorum profundus muscle
27 Recurrent interosseous artery and vein
28 Ulna
29 Anconeus muscle

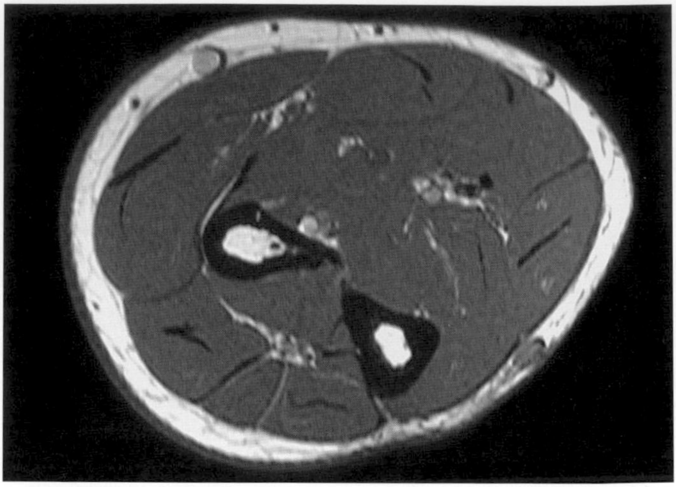

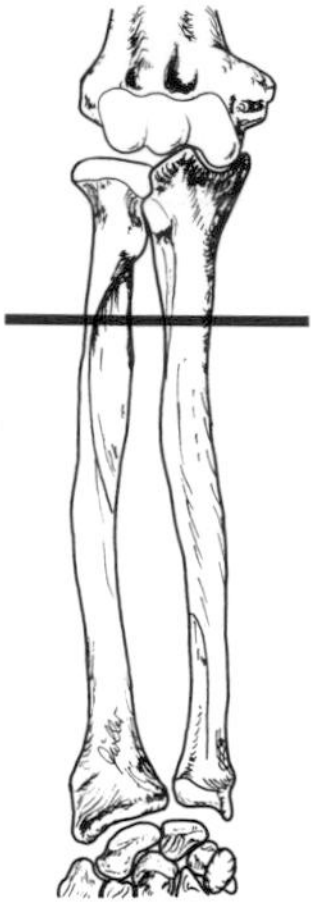

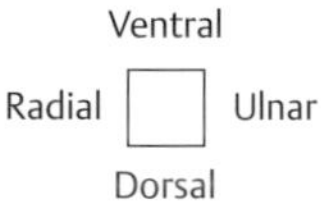
Ventral
Radial
Ulnar
Dorsal

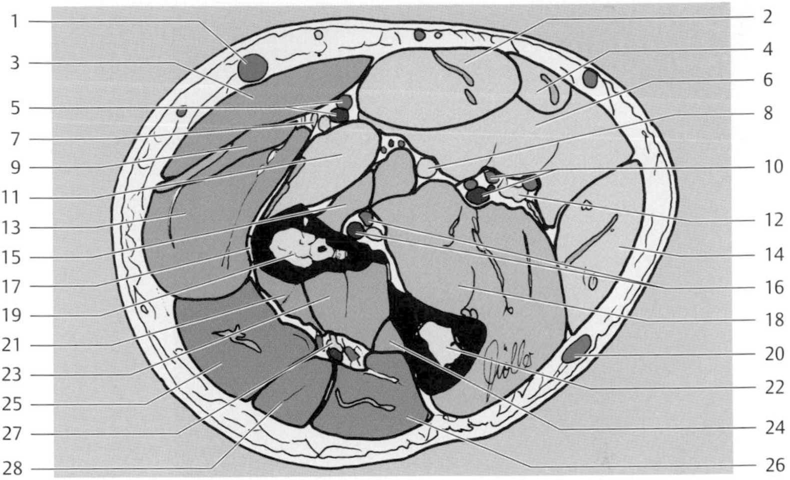

1 Median cubital vein
2 Flexor carpi radialis muscle
3 Brachioradialis muscle
4 Palmaris longus muscle
5 Radial artery and vein
6 Flexor digitorum superficialis muscle
7 Radial nerve (superficial branch)
8 Median nerve
9 Extensor carpi radialis longus muscle (+ tendon)
10 Ulnar artery and vein
11 Pronator teres muscle
12 Ulnar nerve
13 Extensor carpi radialis brevis muscle
14 Flexor carpi ulnaris muscle
15 Flexor pollicis longus muscle
16 Posterior interosseous artery, vein, and nerve
17 Radial nerve (deep branch)
18 Flexor digitorum profundus muscle
19 Radius
20 Cephalic vein
21 Supinator muscle
22 Ulna
23 Abductor pollicis longus muscle
24 Extensor pollicis longus muscle
25 Extensor digitorum muscle
26 Extensor carpi ulnaris muscle
27 Posterior interosseous artery, vein, and nerve
28 Extensor digiti minimi muscle

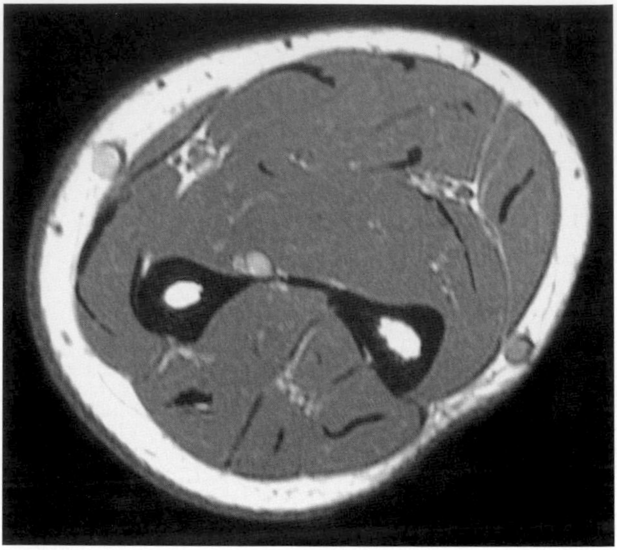

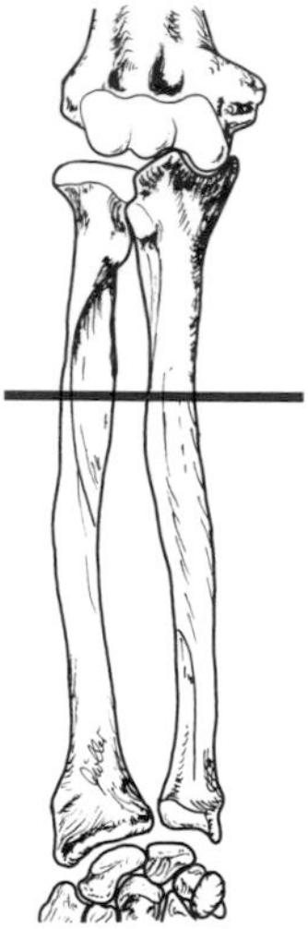

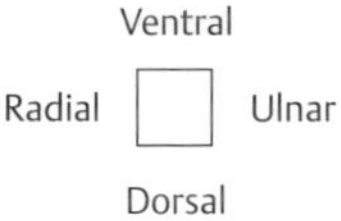
Ventral
Radial
Ulnar
Dorsal

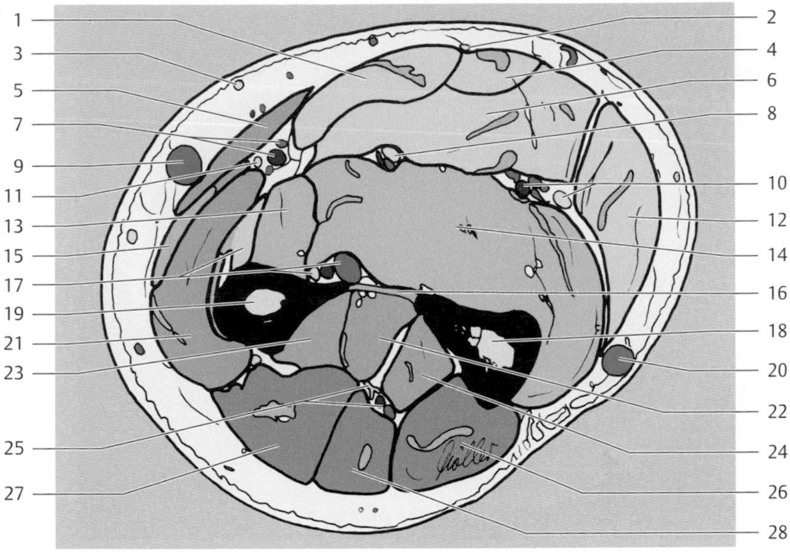

1 Flexor carpi radialis muscle
2 Medial cutaneous nerve of forearm (anterior branch)
3 Lateral cutaneous nerve of forearm (musculocutaneous nerve)
4 Palmaris longus muscle
5 Brachioradialis muscle
6 Flexor digitorum superficialis muscle
7 Radial artery and vein
8 Median nerve
9 Cephalic vein
10 Ulnar artery, vein, and nerve
11 Radial nerve (superficial branch)
12 Flexor carpi ulnaris muscle
13 Flexor pollicis longus muscle
14 Flexor digitorum profundus muscle
15 Extensor carpi radialis longus muscle (and tendon)
16 Interosseous membrane of forearm
17 Pronator teres muscle and anterior interosseous artery, vein, and nerve
18 Ulna
19 Radius
20 Basilic vein
21 Extensor carpi radialis brevis muscle
22 Extensor pollicis brevis muscle
23 Abductor pollicis longus muscle
24 Extensor pollicis longus muscle
25 Posterior interosseous artery, vein, and nerve
26 Extensor carpi ulnaris muscle
27 Extensor digitorum muscle
28 Extensor digiti minimi muscle

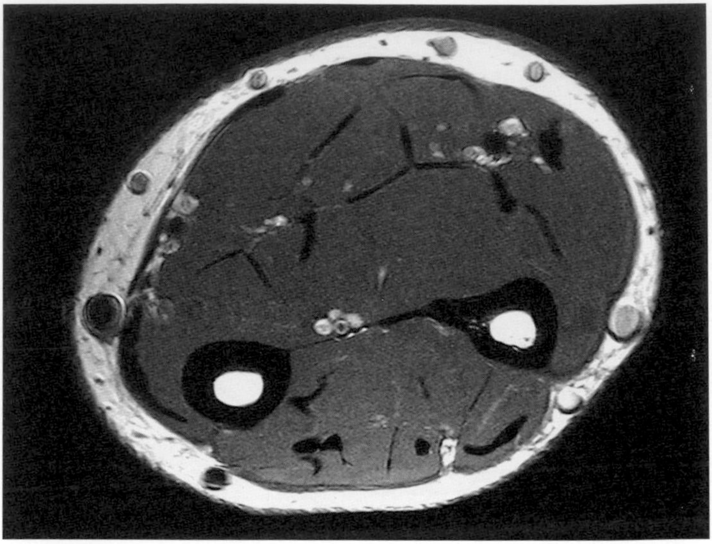

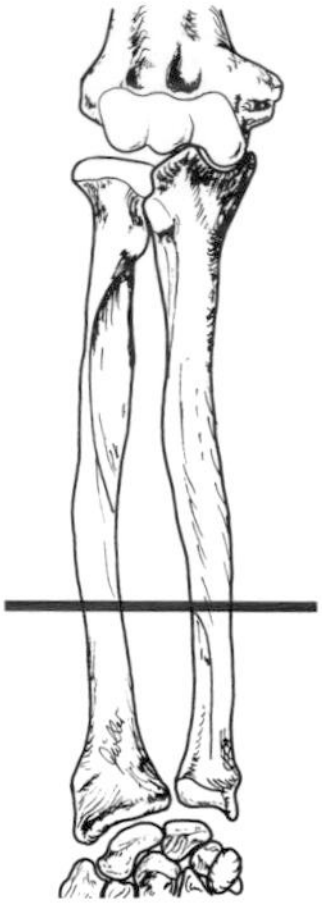

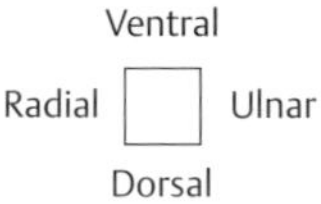
Ventral
Radial
Ulnar
Dorsal

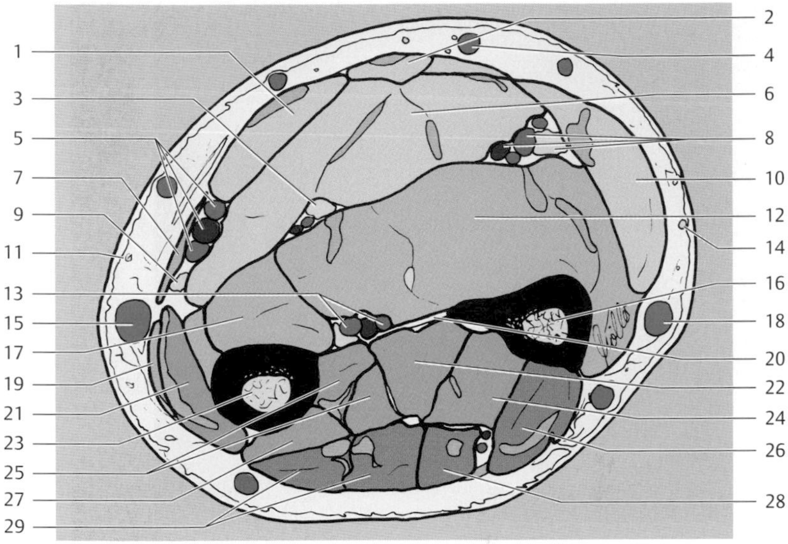

1 Flexor carpi radialis muscle
2 Palmaris longus muscle
3 Median nerve
4 Subcutaneous vein
5 Radial artery and veins
6 Flexor digitorum superficialis muscle
7 Brachioradialis muscle (tendon)
8 Ulnar artery, vein, and nerve
9 Radial nerve (superficial branch)
10 Flexor carpi ulnaris muscle
11 Posterior cutaneous nerve of forearm
12 Flexor digitorum profundus muscle
13 Anterior interosseous artery, vein, and nerve
14 Lateral cutaneous nerve of forearm
15 Cephalic vein
16 Ulna
17 Flexor pollicis longus muscle
18 Basilic vein
19 Extensor carpi radialis longus muscle (tendon)
20 Interosseous membrane of forearm
21 Extensor carpi radialis brevis muscle (+ tendon)
22 Extensor pollicis longus muscle
23 Radius
24 Extensor indicis muscle
25 Extensor pollicis brevis muscle
26 Extensor carpi ulnaris muscle
27 Abductor pollicis longus muscle
28 Extensor digiti minimi muscle
29 Extensor digitorum muscle

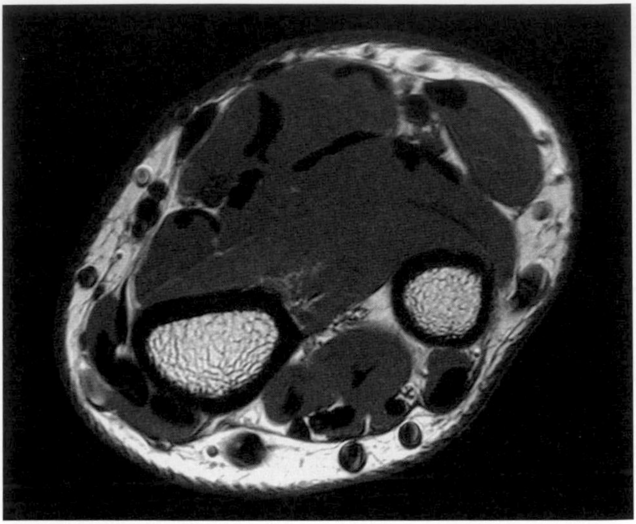

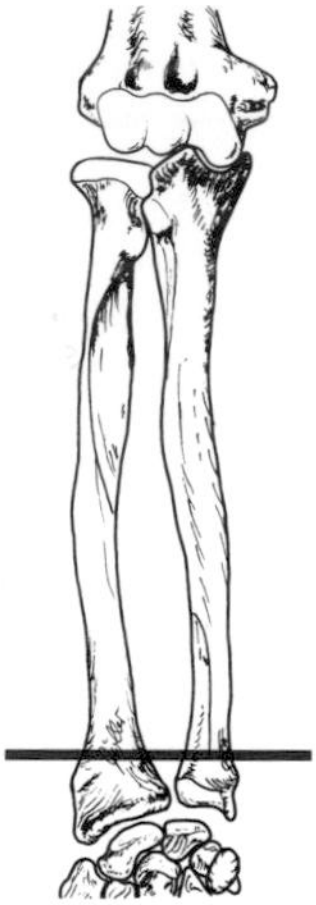

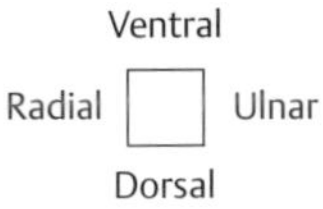
Ventral
Radial
Ulnar
Dorsal

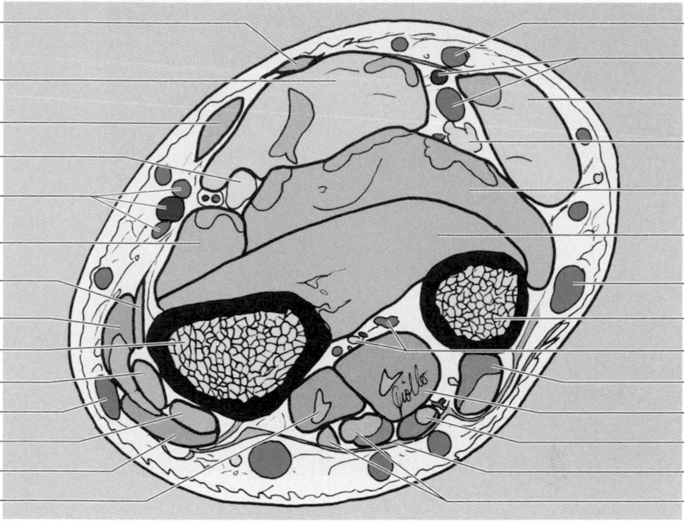

1 Palmaris longus muscle (tendon)
2 Subcutaneous vein
3 Flexor digitorum superficialis muscle
4 Ulnar artery and vein
5 Flexor carpi radialis muscle (tendon)
6 Flexor carpi ulnaris muscle
7 Median nerve
8 Ulnar nerve
9 Radial artery and veins
10 Flexor digitorum profundus muscle
11 Flexor pollicis longus muscle
12 Pronator quadratus muscle
13 Brachioradialis muscle (tendon)
14 Basilic vein
15 Abductor pollicis longus muscle (+ tendon)
16 Ulna
17 Radius
18 Anterior interosseous artery, vein, and nerve
19 Extensor carpi radialis longus muscle (tendon)
20 Extensor carpi ulnaris muscle
21 Cephalic vein
22 Extensor indicis muscle
23 Extensor carpi radialis brevis muscle (tendon)
24 Extensor digiti minimi muscle
25 Extensor pollicis brevis muscle
26 Extensor retinaculum
27 Extensor pollicis longus muscle
28 Extensor digitorum muscle (+ tendon)

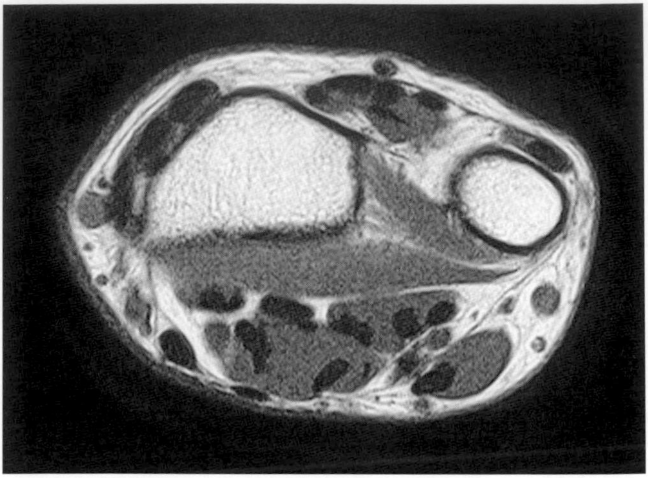

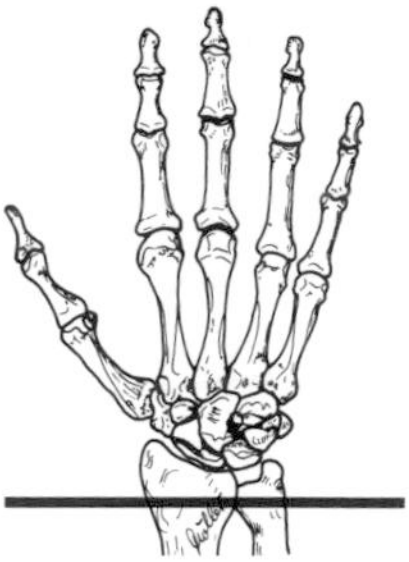

Dorsal

Radial Ulnar

Palmar

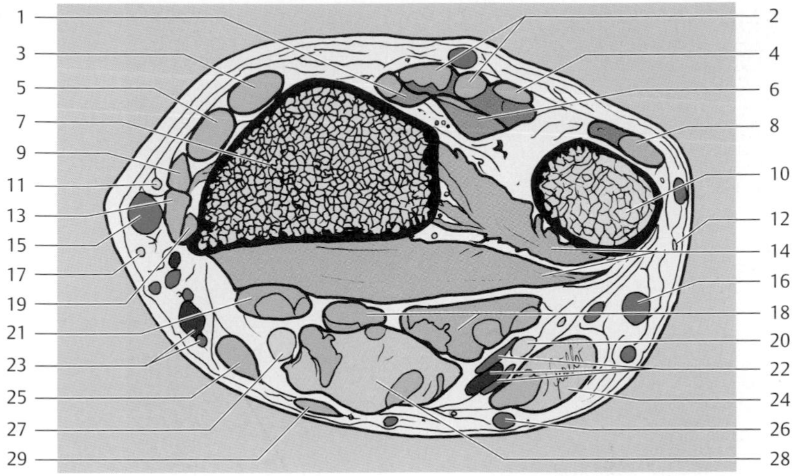

1 Extensor pollicis longus muscle
2 Extensor digitorum muscle
3 Extensor carpi radialis brevis muscle (tendon)
4 Extensor digiti minimi muscle (+ tendon)
5 Extensor carpi radialis longus muscle (tendon)
6 Extensor indicis muscle
7 Radius
8 Extensor carpi ulnaris muscle (+ tendon)
9 Extensor pollicis brevis muscle (tendon)
10 Ulna
11 Radial nerve (superficial branch)
12 Lateral cutaneous nerve of forearm
13 Abductor pollicis longus muscle (tendon)
14 Pronator quadratus muscle
15 Cephalic vein
16 Basilic vein
17 Lateral cutaneous nerve of forearm
18 Flexor digitorum profundus muscle (+ tendon)
19 Brachioradialis muscle (tendon)
20 Ulnar nerve
21 Flexor pollicis longus muscle
22 Ulnar artery and veins
23 Radial artery and veins
24 Flexor carpi ulnaris muscle
25 Flexor carpi radialis muscle (tendon)
26 Subcutaneous vein
27 Median nerve
28 Flexor digitorum superficialis muscle
29 Palmaris longus muscle (+ tendon)

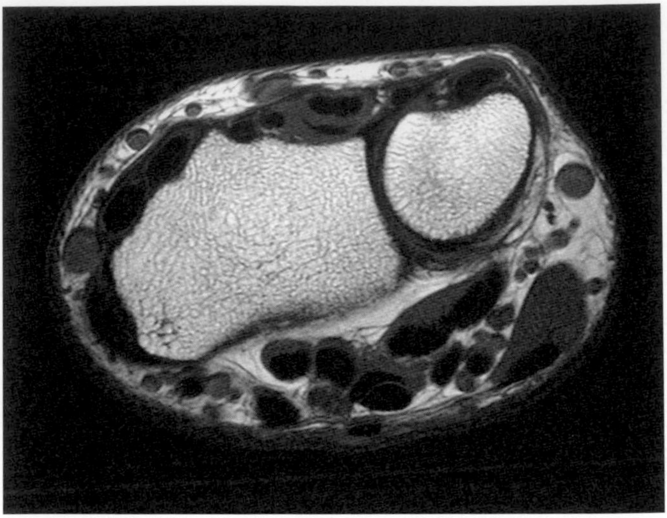

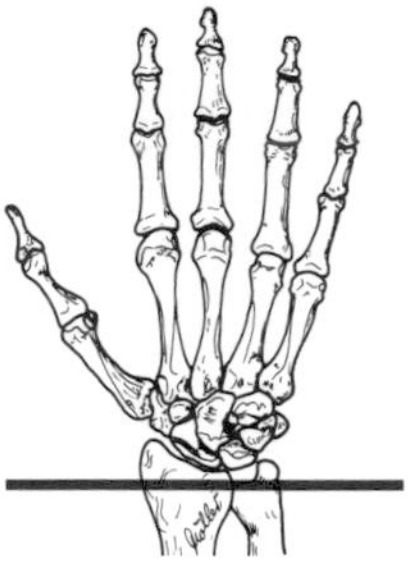

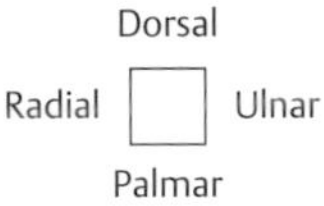
Dorsal
Radial
Ulnar
Palmar

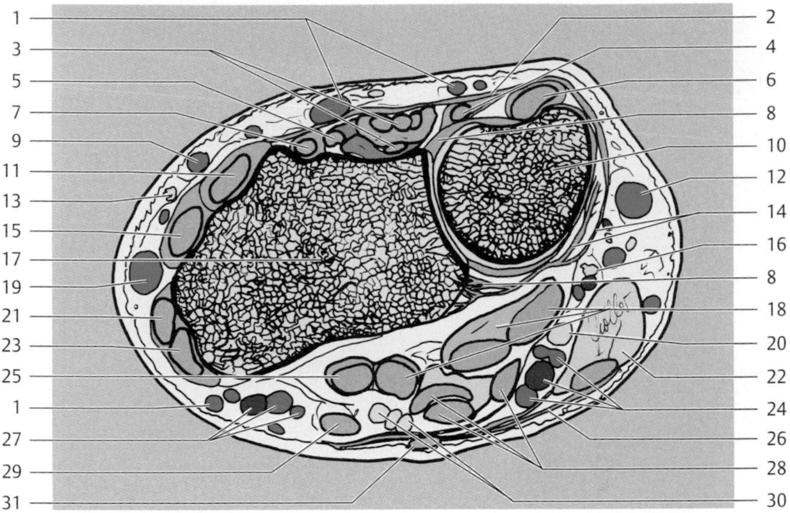

1 Subcutaneous vein
2 Extensor retinaculum
3 Extensor digitorum muscle (+ tendon)
4 Extensor digiti minimi muscle (tendon)
5 Extensor indicis muscle (tendon)
6 Extensor carpi ulnaris muscle (tendon)
7 Extensor pollicis longus muscle (tendon)
8 Joint capsule
9 Accessory cephalic vein
10 Ulna
11 Extensor carpi radialis brevis muscle (tendon)
12 Basilic vein
13 Radial nerve (superficial branch)
14 Palmar ulnocarpal ligament
15 Extensor carpi radialis longus muscle (tendon)
16 Ulnar nerve (dorsal branch)
17 Radius
18 Flexor digitorum profundus muscle (+ tendon)
19 Cephalic vein
20 Ulnar nerve
21 Extensor pollicis brevis muscle (tendon)
22 Flexor carpi ulnaris muscle
23 Abductor pollicis longus muscle (tendon)
24 Ulnar artery and veins
25 Flexor pollicis longus muscle (tendon)
26 Antebrachial fascia
27 Radial artery and veins
28 Flexor digitorum superficialis muscle (+ tendon)
29 Flexor carpi radialis muscle (tendon)
30 Median nerve
31 Palmaris longus muscle (tendon)

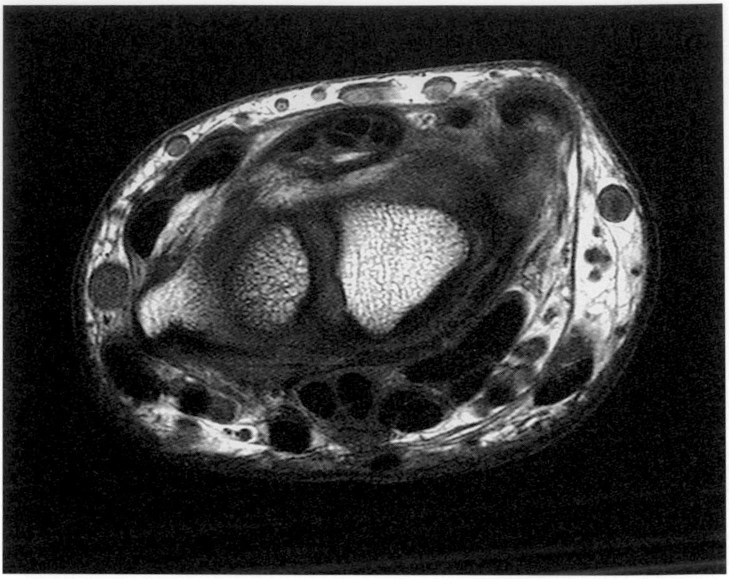

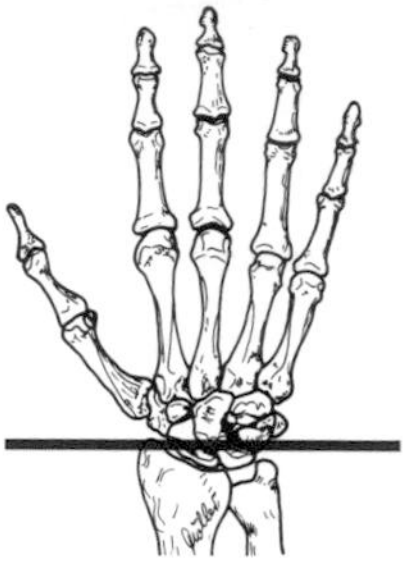

Dorsal

Radial ☐ Ulnar

Palmar

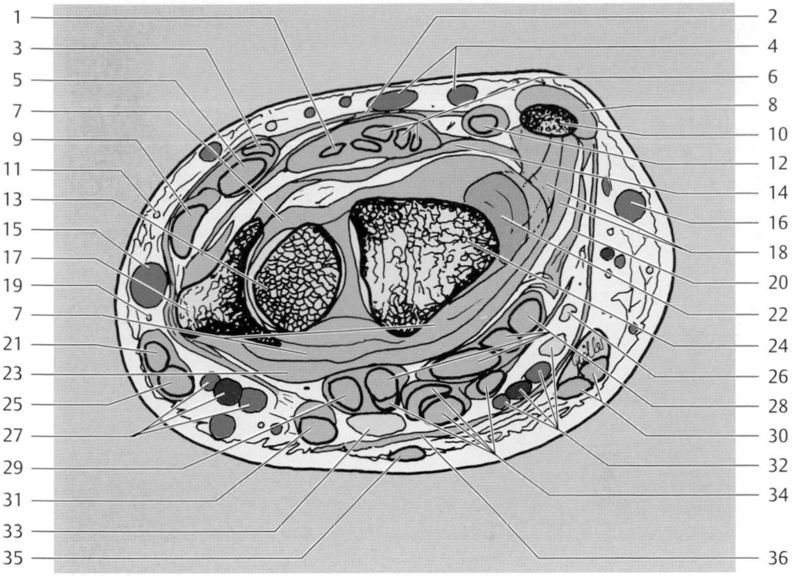

1 Extensor indicis muscle (tendon)
2 Extensor retinaculum
3 Extensor pollicis longus muscle (tendon)
4 Subcutaneous vein
5 Extensor carpi radialis brevis muscle (tendon)
6 Extensor digitorum muscle (tendon)
7 Joint capsule
8 Extensor carpi ulnaris muscle (tendon)
9 Extensor carpi radialis longus muscle (tendon)
10 Ulnar styloid process
11 Posterior cutaneous nerve of forearm (radial nerve)
12 Extensor digiti minimi muscle (tendon)
13 Scaphoid
14 Dorsal radiocarpal ligament
15 Cephalic vein
16 Basilic vein
17 Radius
18 Palmar ulnocarpal ligament
19 Radial nerve (superficial branch)
20 Ulnar collateral ligament of wrist joint
21 Extensor pollicis brevis muscle (tendon)
22 Triangular fibrocartilage
23 Palmar radiocarpal ligament
24 Lunate
25 Abductor pollicis longus muscle (tendon)
26 Ulnar nerve (dorsal branch)
27 Radial artery and veins
28 Flexor digitorum profundus muscle (tendons)
29 Flexor pollicis longus muscle (tendon)
30 Flexor carpi ulnaris muscle (+ tendon)
31 Flexor carpi radialis muscle (tendon)
32 Ulnar nerve, artery, and veins
33 Median nerve
34 Flexor digitorum superficialis muscle (tendons)
35 Palmaris longus muscle (tendon)
36 Flexor retinaculum

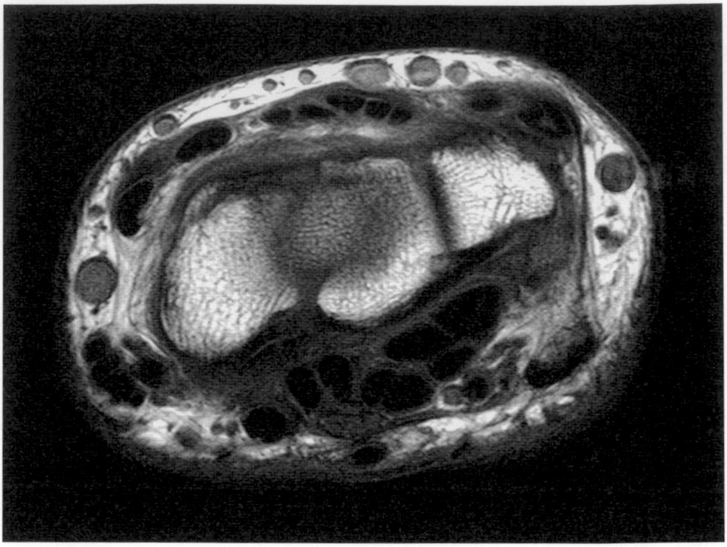

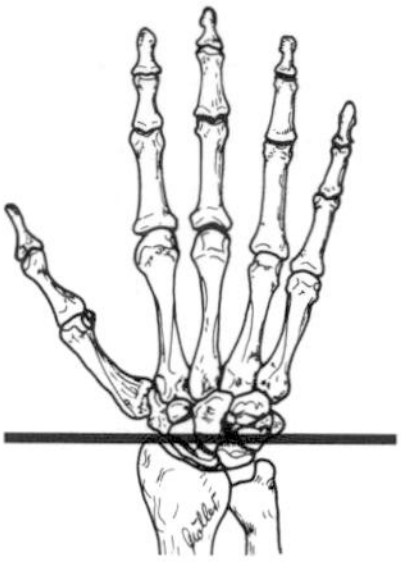

Dorsal

Radial ☐ Ulnar

Palmar

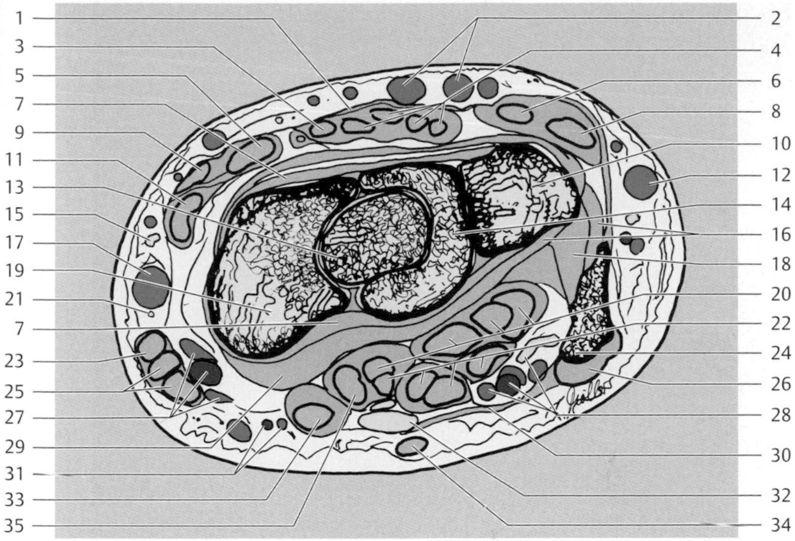

1 Extensor retinaculum
2 Subcutaneous vein
3 Extensor indicis muscle (tendon)
4 Extensor digitorum muscle (tendons)
5 Extensor carpi radialis brevis muscle (tendon)
6 Extensor digiti minimi muscle (tendon)
7 Joint capsule
8 Extensor carpi ulnaris muscle (tendon)
9 Extensor pollicis longus muscle (tendon)
10 Triquetrum
11 Extensor carpi radialis longus muscle (tendon)
12 Basilic vein
13 Capitate
14 Lunate
15 Posterior cutaneous nerve of forearm (radial nerve)
16 Palmar ulnocarpal ligament
17 Cephalic vein
18 Palmar intercarpal ligament
19 Scaphoid
20 Flexor digitorum profundus muscle (tendons)
21 Radial nerve (superficial branch)
22 Flexor digitorum superficialis muscle (tendons)
23 Extensor pollicis brevis muscle (tendon)
24 Pisiform
25 Abductor pollicis longus muscle (tendon)
26 Flexor carpi ulnaris muscle (tendon attachment)
27 Radial artery and veins
28 Ulnar nerve, artery, and veins
29 Ulnar radiocarpal ligament
30 Flexor retinaculum
31 Superficial palmar branch of radial artery and vein
32 Median nerve
33 Flexor carpi radialis muscle (tendon)
34 Palmaris longus muscle (tendon)
35 Flexor pollicis longus muscle (tendon)

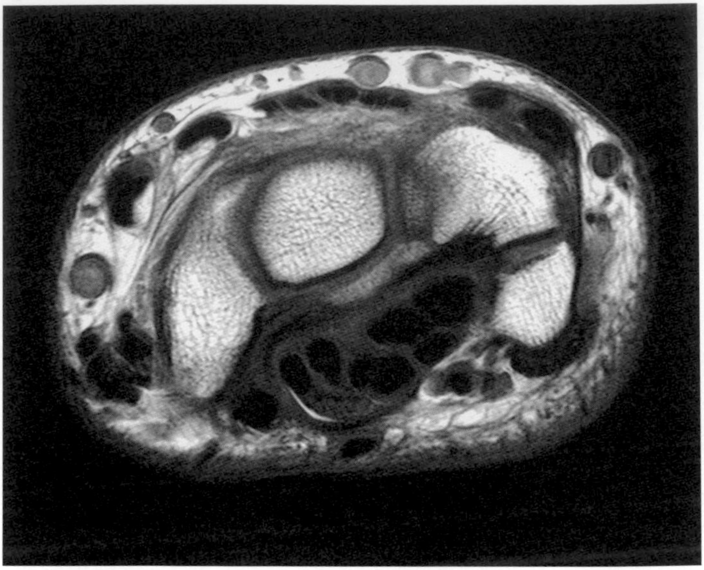

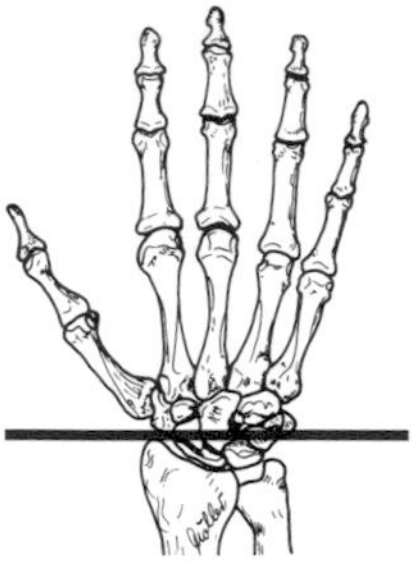

Dorsal

Radial ☐ Ulnar

Palmar

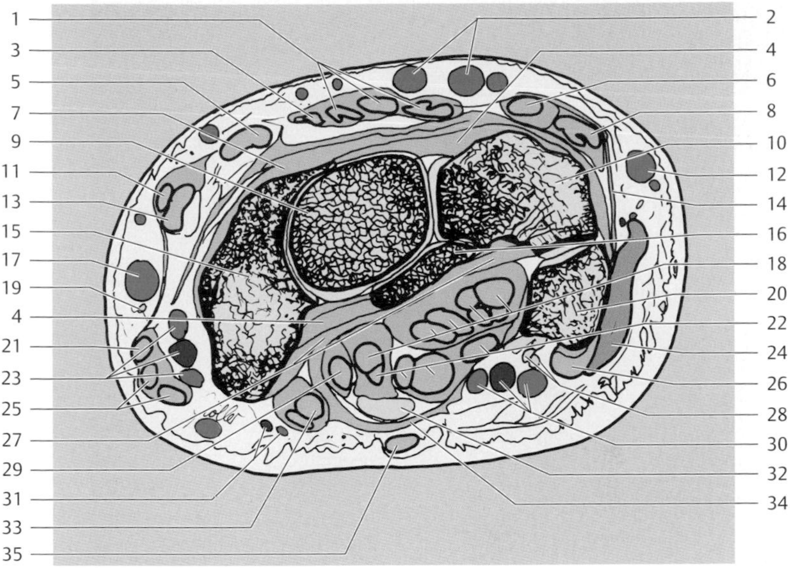

1 Extensor digitorum muscle (tendons)
2 Subcutaneous vein
3 Extensor indicis muscle (tendon)
4 Joint capsule
5 Extensor carpi radialis brevis muscle (tendon)
6 Extensor digiti minimi muscle (tendon)
7 Dorsal intercarpal ligament
8 Extensor carpi ulnaris muscle (tendon)
9 Capitate
10 Triquetrum
11 Extensor pollicis longus muscle (tendon)
12 Basilic vein
13 Extensor carpi radialis longus muscle (tendon)
14 Palmar ulnocarpal ligament
15 Scaphoid
16 Lunate
17 Cephalic vein
18 Flexor digitorum profundus muscle (tendons)
19 Radial nerve (superficial branch)
20 Pisiform
21 Extensor pollicis brevis muscle (tendon)
22 Flexor digitorum superficialis muscle (tendons)
23 Radial artery and veins
24 Abductor digiti minimi muscle
25 Abductor pollicis longus muscle (tendon)
26 Flexor carpi ulnaris muscle (tendon)
27 Palmar radiocarpal ligament
28 Ulnar nerve
29 Flexor pollicis longus muscle (tendon)
30 Ulnar artery and veins
31 Superficial palmar branch of radial artery and vein
32 Median nerve
33 Flexor carpi radialis muscle (tendon)
34 Flexor retinaculum
35 Palmaris longus muscle (tendon)

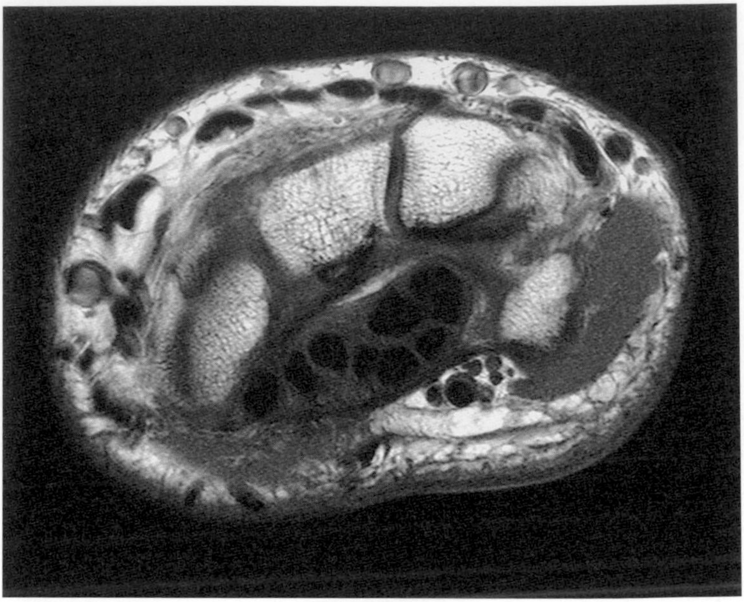

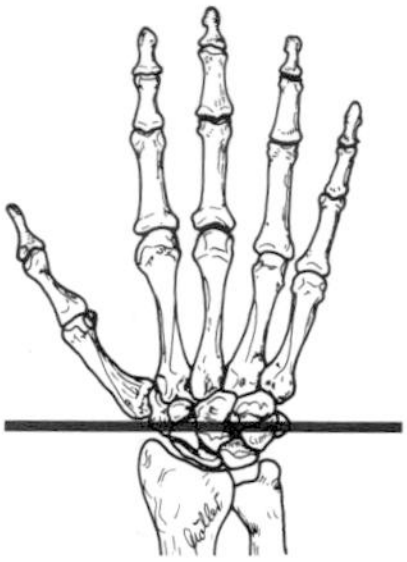

Dorsal

Radial ☐ Ulnar

Palmar

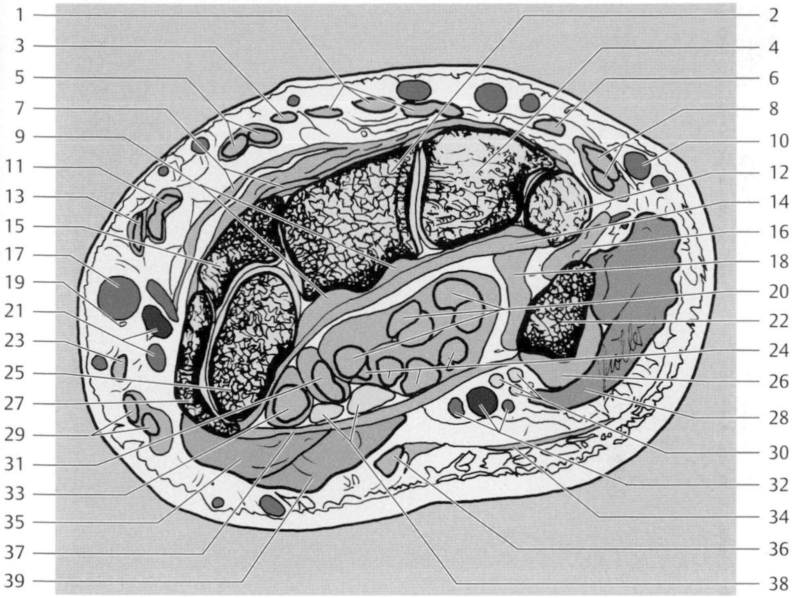

1 Extensor digitorum muscle (tendons)
2 Capitate
3 Extensor indicis muscle (tendon)
4 Hamate
5 Extensor carpi radialis brevis muscle (tendon)
6 Extensor digiti minimi muscle (tendon)
7 Dorsal intercarpal ligament
8 Extensor carpi ulnaris muscle (tendon)
9 Joint capsule
10 Basilic vein
11 Extensor carpi radialis longus muscle (tendon)
12 Triquetrum
13 Extensor pollicis longus muscle (tendon)
14 Palmar intercarpal ligament
15 Trapezoid
16 Pisometacarpal ligament
17 Cephalic vein
18 Pisohamate ligament
19 Radial nerve (superficial branch)
20 Flexor digitorum profundus muscle (tendons)
21 Radial artery and veins
22 Pisiform
23 Extensor pollicis brevis muscle (tendon)
24 Flexor digitorum superficialis muscle (tendons)
25 Scaphoid
26 Flexor carpi ulnaris muscle (tendon)
27 Trapezium
28 Abductor digiti minimi muscle
29 Abductor pollicis longus muscle (tendon)
30 Ulnar nerve
31 Flexor pollicis longus muscle (tendon)
32 Ulnar artery and veins
33 Flexor carpi radialis muscle (tendon)
34 Palmaris brevis muscle (tendon)
35 Opponens pollicis muscle
36 Palmaris longus muscle (tendon)
37 Flexor retinaculum
38 Median nerve
39 Abductor pollicis brevis muscle

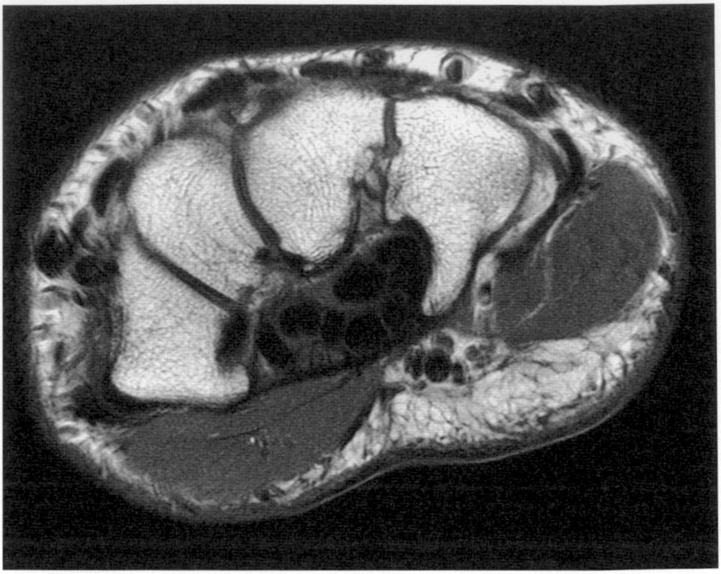

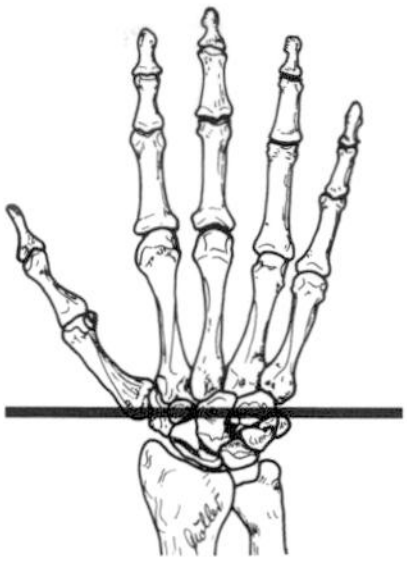

Dorsal

Radial ☐ Ulnar

Palmar

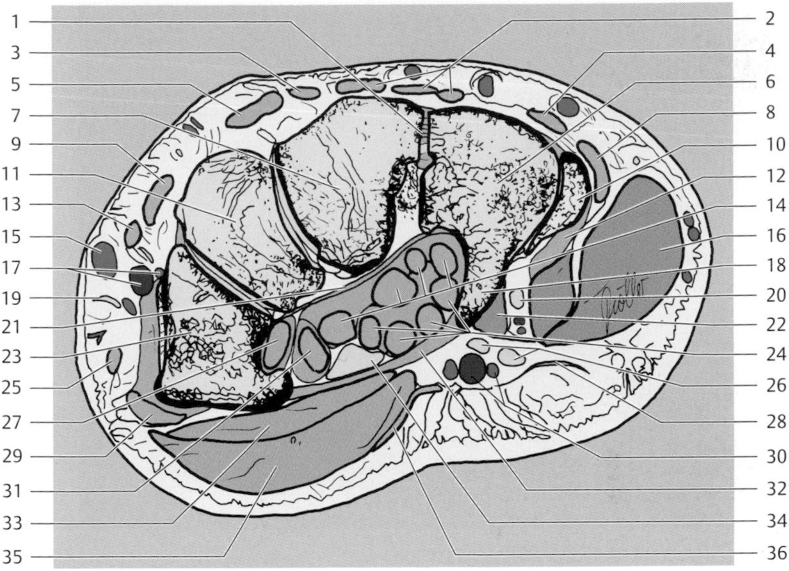

1 Intercarpal (capitohamate) joint
2 Extensor digitorum muscle (tendons)
3 Extensor indicis muscle (tendon)
4 Extensor digiti minimi muscle (tendon)
5 Extensor carpi radialis brevis muscle (tendon)
6 Hamate
7 Capitate
8 Extensor carpi ulnaris muscle (tendon)
9 Extensor carpi radialis longus muscle (tendon)
10 Metacarpal V (base)
11 Trapezoid
12 Pisometacarpal ligament
13 Extensor pollicis longus muscle (tendon)
14 Flexor digitorum profundus muscle (tendons)
15 Cephalic vein
16 Abductor digiti minimi muscle
17 Radial artery and veins
18 Hook of hamate
19 Radial nerve (superficial branch)
20 Ulnar nerve (deep branch)
21 Palmar intercarpal ligament
22 Flexor digiti minimi muscle
23 Trapezium
24 Flexor digitorum superficialis muscle (tendons)
25 Extensor pollicis brevis muscle (tendon)
26 Ulnar nerve
27 Flexor carpi radialis muscle (tendon)
28 Palmaris brevis muscle
29 Flexor pollicis longus muscle (tendon)
30 Ulnar artery and veins
31 Abductor pollicis longus muscle (tendon)
32 Flexor retinaculum
33 Opponens pollicis muscle
34 Median nerve
35 Abductor pollicis brevis muscle
36 Palmar aponeurosis

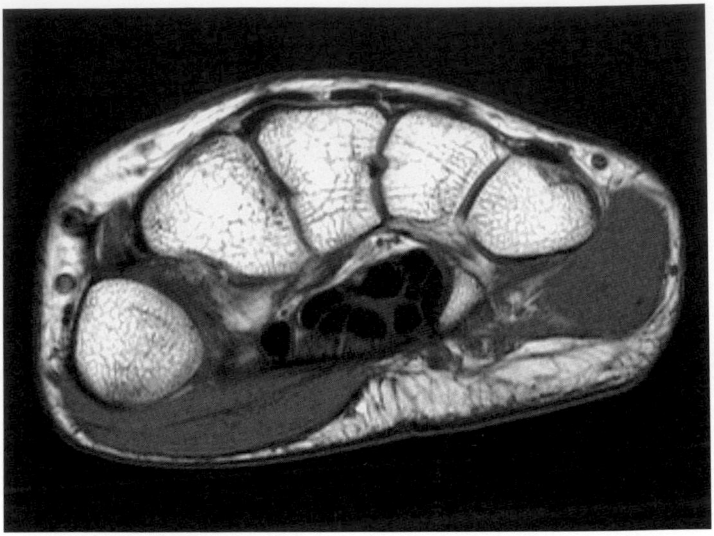

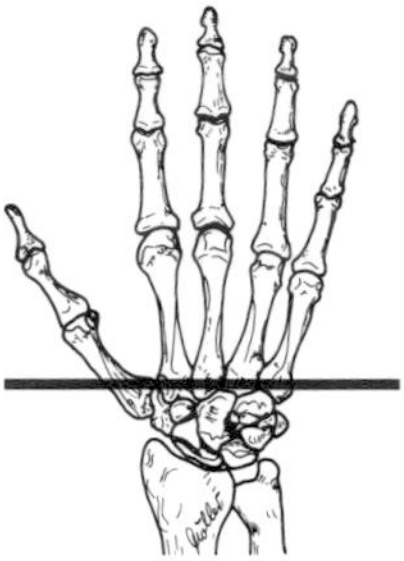

Dorsal

Radial ☐ Ulnar

Palmar

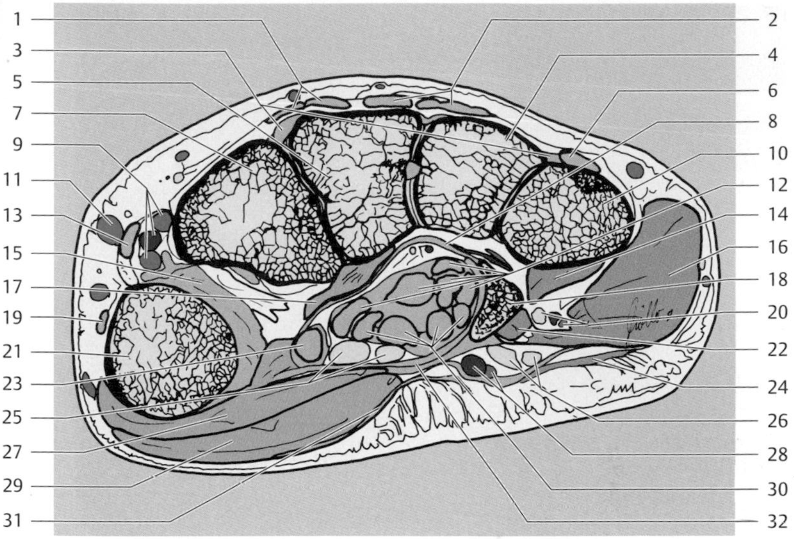

1 Extensor indicis muscle (tendon)
2 Extensor digitorum muscle (tendons)
3 Dorsal metacarpal ligament
4 Metacarpal IV (base)
5 Metacarpal III (base)
6 Extensor digiti minimi muscle (tendon)
7 Metacarpal II (base)
8 Palmar intercarpal ligament
9 Radial artery and veins
10 Metacarpal V (base)
11 Cephalic vein
12 Flexor digitorum profundus muscle (tendons)
13 Extensor pollicis longus muscle (tendon)
14 Opponens digiti minimi muscle
15 Joint capsule
16 Abductor digiti minimi muscle
17 Adductor pollicis muscle (oblique head)
18 Hamate (hook)
19 Extensor pollicis brevis muscle (tendon)
20 Ulnar nerve, artery, and vein (deep branch)
21 Metacarpal I (base)
22 Flexor digiti minimi muscle
23 Flexor pollicis longus muscle (tendon)
24 Palmaris brevis muscle
25 Median nerve
26 Ulnar nerve
27 Opponens pollicis muscle
28 Ulnar artery and vein
29 Abductor pollicis brevis muscle
30 Flexor digitorum superficialis muscle (tendons)
31 Palmar aponeurosis
32 Flexor retinaculum

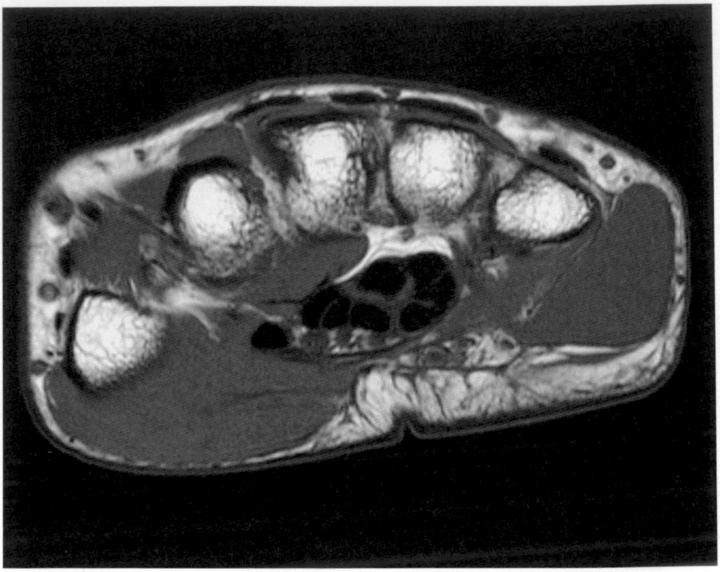

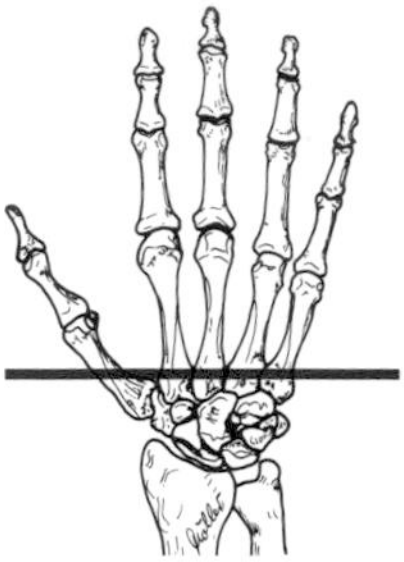

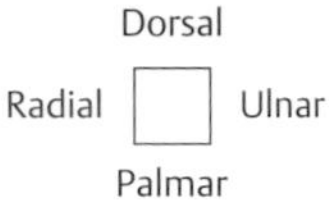
Dorsal
Radial
Ulnar
Palmar

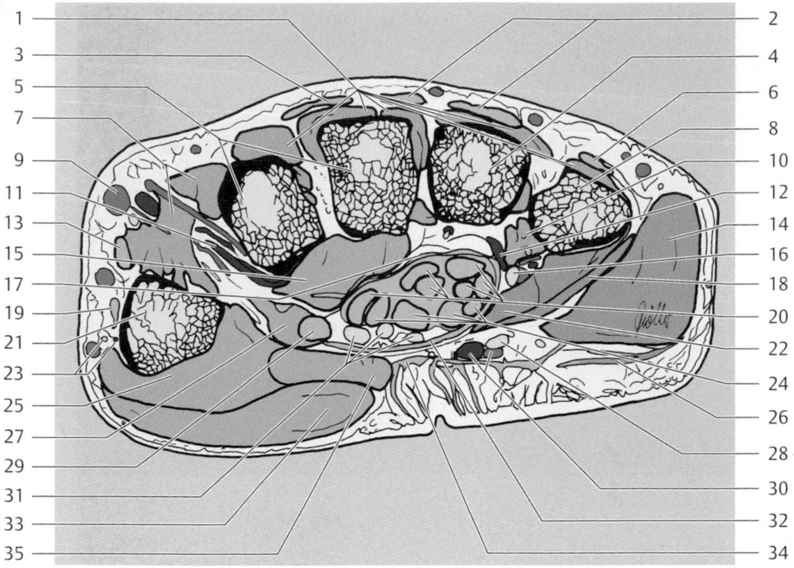

1 Dorsal interosseous muscles
2 Extensor digitorum muscle (tendons)
3 Extensor indicis muscle (tendon)
4 Metacarpal IV (base)
5 Metacarpals II and III (bases)
6 Extensor digiti minimi muscle (tendon)
7 Dorsal interosseous muscle I
8 Metacarpal V
9 Cephalic vein
10 Palmar interosseous muscles
11 Deep palmar arch (from radial artery)
12 Deep palmar arch (from deep ulnar artery)
13 Extensor pollicis longus muscle (tendon)
14 Abductor digiti minimi muscle
15 Adductor pollicis muscle (oblique head)
16 Ulnar nerve (deep branch)
17 Palmar intercarpal ligament
18 Flexor digiti minimi muscle
19 Extensor pollicis brevis muscle (tendon)
20 Flexor digitorum profundus muscle (tendons)
21 Metacarpal I (head)
22 Opponens digiti minimi muscle
23 Dorsal nerve and artery of thumb
24 Flexor digitorum superficialis muscle (tendons)
25 Opponens pollicis muscle
26 Palmaris brevis muscle
27 Flexor pollicis brevis muscle (deep head)
28 Ulnar nerve
29 Flexor pollicis longus muscle (tendon)
30 Ulnar artery and veins
31 Median nerve
32 Flexor retinaculum
33 Abductor pollicis brevis muscle
34 Palmar aponeurosis
35 Flexor pollicis brevis muscle (superficial head)

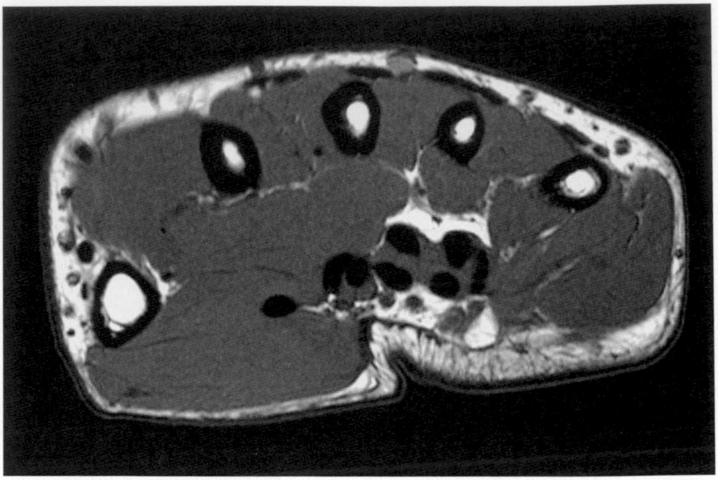

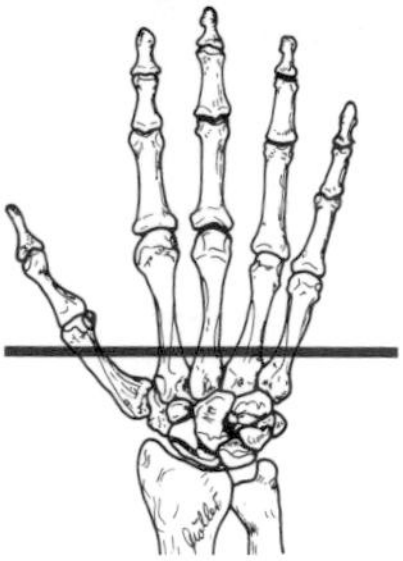

Dorsal

Radial ☐ Ulnar

Palmar

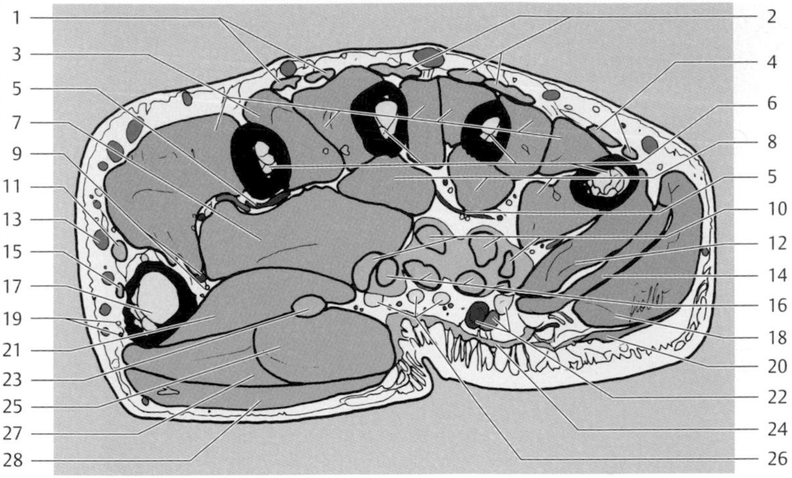

1 Extensor indicis muscle (tendon)
2 Extensor digitorum muscle (tendons)
3 Dorsal interosseous muscles
4 Extensor digiti minimi muscle (tendon)
5 Deep palmar arch
6 Metacarpals II–V (shafts)
7 Adductor pollicis muscle (oblique head)
8 Palmar interosseous muscles
9 Princeps pollicis artery and palmar digital nerve (of thumb)
10 Flexor digitorum profundus muscle (tendons)
11 Extensor pollicis longus muscle (tendon)
12 Opponens digiti minimi muscle
13 Cephalic vein (of thumb)
14 Flexor digiti minimi brevis muscle
15 Extensor pollicis brevis muscle (tendon)
16 Flexor digitorum superficialis muscle (tendons)
17 Metacarpal I (shaft)
18 Abductor digiti minimi muscle
19 Dorsal digital artery and nerve of thumb
20 Palmaris brevis muscle
21 Flexor pollicis brevis muscle (deep head)
22 Ulnar nerve, artery, and vein
23 Flexor pollicis longus muscle (tendon)
24 Palmar aponeurosis
25 Flexor pollicis brevis muscle (superficial head)
26 Median nerve
27 Opponens pollicis muscle
28 Abductor pollicis brevis muscle

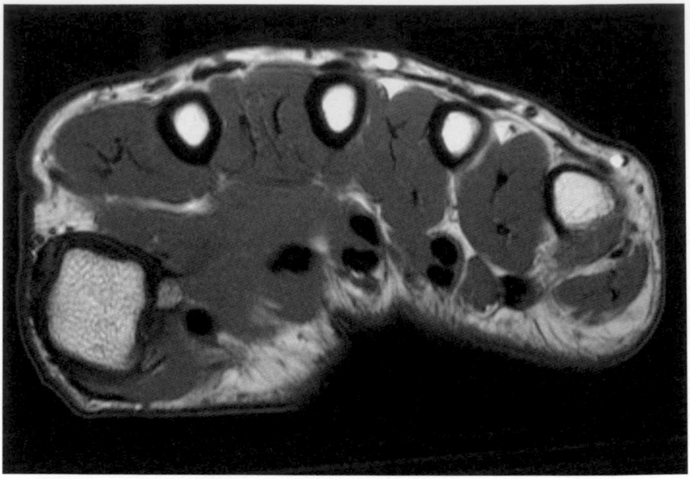

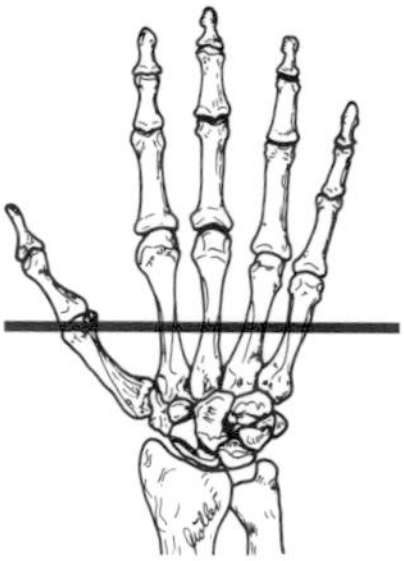

Dorsal

Radial ☐ Ulnar

Palmar

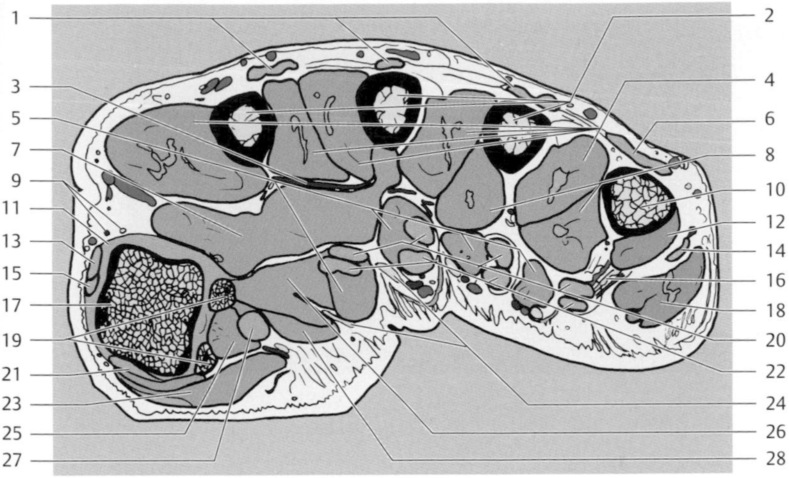

1 Extensor digitorum muscle (tendons)
2 Metacarpals II–IV (shafts)
3 Deep palmar arch
4 Dorsal interosseous muscles
5 Lumbrical muscles
6 Extensor digiti minimi muscle (tendon)
7 Adductor pollicis muscle (transverse head)
8 Palmar interosseous muscles
9 Dorsal digital nerve and artery of thumb
10 Metacarpal V (head)
11 Collateral ligament
12 Opponens digiti minimi muscle
13 Extensor pollicis brevis muscle (tendon)
14 Flexor digiti minimi brevis muscle (+ tendon)
15 Extensor pollicis brevis muscle (tendon)
16 Ulnar nerve (superficial branch)
17 Metacarpal I (head)
18 Abductor digiti minimi muscle
19 Sesamoid bones
20 Flexor digitorum profundus muscle (tendons)
21 Opponens pollicis muscle (+ tendon attachment)
22 Flexor digitorum superficialis muscle (tendons)
23 Abductor pollicis brevis muscle
24 Common palmar digital nerves of median nerve
25 Flexor pollicis brevis muscle (superficial head)
26 Adductor pollicis muscle (oblique head)
27 Flexor pollicis longus muscle (tendon)
28 Flexor pollicis brevis muscle (deep head)

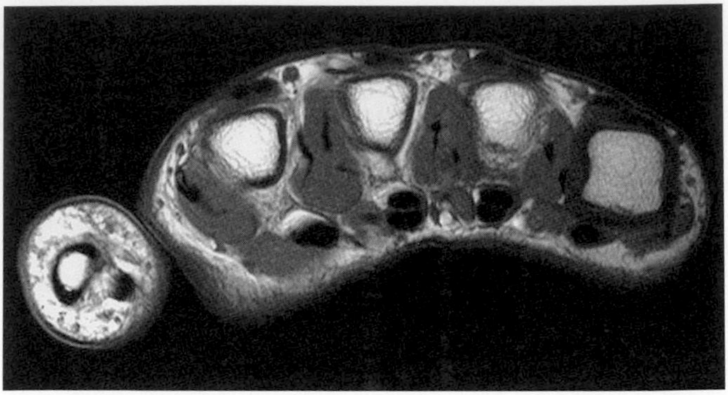

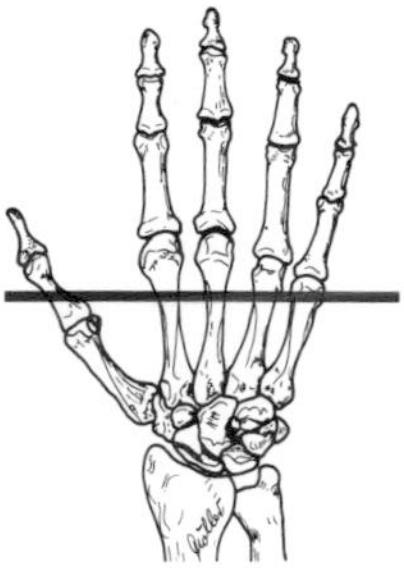

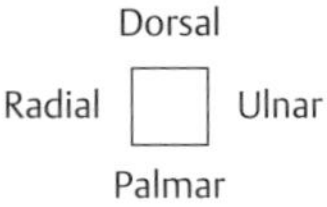
Dorsal
Radial
Ulnar
Palmar

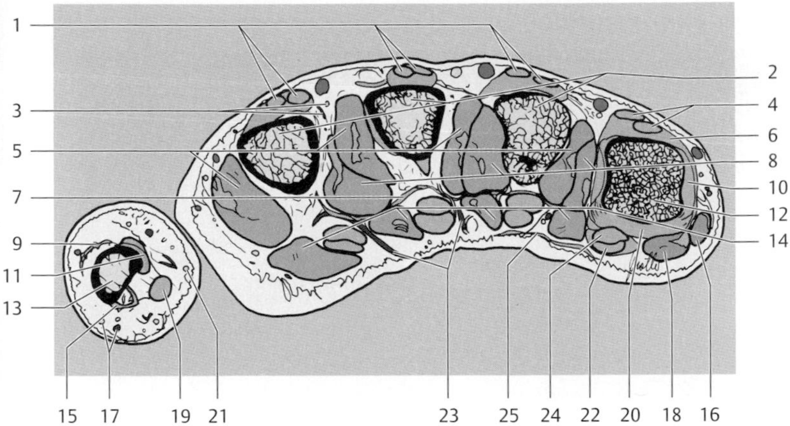

1 Extensor digitorum muscle (tendons)
2 Metacarpals II–IV (shafts)
3 Dorsal digital artery and nerve
4 Extensor digiti minimi muscle (tendon)
5 Dorsal interosseous muscles
6 Dorsal (extensor) expansion
7 Deep transverse metacarpal ligament
8 Palmar interosseous muscles
9 Extensor pollicis muscle (aponeurosis)
10 Collateral ligament
11 Adductor pollicis muscle (tendon attachment)
12 Metacarpal V (head)
13 First proximal phalanx
14 Lumbrical muscles
15 Flexor pollicis brevis muscle and abductor pollicis brevis muscle (tendon attachment)
16 Abductor digiti minimi muscle
17 Dorsal digital nerve and artery of thumb
18 Flexor digiti minimi brevis muscle
19 Flexor pollicis longus muscle (tendon)
20 Palmar ligament
21 Palmar digital artery and nerve of thumb
22 Flexor digitorum superficialis muscle (tendons)
23 Palmar digital arteries and nerves
24 Flexor digitorum profundus muscle (tendons)
25 Palmar aponeurosis with longitudinal fasciculi

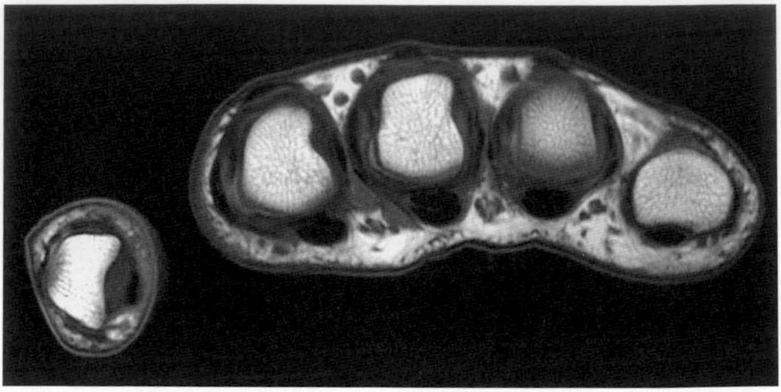

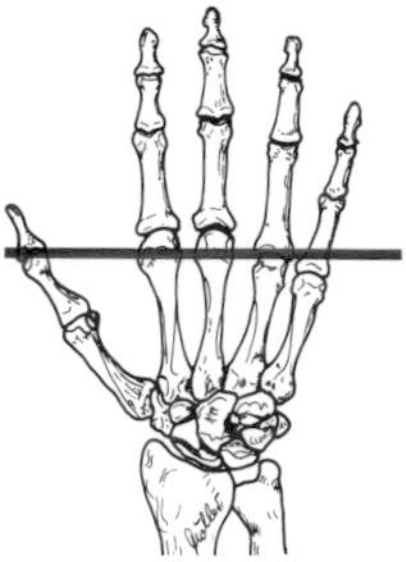

Dorsal

Radial ☐ Ulnar

Palmar

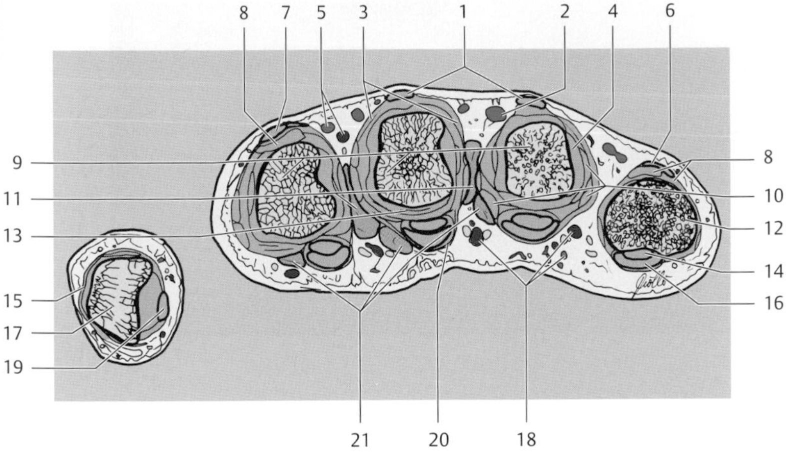

1 Extensor digitorum muscle (tendons)
2 Dorsal digital vein
3 Sagittal ligament
4 Collateral ligament
5 Dorsal digital artery, vein and nerve
6 Extensor digiti minimi muscle (tendon)
7 Extensor indicis muscle (tendon)
8 Dorsal (extensor) expansion ("dorsal aponeurosis")
9 Metacarpals (shafts)
10 Interosseous muscle (tendon)
11 Interosseous muscle
12 Proximal phalanx V (base)
13 Palmar ligament
14 Flexor digitorum profundus muscle (tendons)
15 Extensor pollicis muscle (aponeurosis)
16 Flexor digitorum superficialis muscle (tendon)
17 Proximal phalanx I
18 Palmar digital arteries and nerves
19 Flexor pollicis longus muscle (tendon)
20 Anular ligament
21 Lumbrical muscle

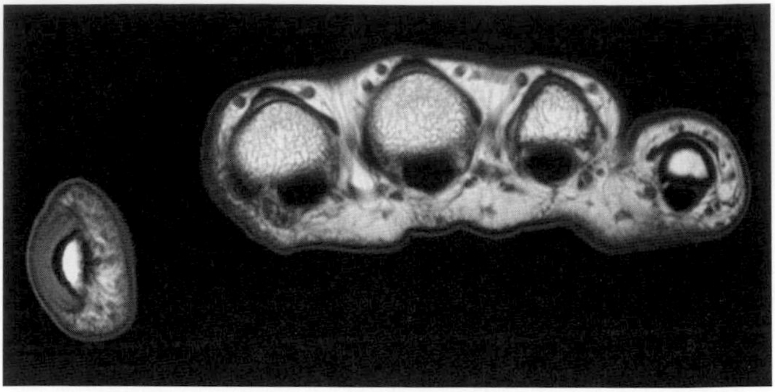

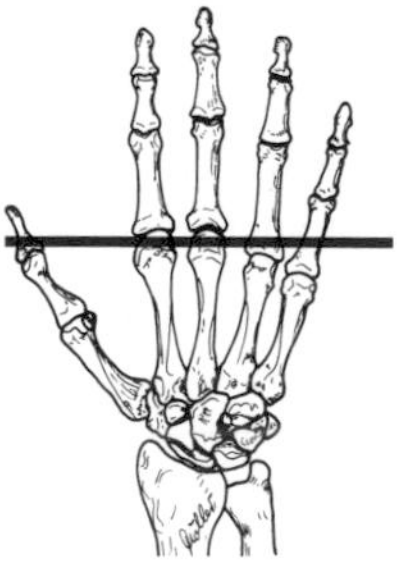

Dorsal

Radial ☐ Ulnar

Palmar

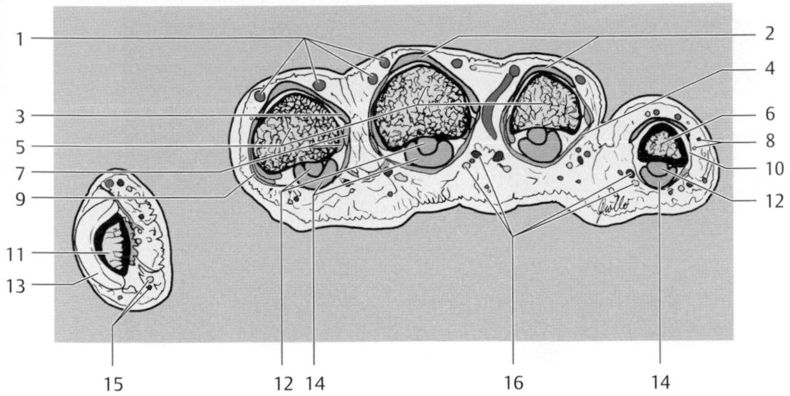

1 Dorsal digital vein
2 Extensor digitorum muscle (aponeurosis)
3 Lateral band
4 Anular ligament
5 Proximal phalanges II–IV (bases)
6 Proximal phalanx V (shaft)
7 Interossei muscles (tendon)
8 Dorsal digital artery and nerve
9 Sagittal ligament
10 Collateral ligament
11 Distal phalanx of thumb
12 Flexor digitorum profundus muscle (tendons)
13 Body of fingernail
14 Flexor digitorum superficialis muscle (tendons)
15 Palmar digital arteries and nerves of thumb
16 Palmar digital arteries and nerves

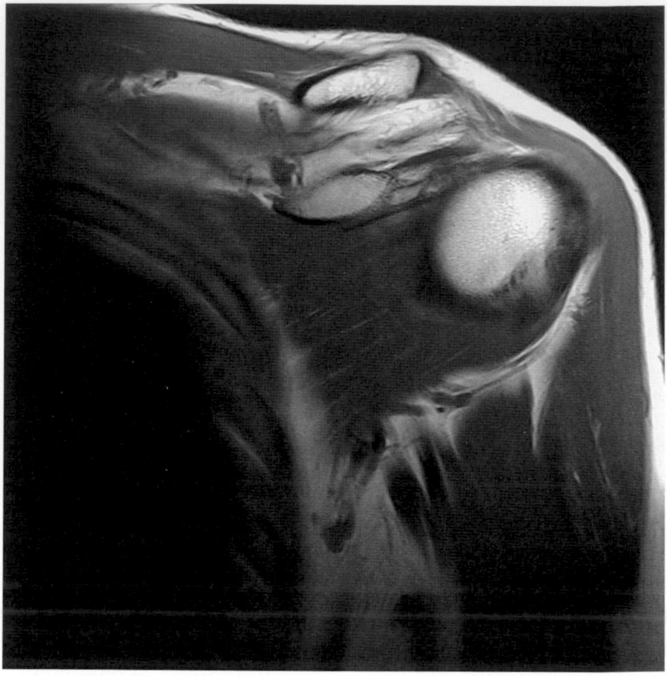

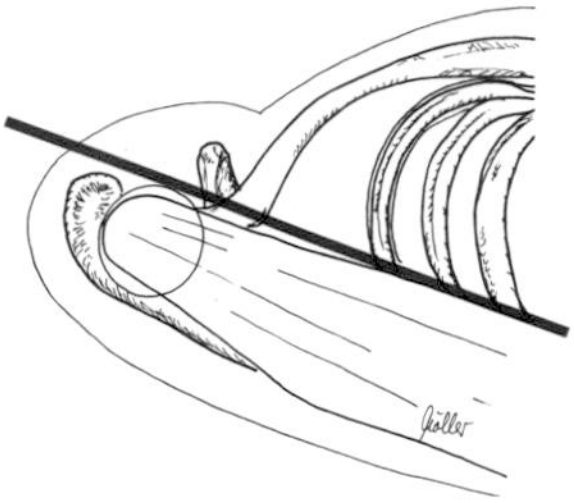

Cranial

Medial | Lateral

Caudal

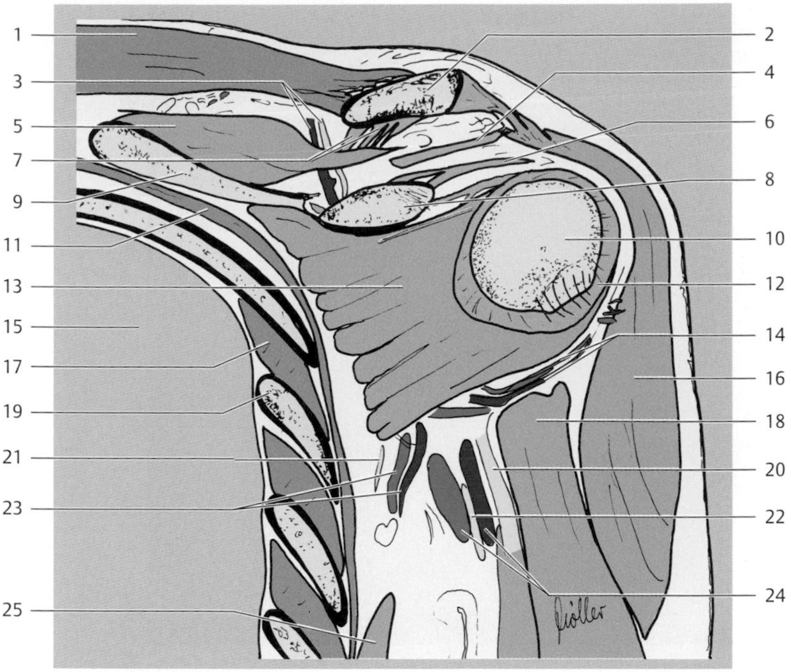

1 Trapezius muscle
2 Clavicle
3 Suprascapular artery (+ vein) and nerve
4 Coracoacromial ligament
5 Supraspinatus muscle
6 Coracohumeral ligament
7 Coracoclavicular ligament
8 Coracoid process
9 Scapula (superior border)
10 Humerus (head)
11 Serratus anterior muscle
12 Joint capsule
13 Subscapularis muscle
14 Anterior circumflex humeral artery and vein
15 Lung
16 Deltoid muscle
17 Intercostal muscle
18 Coracobrachialis muscle
19 Rib
20 Radial nerve
21 Thoracodorsal nerve
22 Median nerve
23 Suprascapular artery and vein
24 Brachial artery and vein
25 Latissimus dorsi muscle

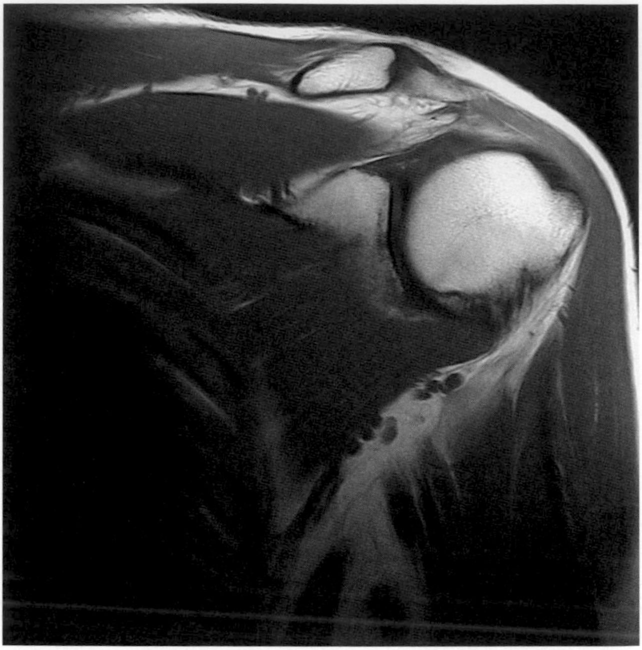

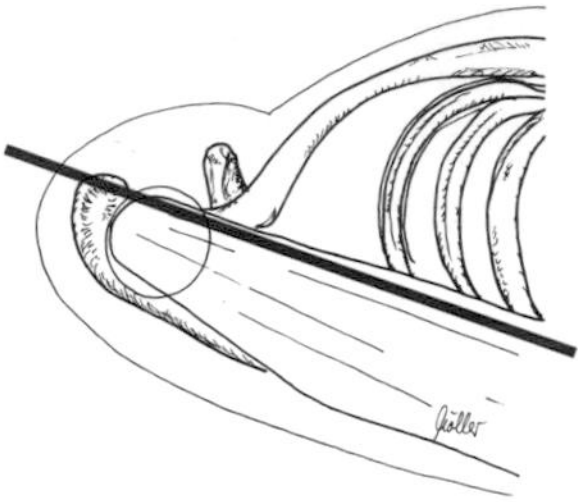

Cranial

Medial ☐ Lateral

Caudal

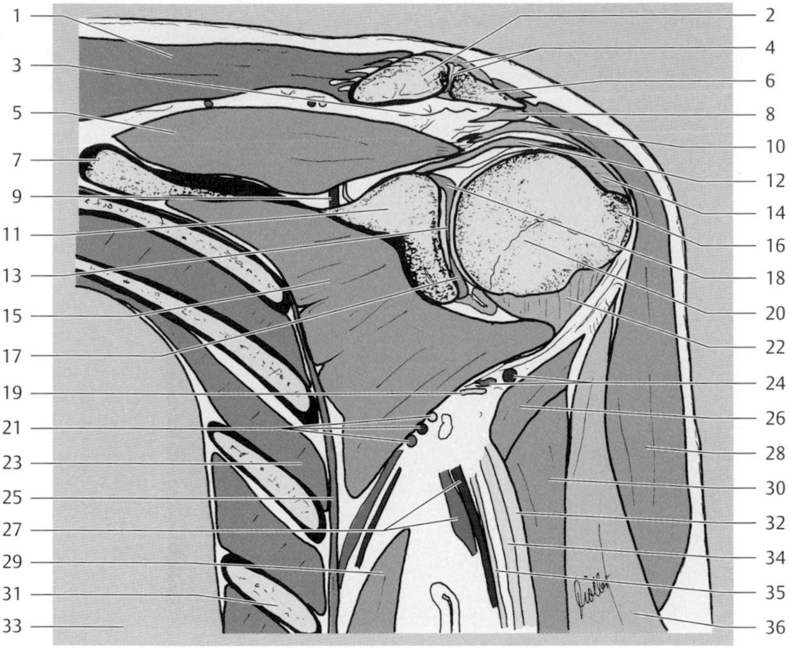

1 Trapezius muscle
2 Clavicle
3 Subacromial bursa
4 Acromioclavicular joint and acromioclavicular ligament
5 Supraspinatus muscle
6 Acromion
7 Scapula
8 Coracoacromial ligament
9 Suprascapular artery (+ vein) and nerve
10 Coracohumeral ligament
11 Glenoid
12 Biceps brachii muscle (long head, tendon)
13 Glenohumeral joint
14 Supraspinatus muscle (tendon attachment)
15 Subscapularis muscle
16 Greater tubercle
17 Glenoid labrum (inferior)
18 Glenoid labrum (superior)
19 Axillary nerve
20 Humerus (head)
21 Subscapular artery, vein, and nerve
22 Glenohumeral ligament
23 Intercostal muscle
24 Posterior circumflex humeral artery and vein
25 Serratus anterior muscle
26 Teres major muscle
27 Axillary artery and vein
28 Deltoid muscle
29 Latissimus dorsi muscle
30 Coracobrachialis muscle
31 Rib
32 Radial nerve
33 Lung
34 Median nerve
35 Ulnar nerve
36 Biceps muscle (long head)

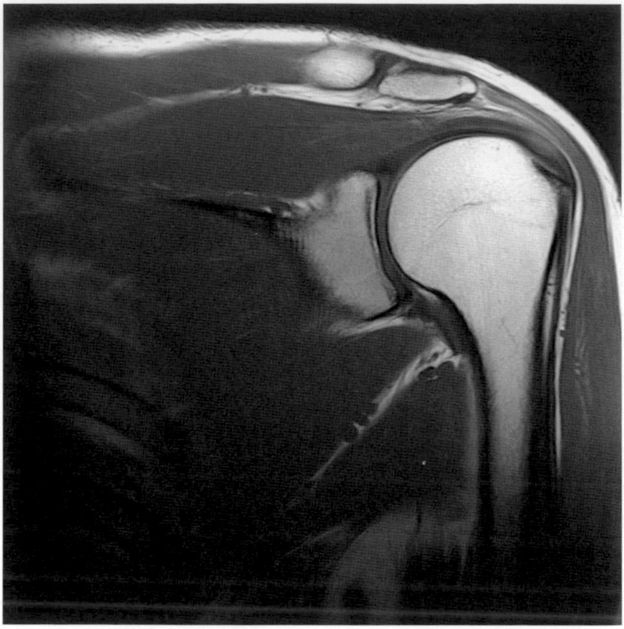

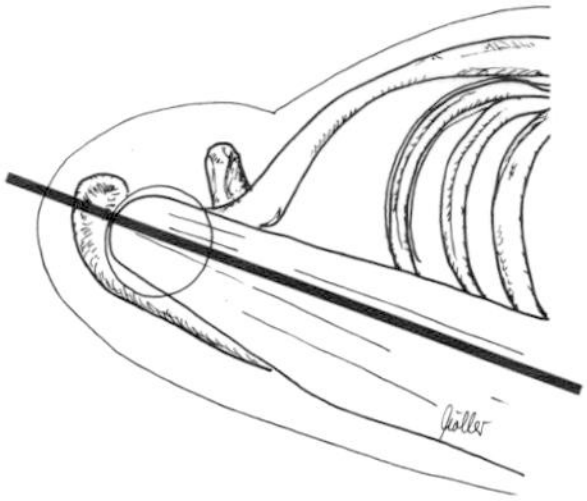

Cranial

Medial Lateral

Caudal

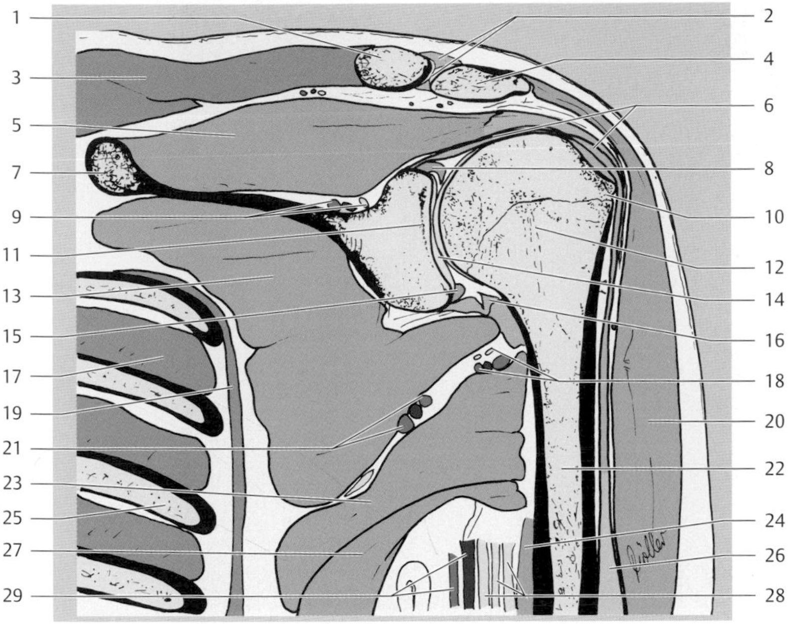

1 Clavicle
2 Acromioclavicular joint and acromioclavicular ligament
3 Trapezius muscle
4 Acromion
5 Supraspinatus muscle
6 Biceps brachii muscle (long head, tendon)
7 Scapula
8 Glenoid labrum (superior)
9 Suprascapular artery, vein, and nerve
10 Greater tubercle
11 Glenoid
12 Humerus (head)
13 Subscapularis muscle
14 Glenohumeral joint
15 Glenoid labrum (inferior)
16 Axillary recess
17 Intercostal muscle
18 Posterior circumflex humeral artery and vein and axillary nerve
19 Serratus anterior muscle
20 Deltoid muscle
21 Subscapular artery and vein
22 Humerus (shaft)
23 Teres major muscle
24 Coracobrachialis muscle
25 Rib
26 Biceps brachii muscle (long head)
27 Latissimus dorsi muscle
28 Ulnar, medial, and radial nerves
29 Brachial artery and vein

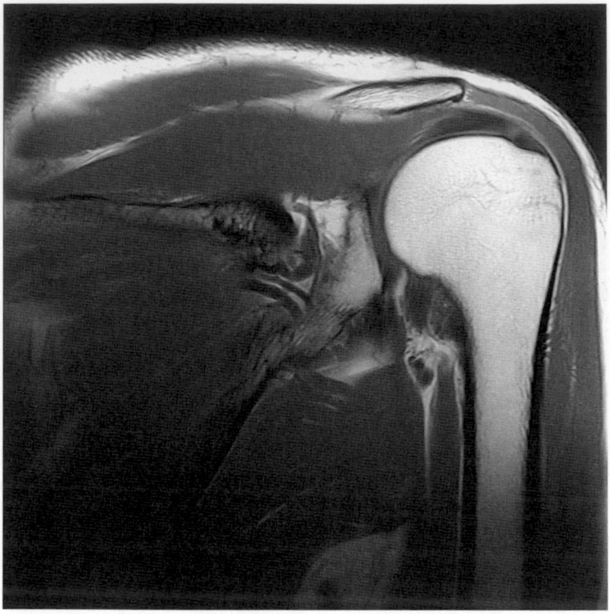

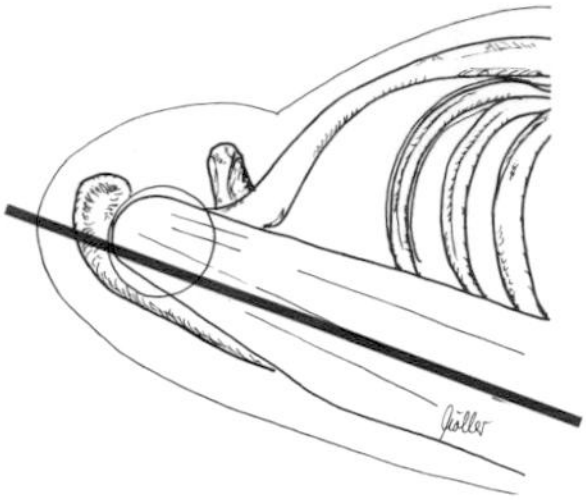

Cranial

Medial Lateral

Caudal

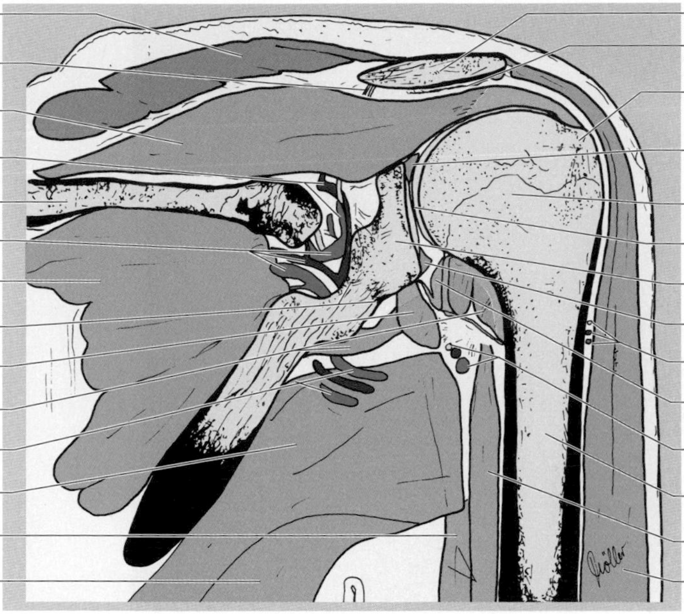

1 Trapezius muscle
2 Acromion
3 Suprascapular artery and vein (acromial branch)
4 Subacromial bursa
5 Supraspinatus muscle
6 Lesser tubercle
7 Suprascapular artery, vein, and nerve
8 Glenoid labrum (superior)
9 Scapula
10 Humerus (head)
11 Circumflex scapular artery and vein
12 Glenohumeral joint
13 Infraspinatus muscle
14 Glenoid
15 Neck of scapula
16 Glenoid labrum (inferior)
17 Triceps brachii muscle (long head, tendon attachment)
18 Posterior circumflex humeral artery and vein and axillary nerve (muscular branches)
19 Teres minor muscle
20 Axillary recess
21 Subscapular artery and vein
22 Posterior circumflex humeral artery and vein and axillary nerve
23 Teres major muscle
24 Humerus (shaft)
25 Triceps brachii muscle (long head)
26 Triceps brachii muscle (lateral head)
27 Latissimus dorsi muscle
28 Deltoid muscle

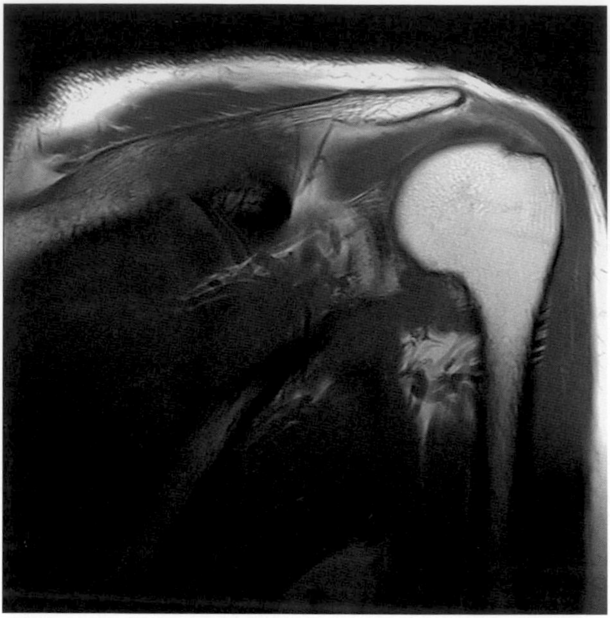

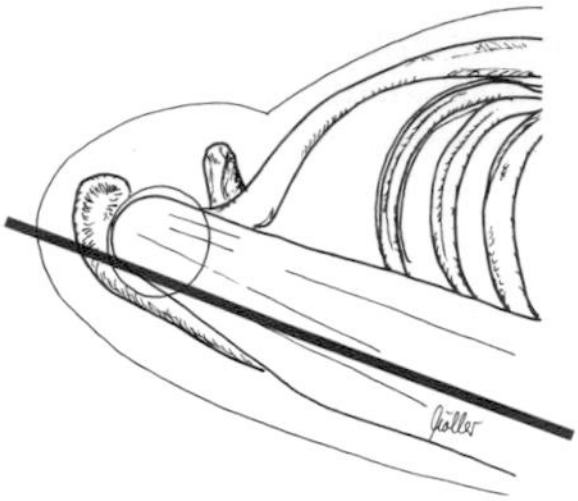

Cranial

Medial Lateral

Caudal

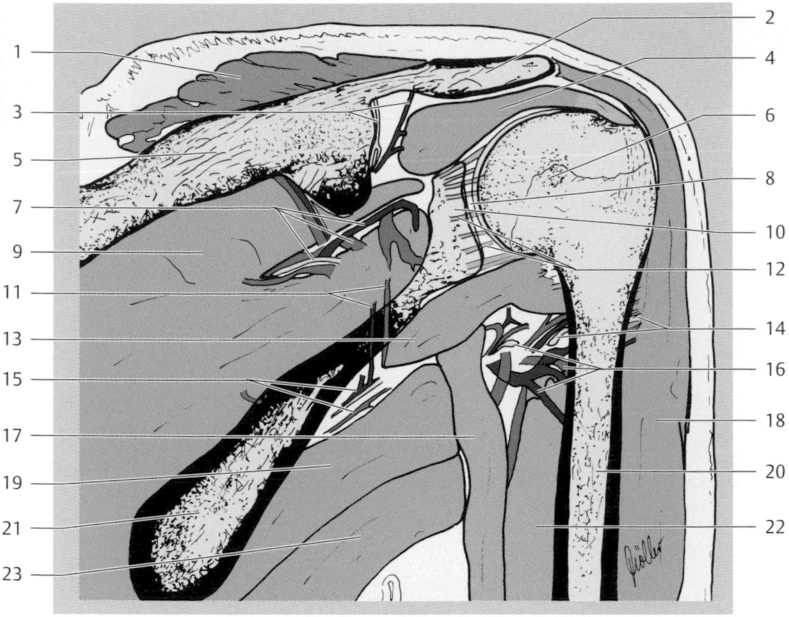

1 Trapezius muscle
2 Acromion
3 Subscapular artery, vein, and nerve (acromial branch)
4 Supraspinatus muscle
5 Spine of scapula
6 Humerus (head)
7 Scapular artery, vein, and nerve
8 Glenohumeral joint
9 Infraspinatus muscle
10 Glenoid
11 Circumflex scapular artery and vein
12 Joint capsule
13 Teres minor muscle
14 Posterior circumflex humeral artery and vein and axillary nerve (muscular branches)
15 Subscapular artery and vein
16 Posterior circumflex humeral artery and vein and axillary nerve
17 Triceps brachii muscle (long head)
18 Deltoid muscle
19 Teres major muscle
20 Humerus (shaft)
21 Scapula
22 Triceps brachii muscle (lateral head)
23 Latissimus dorsi muscle

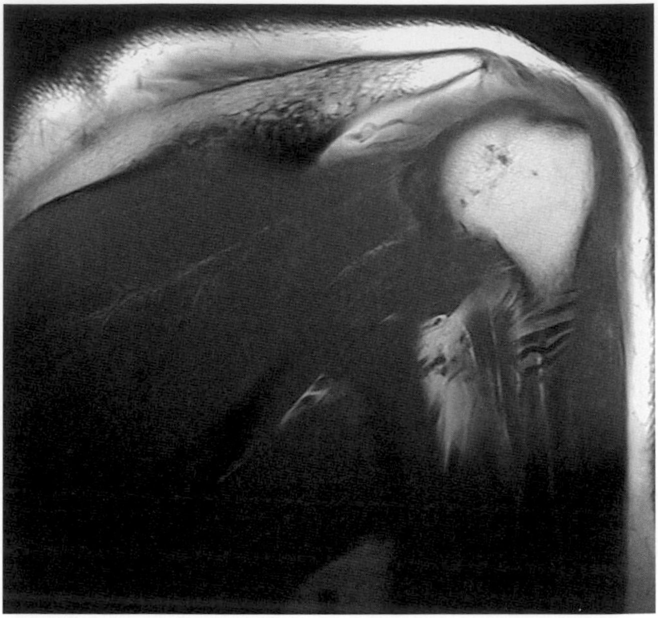

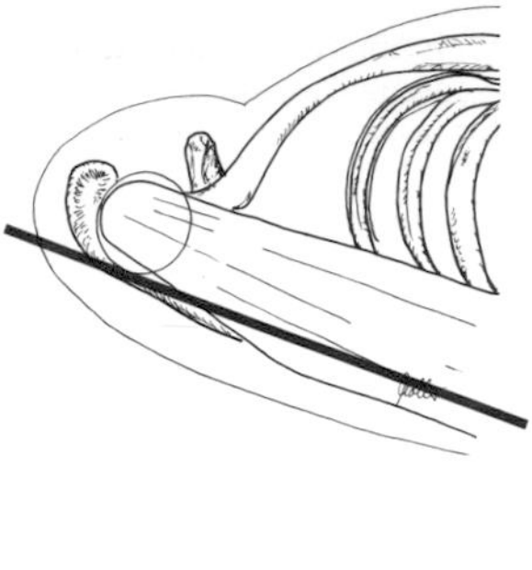

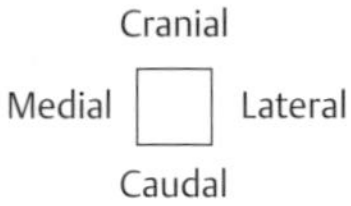
Cranial
Medial
Lateral
Caudal

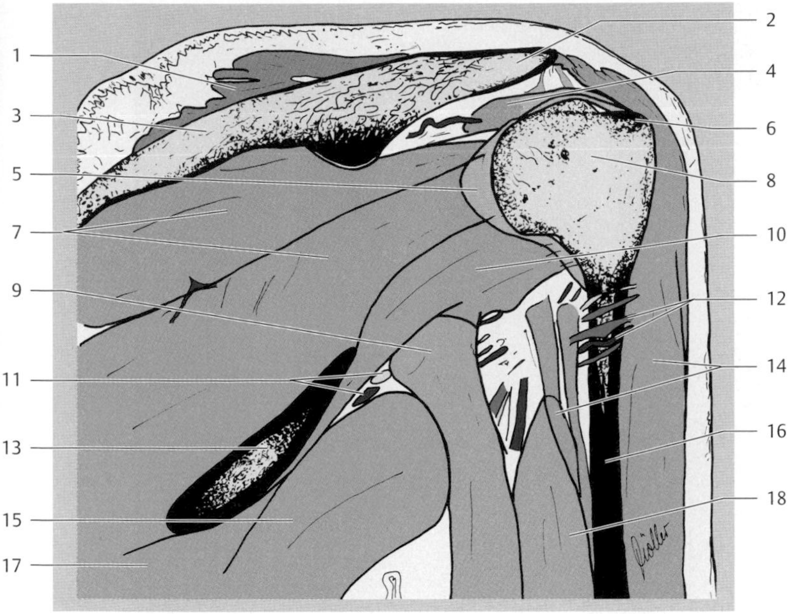

1 Trapezius muscle
2 Acromion
3 Spine of scapula
4 Supraspinatus muscle
5 Joint capsule
6 Lesser tubercle
7 Infraspinatus muscle
8 Humerus (head)
9 Triceps brachii muscle (long head)
10 Teres minor muscle
11 Subscapular artery (+ vein) and nerve
12 Posterior circumflex humeral artery and vein and axillary nerve
13 Scapula
14 Deltoid muscle
15 Teres major muscle
16 Humerus (shaft)
17 Latissimus dorsi muscle
18 Triceps brachii muscle (lateral head)

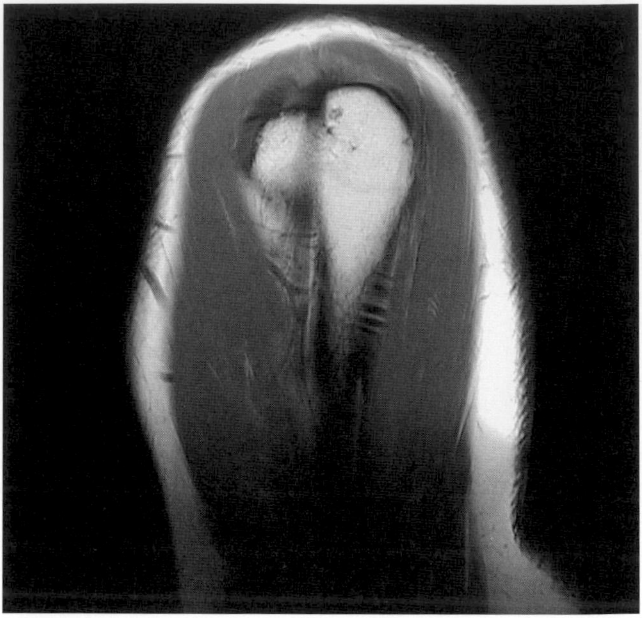

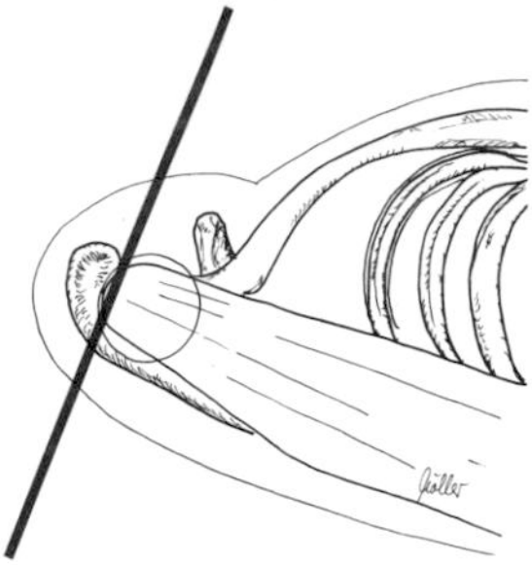

Cranial

Ventral Dorsal

Caudal

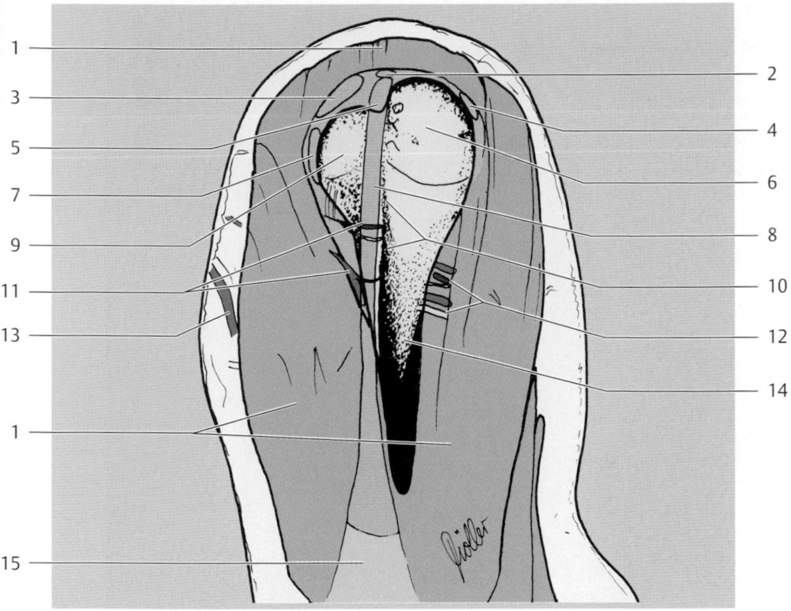

1 Deltoid muscle (acromial part)
2 Supraspinatus muscle (tendon)
3 Glenohumeral ligament (superior)
4 Infraspinatus muscle (tendon)
5 Intertubercular sulcus (bicipital groove)
6 Greater tubercle
7 Glenohumeral ligament (middle)
8 Biceps brachii muscle (long head, tendon)
9 Lesser tubercle
10 Crest of greater tubercle
11 Anterior circumflex humeral artery and vein
12 Posterior circumflex humeral artery and vein and axillary nerve (branch)
13 Cephalic vein
14 Humerus (shaft)
15 Biceps brachii muscle (long head)

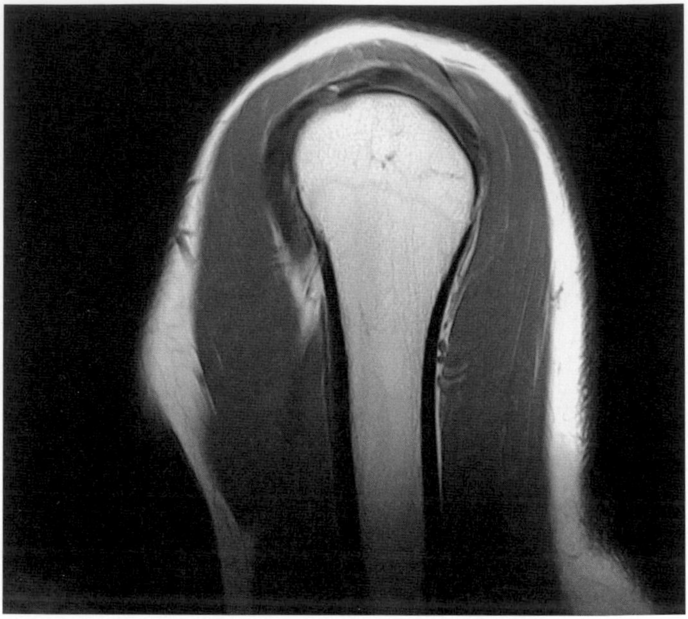

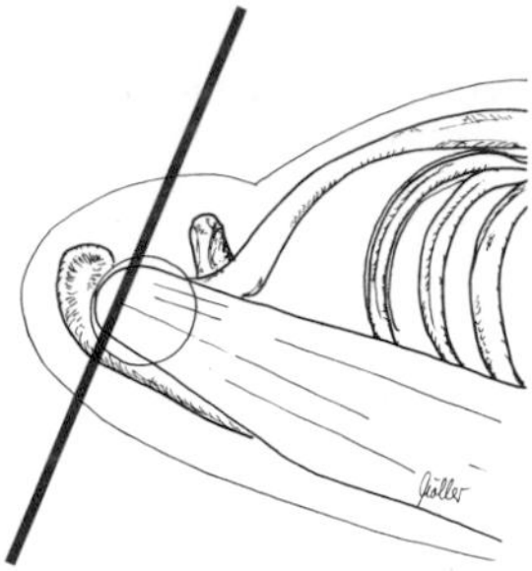

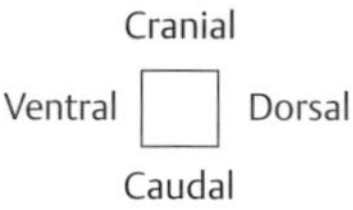
Cranial
Ventral
Dorsal
Caudal

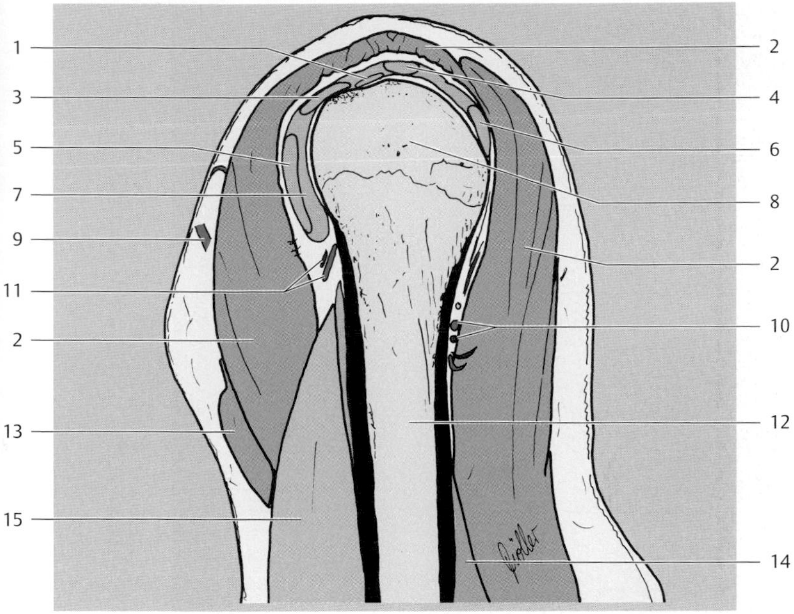

1 Biceps brachii muscle (long head, tendon)
2 Deltoid muscle (acromial part)
3 Glenohumeral ligament (superior)
4 Supraspinatus muscle (tendon)
5 Glenohumeral ligament (middle)
6 Infraspinatus muscle (tendon)
7 Joint capsule
8 Humerus (head)
9 Cephalic vein
10 Posterior circumflex humeral artery and vein
11 Anterior circumflex humeral artery and vein
12 Humerus (shaft)
13 Pectoralis major muscle
14 Triceps brachii muscle (medial head)
15 Biceps brachii muscle (long head)

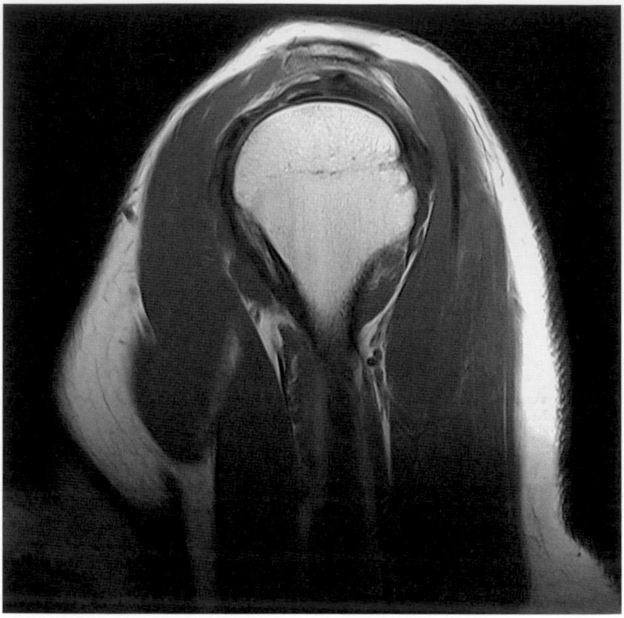

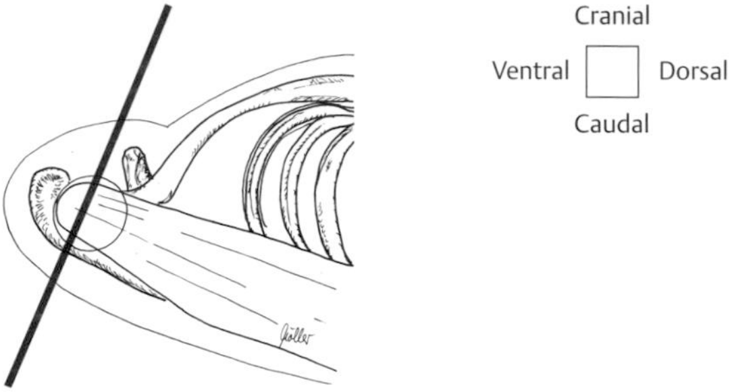
Cranial
Ventral
Dorsal
Caudal

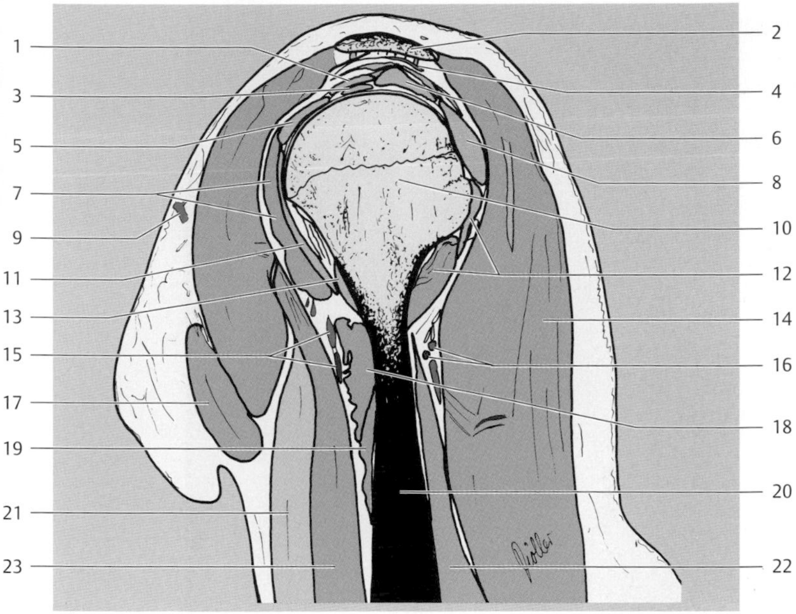

1 Transverse humeral ligament
2 Acromion
3 Biceps brachii muscle (long head, tendon)
4 Subdeltoid bursa
5 Glenohumeral ligament (superior)
6 Supraspinatus muscle (tendon)
7 Subscapularis muscle
8 Infraspinatus muscle (tendon)
9 Cephalic vein
10 Humerus (head)
11 Glenohumeral ligament (middle)
12 Teres minor muscle (+ tendon attachment)
13 Glenohumeral ligament (inferior)
14 Deltoid muscle (acromial part)
15 Anterior circumflex humeral artery and vein
16 Posterior circumflex humeral artery and vein
17 Pectoralis major muscle
18 Latissimus dorsi muscle
19 Teres major muscle
20 Humerus (shaft)
21 Biceps brachii muscle (long head)
22 Triceps brachii muscle (medial head)
23 Coracobrachialis muscle

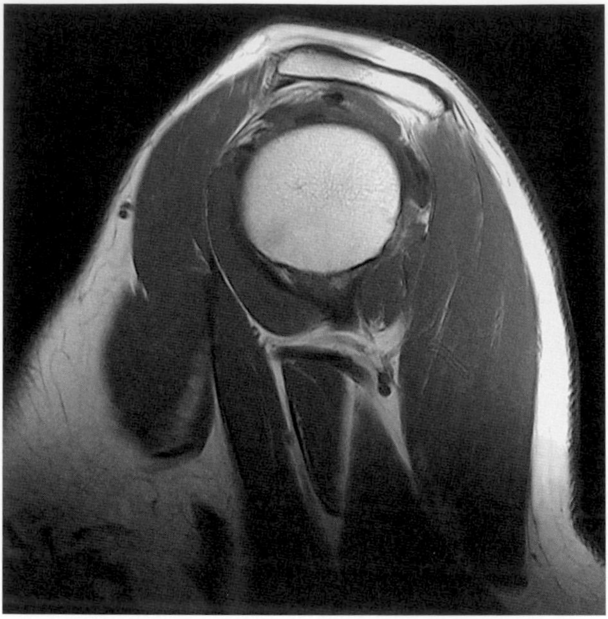

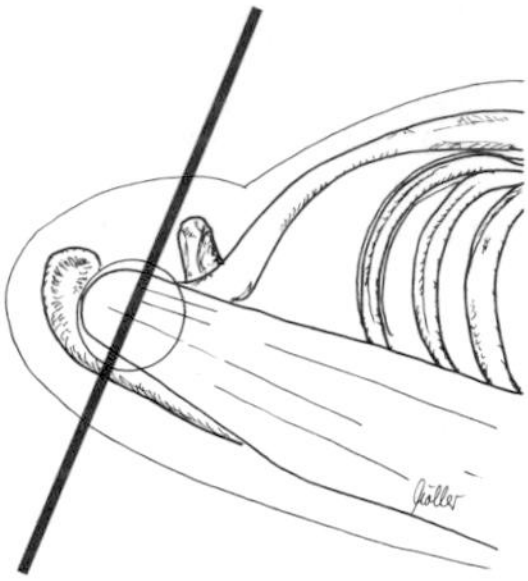

Cranial

Ventral Dorsal

Caudal

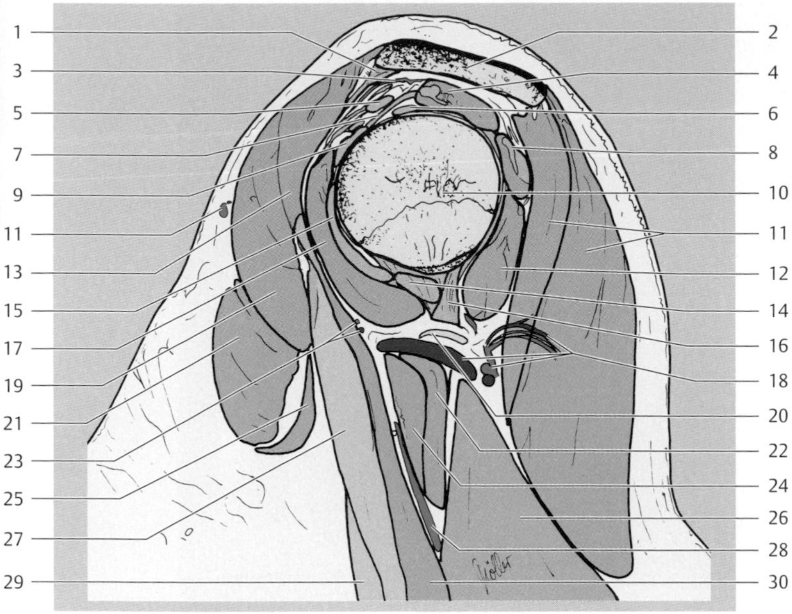

1 Coracoacromial ligament
2 Acromion
3 Subacromial bursa
4 Supraspinatus muscle (+ tendon)
5 Coracohumeral ligament
6 Biceps brachii muscle (long head, tendon)
7 Transverse humeral ligament
8 Infraspinatus muscle (+ tendon)
9 Superior glenohumeral ligament
10 Humerus (head)
11 Cephalic vein
12 Teres minor muscle
13 Deltoid muscle (acromial part)
14 Inferior glenohumeral ligament
15 Middle glenohumeral ligament
16 Teres major muscle (tendon)
17 Subscapularis muscle
18 Posterior circumflex humeral artery and vein + muscular branches
19 Deltoid muscle (clavicular part)
20 Axillary nerve
21 Pectoralis major muscle
22 Teres major muscle
23 Anterior circumflex humeral artery and vein
24 Latissimus dorsi muscle
25 Pectoralis minor muscle
26 Triceps brachii muscle (long head)
27 Biceps brachii muscle (short head + tendon)
28 Basilic vein
29 Biceps brachii muscle (long head)
30 Coracobrachialis muscle

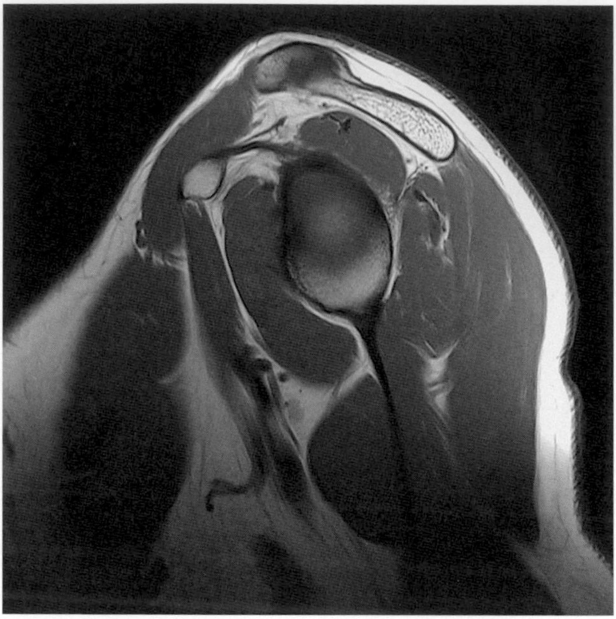

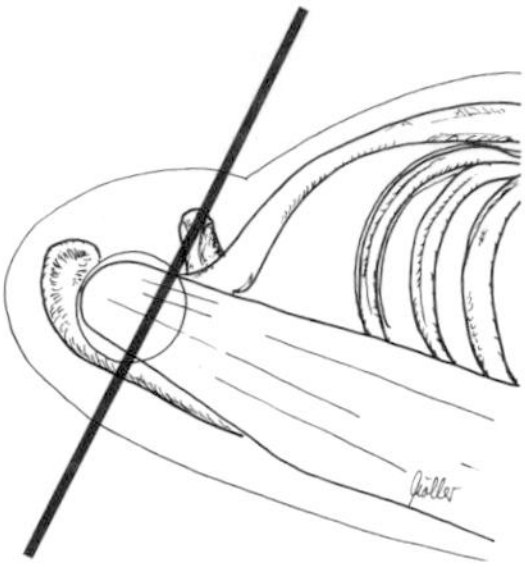

Cranial

Ventral ☐ Dorsal

Caudal

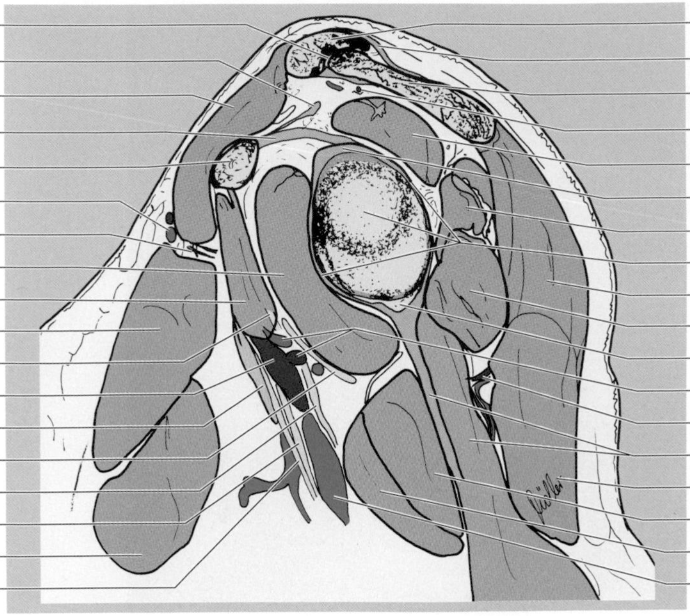

1 Acromioclavicular joint
2 Clavicle
3 Coracoacromial ligament
4 Acromioclavicular ligament
5 Deltoid muscle (clavicular part)
6 Acromion
7 Coracohumeral ligament
8 Thoracoacromial artery (acromial branch)
9 Coracoid process
10 Supraspinatus muscle (+ tendon)
11 Cephalic vein
12 Biceps brachii muscle (long head, tendon attachment)
13 Thoracoacromial artery (deltoid branch)
14 Infraspinatus muscle (+ tendon)
15 Subscapularis muscle
16 Glenohumeral joint and joint capsule
17 Coracobrachialis muscle
18 Deltoid muscle (acromial part)
19 Pectoralis major muscle
20 Teres major muscle
21 Musculocutaneous nerve
22 Infraglenoid tubercle
23 Brachial artery
24 Posterior circumflex humeral artery and vein
25 Biceps brachii muscle (short head)
26 Posterior circumflex humeral artery and vein (muscular branches)
27 Axillary nerve
28 Triceps brachii muscle (long head + tendon)
29 Radial nerve
30 Deltoid muscle (spinal part)
31 Ulnar nerve
32 Teres major muscle
33 Pectoralis minor muscle
34 Latissimus dorsi muscle
35 Median nerve
36 Brachial vein

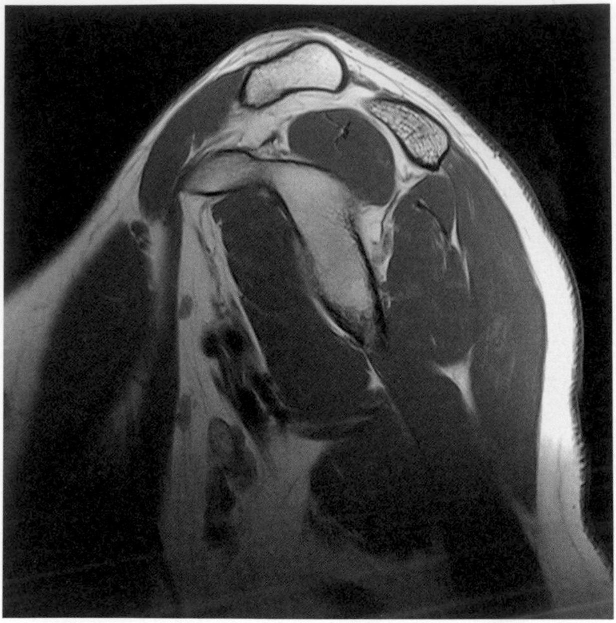

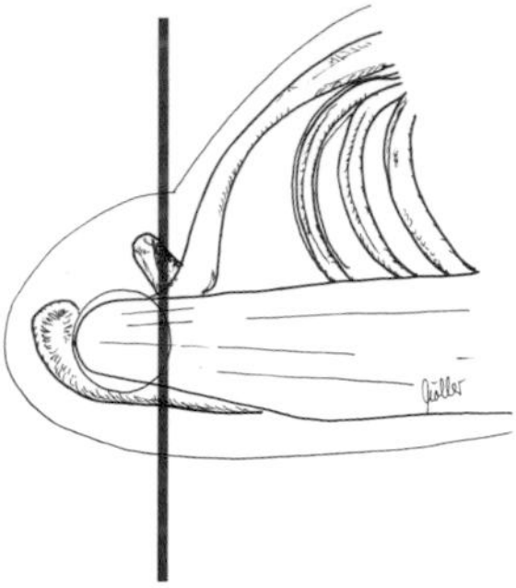

Cranial

Ventral Dorsal

Caudal

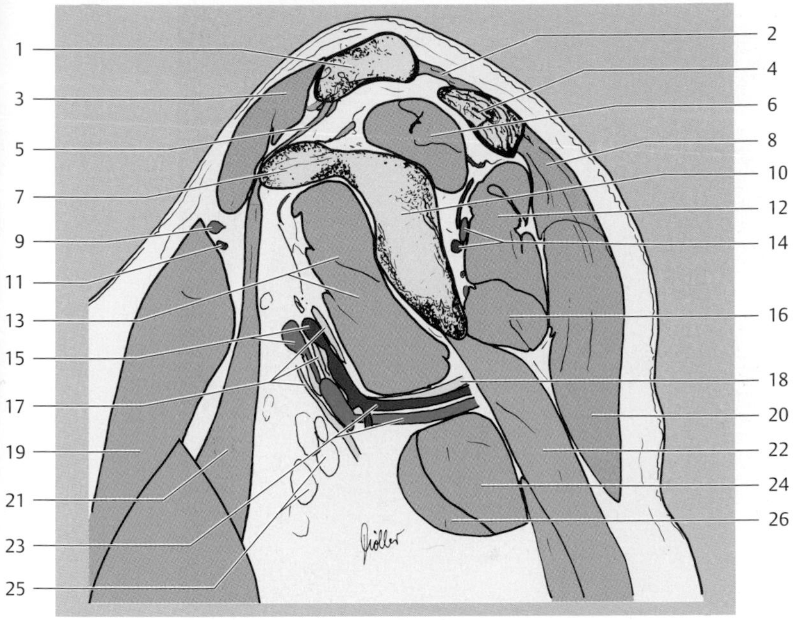

1 Clavicle
2 Trapezius muscle
3 Deltoid muscle (clavicular part)
4 Acromion
5 Coracoclavicular ligament
6 Supraspinatus muscle
7 Coracoid process
8 Deltoid muscle (acromial part)
9 Cephalic vein
10 Scapula
11 Thoracoacromial artery (pectoralis branch)
12 Infraspinatus muscle (and tendon)
13 Subscapularis muscle
14 Circumflex scapular artery and vein
15 Axillary artery and vein
16 Teres minor muscle
17 Brachial plexus
18 Axillary nerve
19 Pectoralis major muscle
20 Deltoid muscle (spinal part)
21 Pectoralis minor muscle
22 Triceps brachii muscle (long head and tendon)
23 Posterior circumflex humeral artery and vein
24 Teres major muscle
25 Axillary lymph node
26 Latissimus dorsi muscle

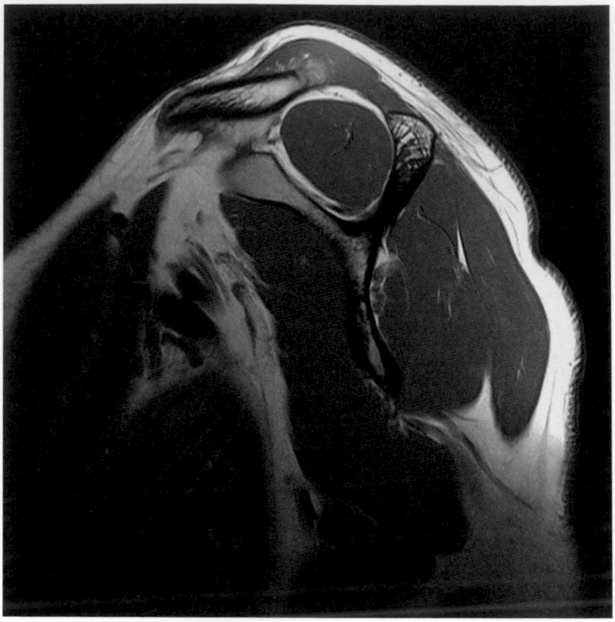

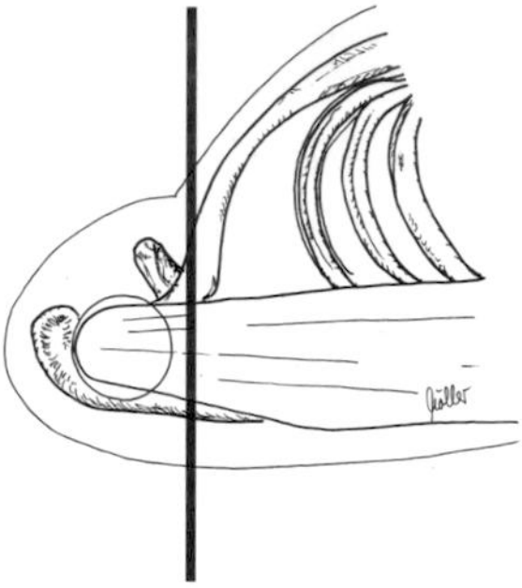

Cranial

Ventral Dorsal

Caudal

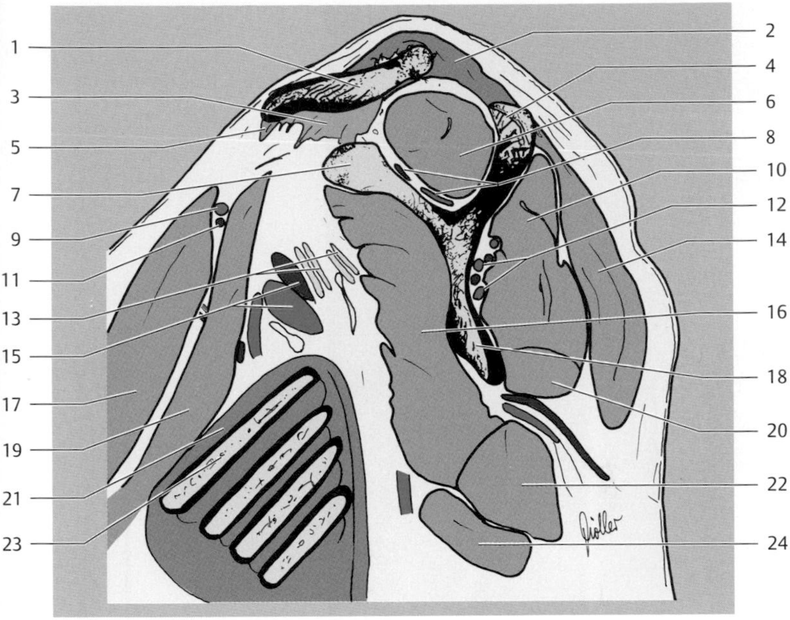

1 Clavicle
2 Trapezius muscle
3 Coracoclavicular ligament
4 Acromion
5 Deltoid muscle (clavicular part)
6 Supraspinatus muscle
7 Scapula (spine)
8 Suprascapular artery and vein
9 Cephalic vein
10 Infraspinatus muscle
11 Thoracoacromial artery (pectoral branch)
12 Circumflex scapular artery and vein
13 Brachial plexus
14 Deltoid muscle (spinal part)
15 Axillary artery and vein
16 Subscapularis muscle
17 Pectoralis major muscle
18 Scapula (body)
19 Pectoralis minor muscle
20 Teres minor muscle
21 Serratus anterior muscle
22 Teres major muscle
23 Ribs
24 Latissimus dorsi muscle

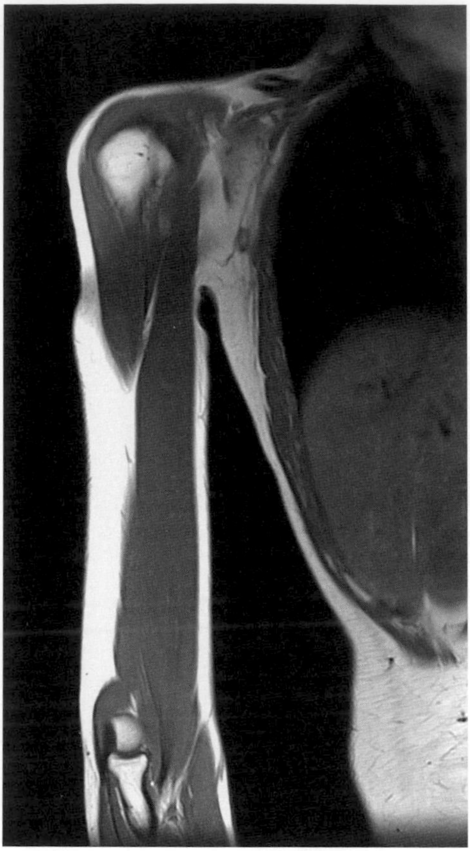

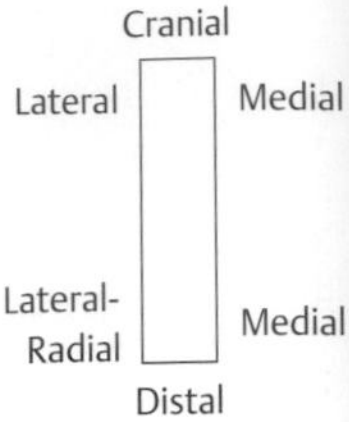

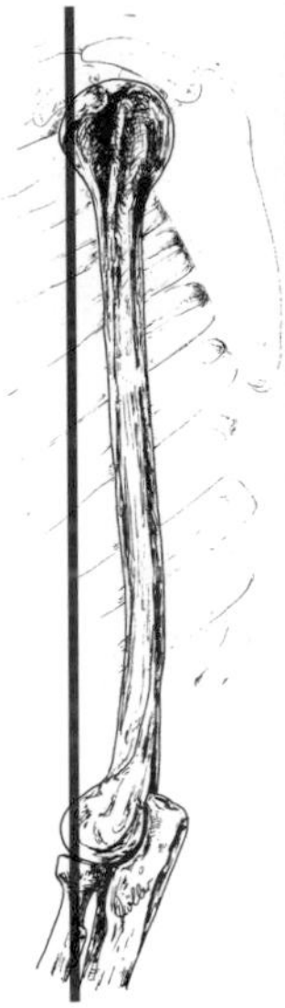

1 Clavicle
2 Subclavian vein
3 Coracoid process
4 Internal jugular vein
5 Biceps brachii muscle (long head, tendon)

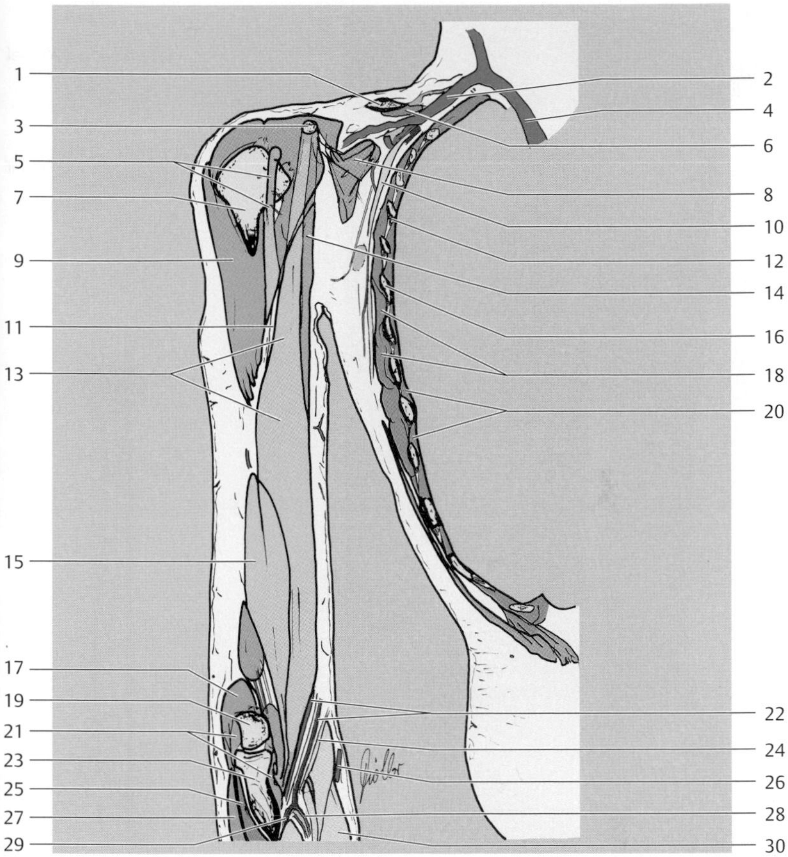

6 Subclavius muscle
7 Humerus (head, collum)
8 Pectoralis minor muscle
9 Deltoid muscle
10 Long thoracic nerve
11 Pectoralis major muscle (tendon)
12 Intercostal artery, vein, and nerve
13 Biceps brachii muscle (short head)
14 Coracobrachialis muscle
15 Brachialis muscle
16 Rib
17 Brachioradialis muscle
18 Serratus anterior muscle
19 Humerus (capitulum)
20 Intercostal muscles
21 Supinator muscle
22 Brachial artery and vein
23 Radius (head)
24 Median nerve
25 Extensor digitorum muscle
26 Cephalic vein
27 Extensor carpi radialis brevis muscle
28 Ulnar artery
29 Radial artery
30 Pronator teres muscle

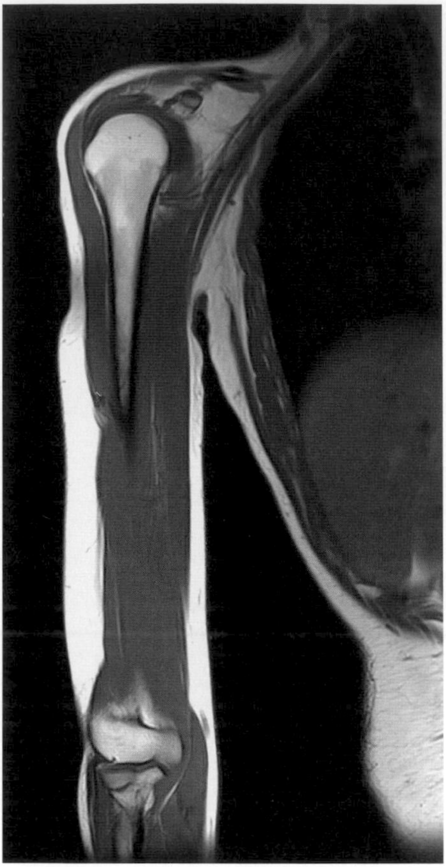

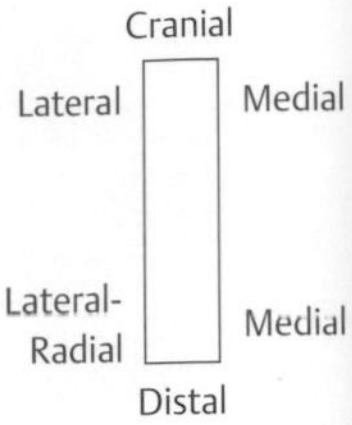

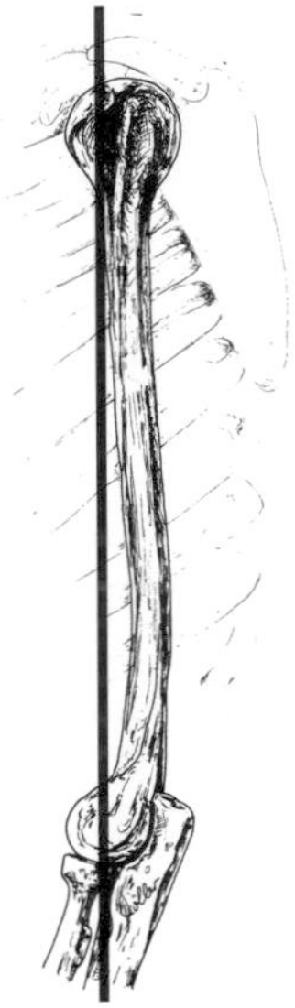

1 Clavicle
2 Scalenus muscle
3 Trapezius muscle
4 Subclavian artery
5 Supraspinatus muscle (tendon)
6 Subclavian vein
7 Coracohumeral ligament
8 Subclavius muscle
9 Biceps brachii muscle (long head, tendon)
10 Coracoclavicular ligament
11 Humerus (head)
12 Coracoid process
13 Greater tubercle
14 Median nerve
15 Anterior circumflex humeral artery and vein
16 Glenoid
17 Deltoid muscle
18 Axillary artery and vein

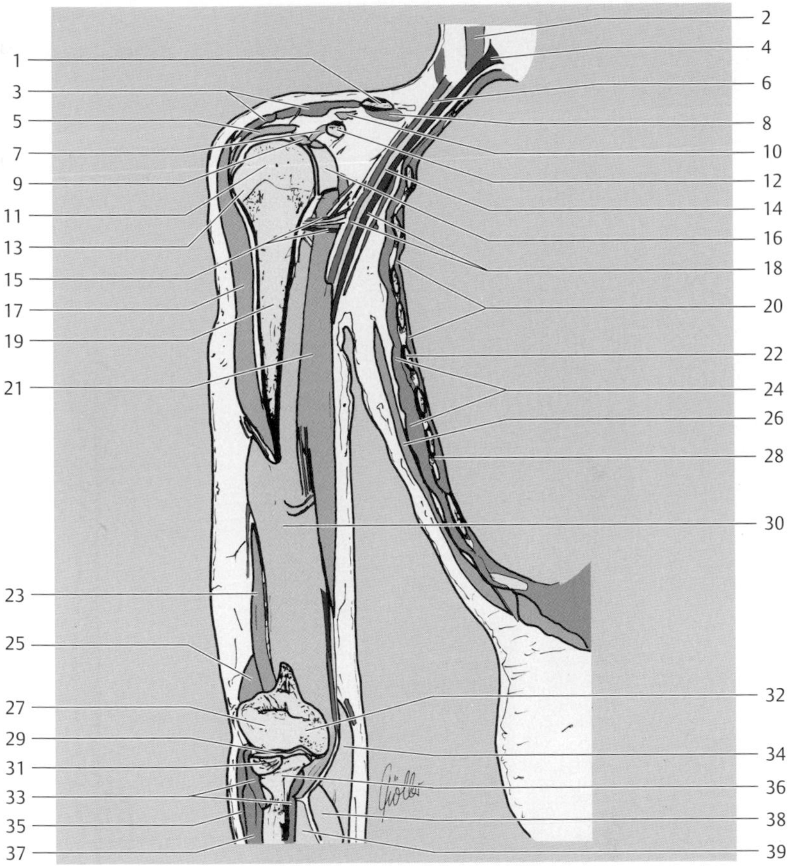

19 Humerus (shaft)
20 Intercostal muscles
21 Coracobrachialis muscle
22 Rib
23 Brachioradialis muscle
24 Serratus anterior muscle
25 Extensor carpi radialis longus muscle
26 Latissimus dorsi muscle
27 Humerus (capitulum)
28 Intercostal artery, vein, and nerve
29 Humeroradial joint
30 Brachialis muscle
31 Radius (head)
32 Humerus (trochlea)
33 Supinator muscle
34 Pronator teres muscle
35 Extensor carpi ulnaris muscle
36 Ulna
37 Extensor digitorum muscle
38 Flexor carpi radialis muscle
39 Flexor digitorum superficialis muscle

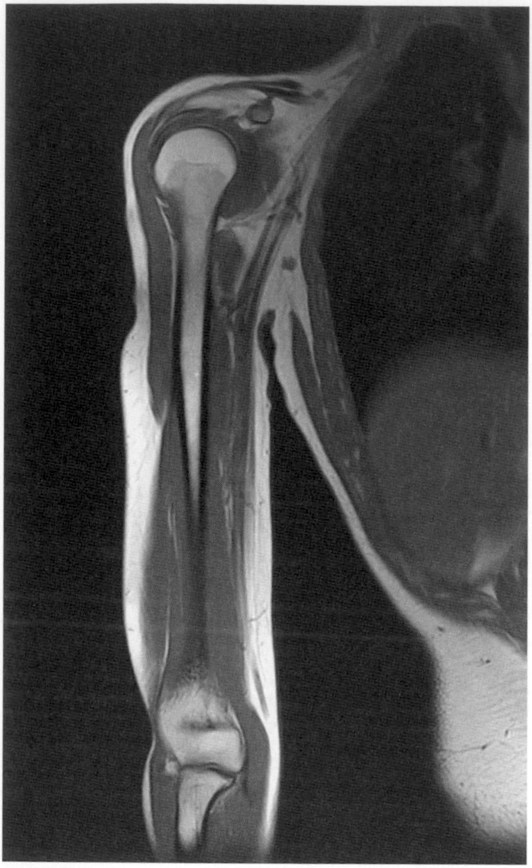

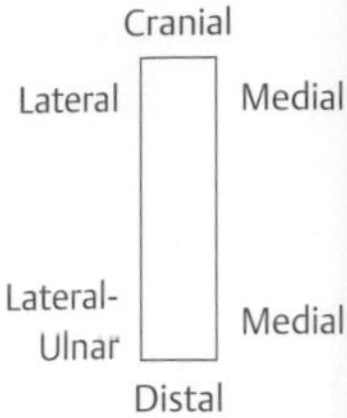

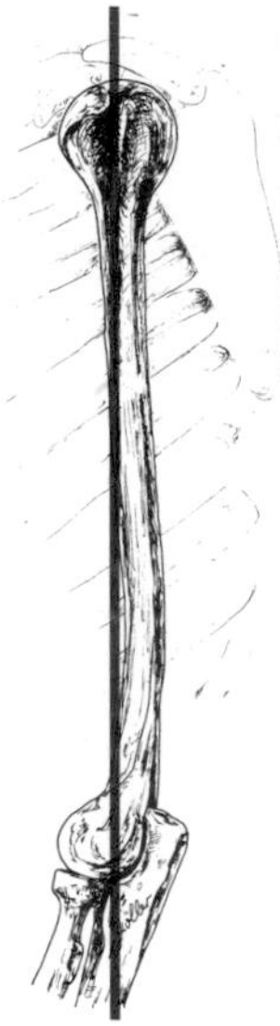

1 Scalenus muscle
2 Brachial plexus
3 Trapezius muscle
4 Posterior (dorsal) funiculus
5 Acromion
6 Clavicle
7 Supraspinatus muscle (tendon)
8 Coracoclavicular ligament
9 Biceps brachii muscle (long head, tendon)
10 Coracoid process
11 Humerus (head)
12 Glenoid
13 Deltoid muscle
14 Subscapularis muscle
15 Humerus (shaft)
16 Anterior circumflex humeral artery and vein
17 Coracobrachialis muscle
18 Teres major muscle

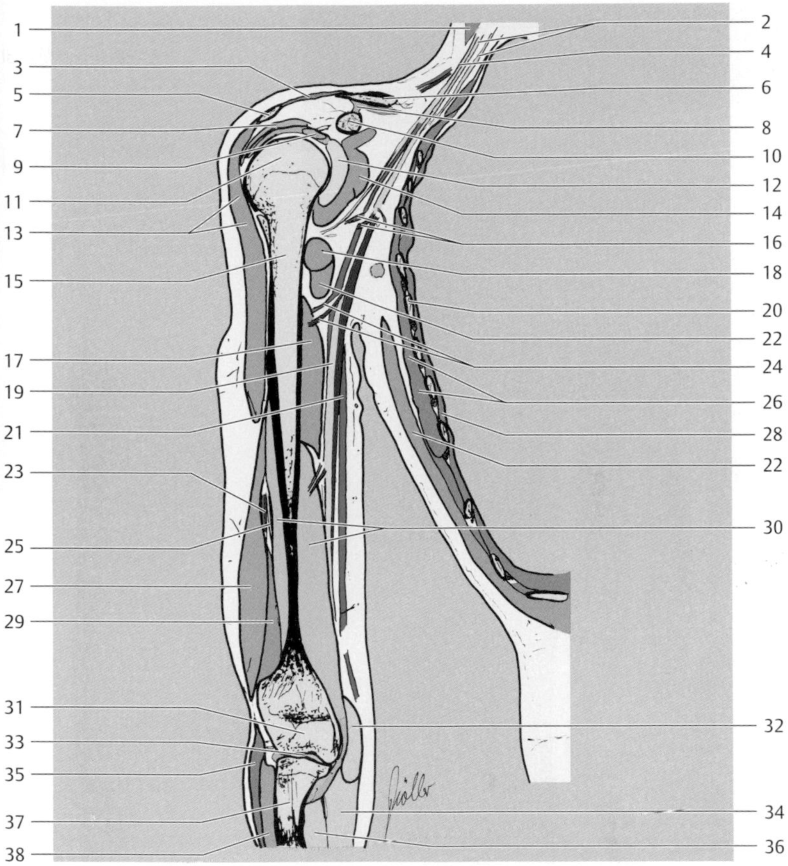

19 Median nerve
20 Rib
21 Basilic vein
22 Latissimus dorsi muscle
23 Deep brachial artery and vein
24 Intercostal artery, vein, and nerve
25 Radial nerve
26 Serratus anterior muscle
27 Triceps brachii muscle (lateral head)
28 Intercostal muscles
29 Brachioradialis muscle
30 Brachialis muscle
31 Humerus (trochlea)
32 Pronator teres muscle
33 Humero-ulnar joint
34 Flexor carpi radialis muscle
35 Extensor carpi ulnaris muscle
36 Flexor digitorum superficialis muscle
37 Ulna
38 Anconeus muscle

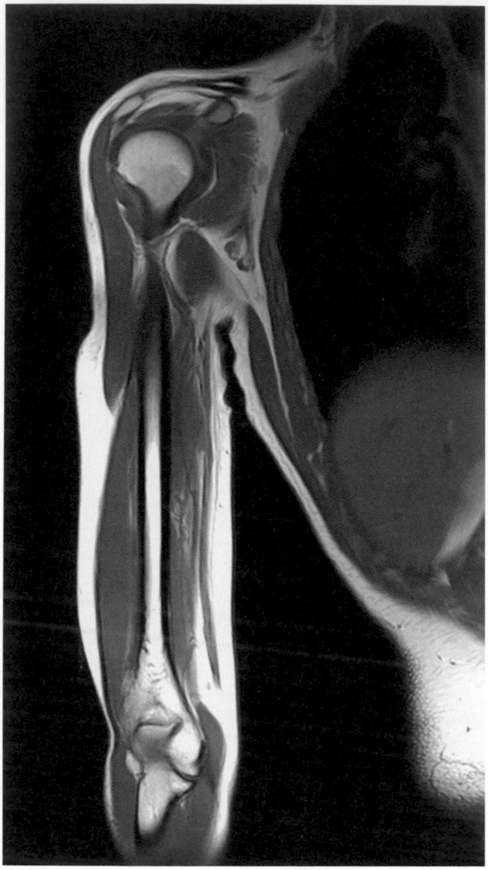

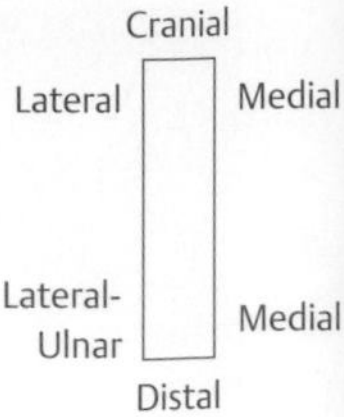

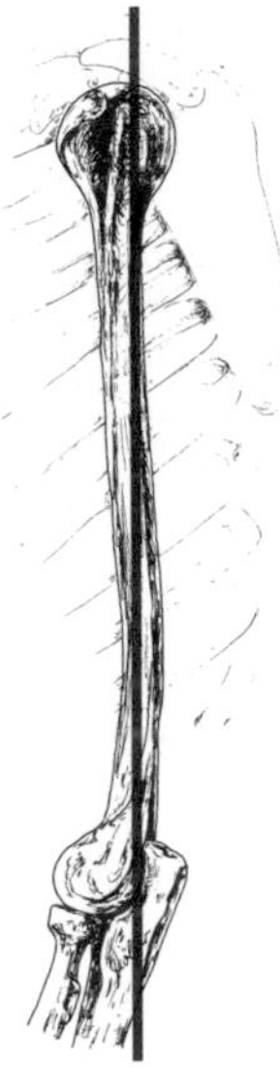

1 Clavicle
2 Scalenus muscle
3 Trapezius muscle
4 Subclavius muscle
5 Coracoclavicular ligament
6 Serratus anterior muscle
7 Acromion
8 Coracoid process
9 Biceps brachii muscle (long head, tendon)
10 Glenoid
11 Supraspinatus muscle (tendon)
12 Subscapularis muscle
13 Humerus (head)
14 Intercostal muscles
15 Infraspinatus muscle
16 Serratus anterior muscle
17 Teres minor muscle
18 Thoracodorsal artery and vein

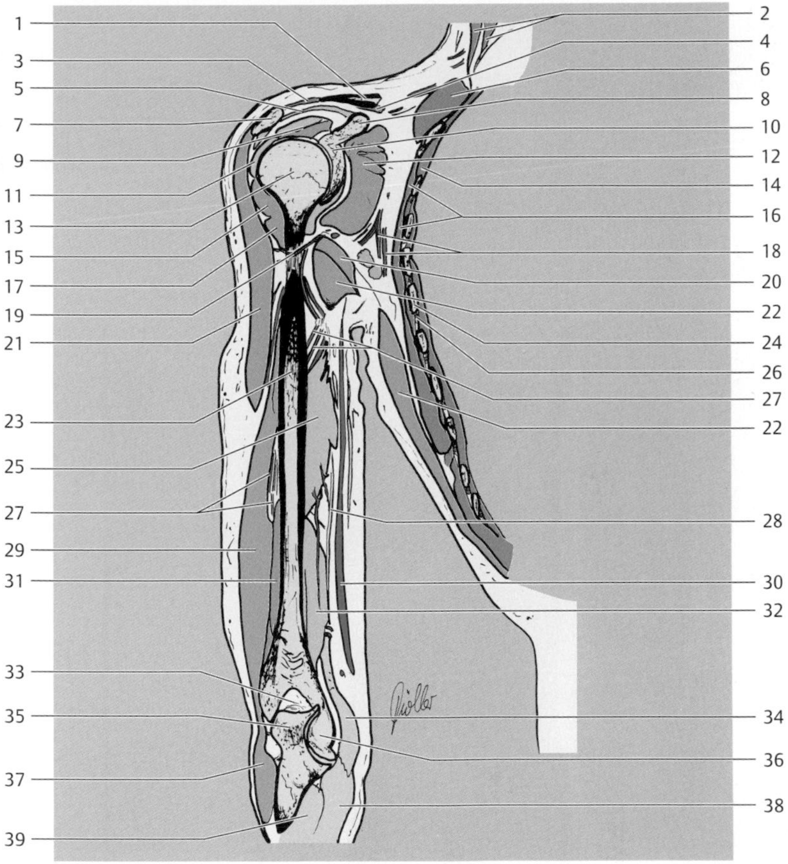

19 Posterior circumflex humeral artery and vein
20 Teres major muscle
21 Deltoid muscle
22 Latissimus dorsi muscle
23 Humerus (shaft)
24 Rib
25 Brachialis muscle
26 Intercostal artery, vein, and nerve
27 Deep brachial artery and vein
28 Ulnar nerve
29 Triceps brachii muscle (lateral head)
30 Basilic vein
31 Brachioradialis muscle
32 Brachialis muscle
33 Olecranon fossa
34 Pronator teres muscle
35 Olecranon
36 Medial epicondyle of humerus
37 Anconeus muscle
38 Flexor digitorum superficialis muscle
39 Flexor digitorum profundus muscle

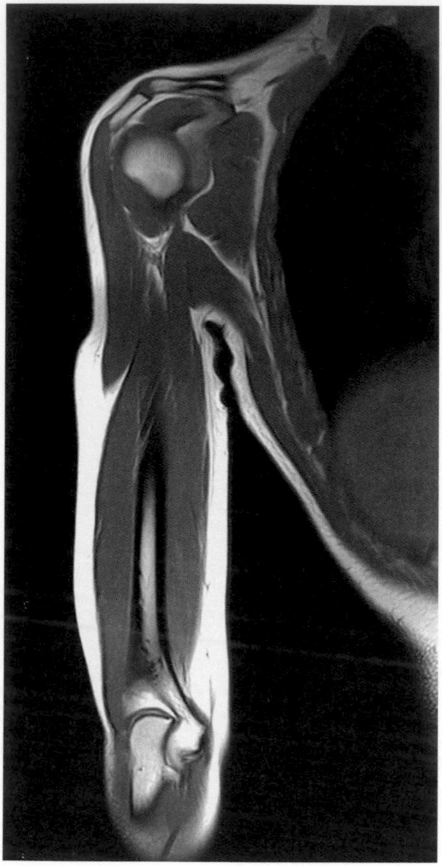

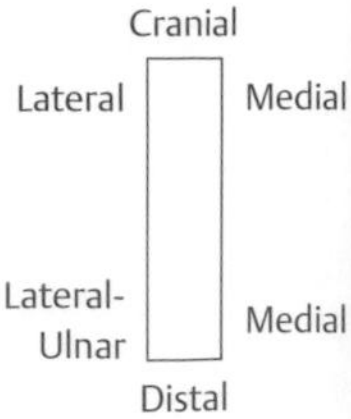

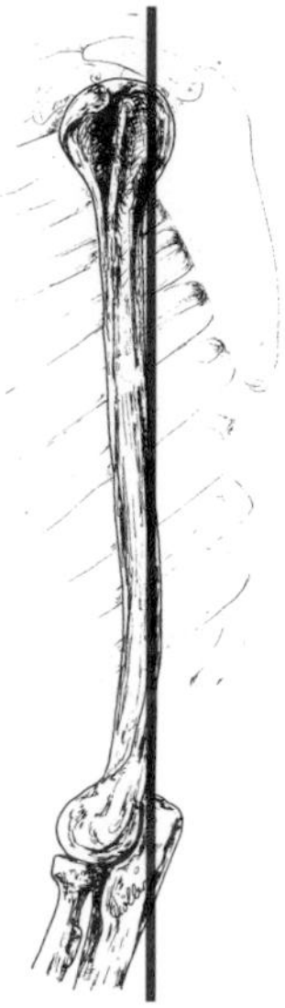

1 Trapezius muscle
2 Scalenus muscle
3 Clavicle
4 Subscapular artery and vein
5 Acromioclavicular joint
6 Serratus anterior muscle
7 Acromion
8 Infraspinatus muscle
9 Biceps brachii muscle (long head, tendon)
10 Intercostal muscles
11 Supraspinatus muscle (tendon)
12 Glenoid
13 Coracoid process

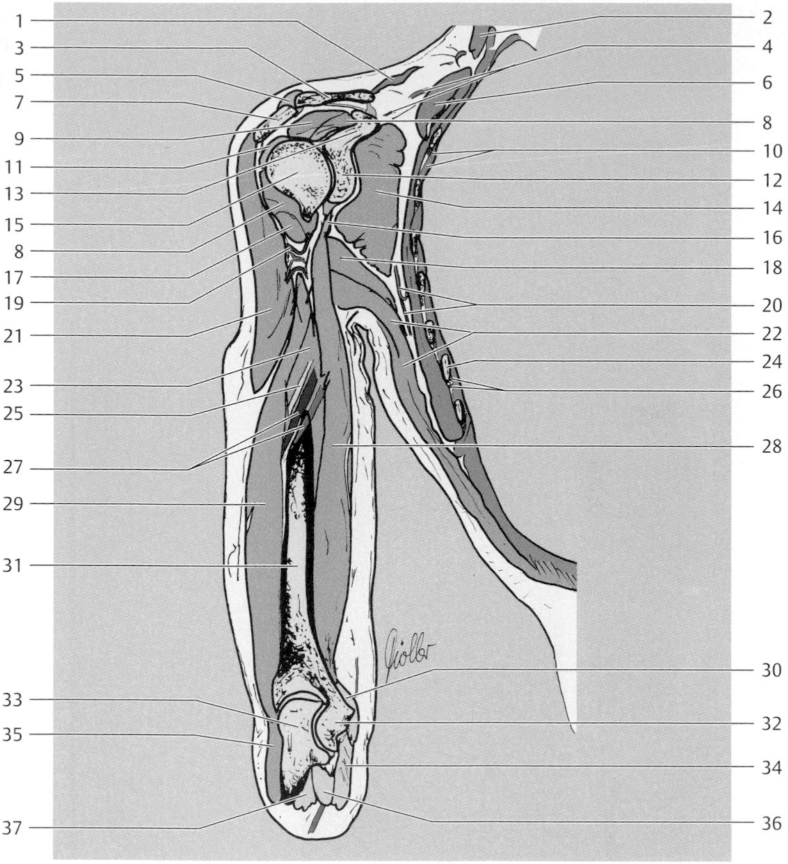

14 Subscapularis muscle
15 Humerus (head)
16 Triceps brachii muscle (long head, tendon attachment)
17 Teres minor muscle
18 Teres major muscle
19 Posterior circumflex humeral artery and vein
20 Thoracodorsal artery and vein
21 Deltoid muscle
22 Latissimus dorsi muscle
23 Triceps brachii muscle (medial head)
24 Rib
25 Radial nerve
26 Intercostal artery, vein, and nerve
27 Deep brachial artery and vein
28 Triceps brachii muscle (long head)
29 Triceps brachii muscle (lateral head)
30 Pronator teres muscle
31 Humerus (shaft)
32 Medial epicondyle of humerus
33 Olecranon
34 Flexor digitorum superficialis muscle
35 Anconeus muscle
36 Flexor carpi ulnaris muscle
37 Flexor digitorum profundus muscle

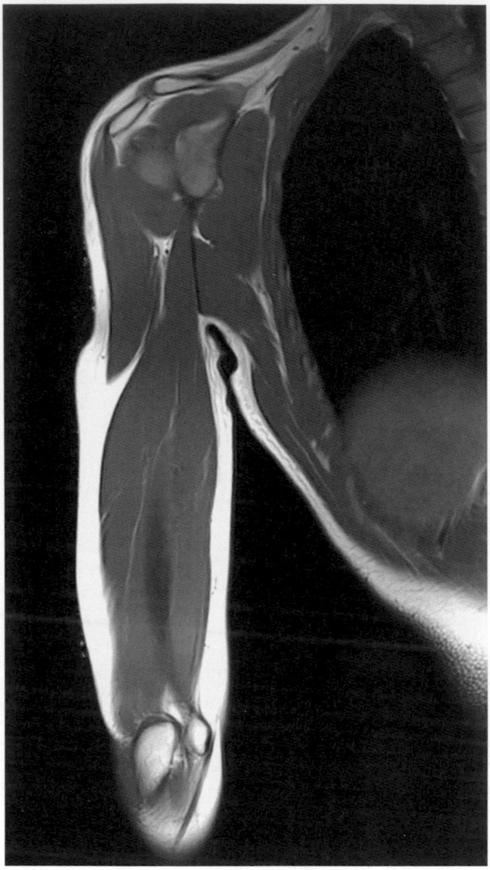

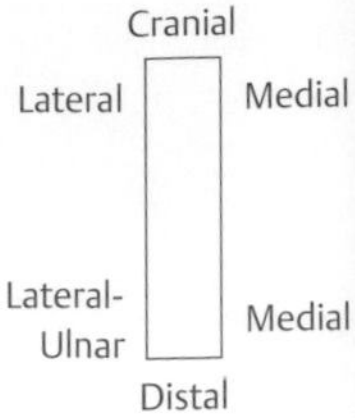

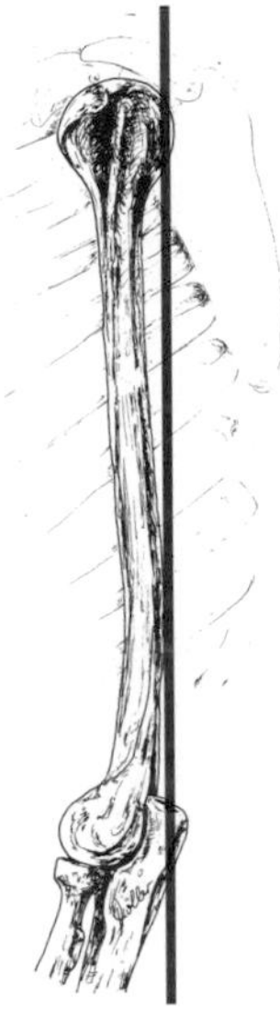

1 Clavicle
2 Scaleni muscles
3 Acromioclavicular joint
4 Trapezius muscle
5 Supraspinatus muscle
6 Serratus anterior muscle
7 Acromion
8 Infraspinatus muscle
9 Teres minor muscle
10 Glenoid

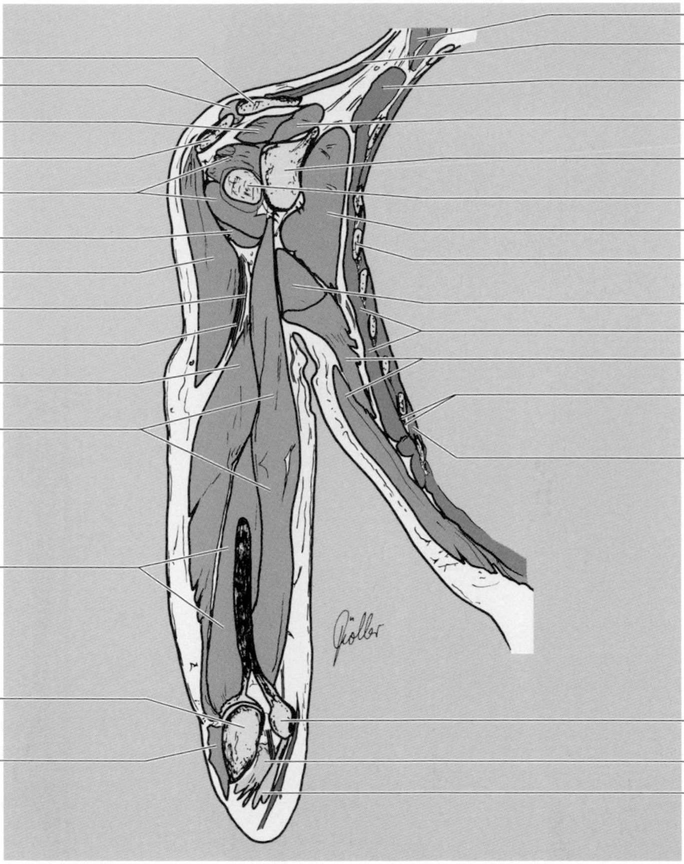

11 Deltoid muscle
12 Humerus (head)
13 Radial nerve
14 Subscapularis muscle
15 Deep brachial artery and vein
16 Rib
17 Triceps brachii muscle (lateral head)
18 Teres major muscle
19 Biceps brachii muscle (long head)
20 Latissimus dorsi muscle
21 Triceps brachii muscle (medial head)
22 Intercostal artery, vein, and nerve
23 Olecranon
24 Intercostal muscles
25 Anconeus muscle
26 Medial epicondyle of humerus
27 Flexor digitorum profundus muscle
28 Flexor carpi ulnaris muscle

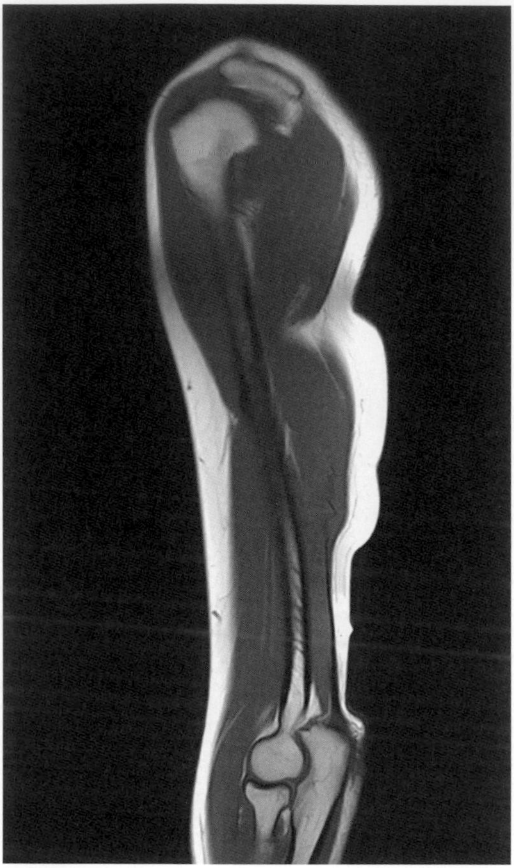

Proximal/
Cranial
Ventral Dorsal
Distal

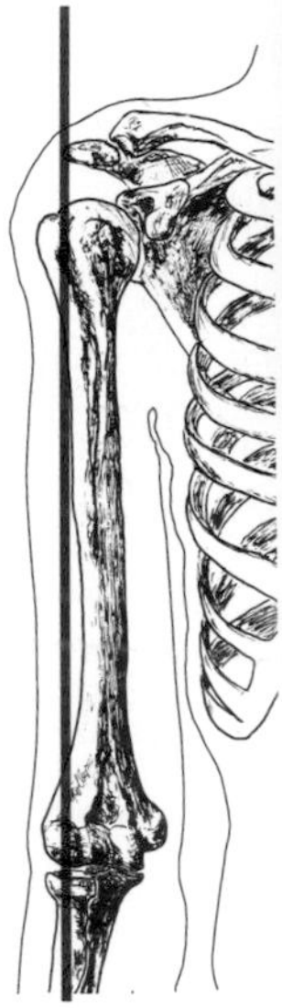

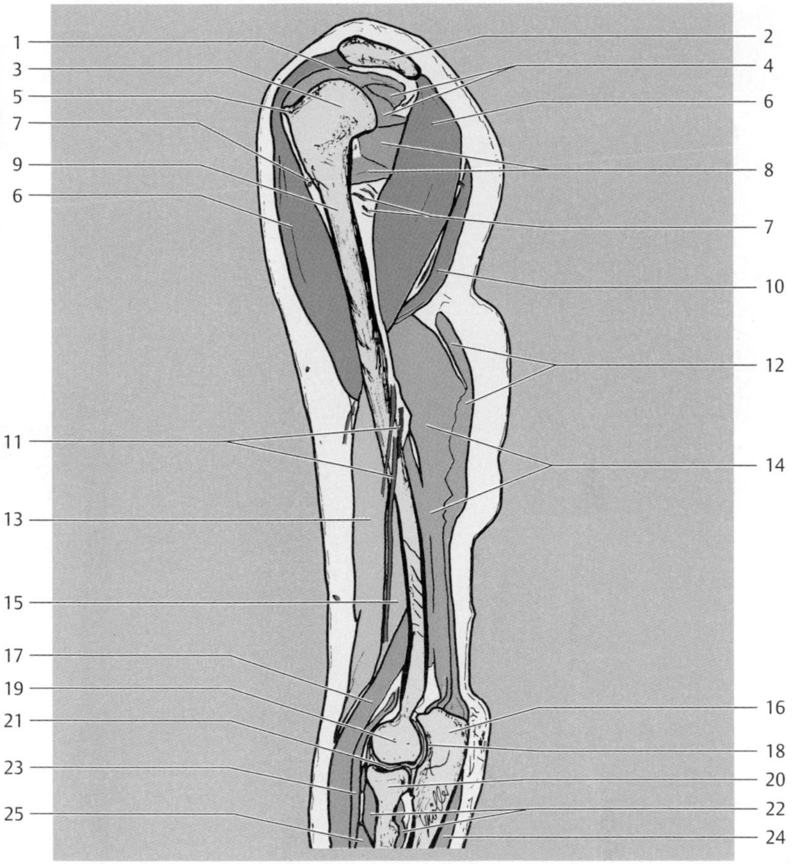

1 Supraspinatus muscle (tendon)
2 Acromion
3 Humerus (head)
4 Infraspinatus muscle
5 Greater tubercle
6 Deltoid muscle (acromial part)
7 Posterior circumflex humeral artery and vein
8 Teres minor muscle
9 Humerus (shaft)
10 Deltoid muscle
11 Deep brachial artery and vein
12 Triceps brachii muscle (long head)
13 Biceps brachii muscle (long head)
14 Triceps brachii muscle (lateral head)
15 Brachialis muscle
16 Olecranon
17 Brachioradialis muscle
18 Humero-ulnar joint
19 Humerus (capitulum)
20 Radius (head)
21 Humeroradial joint
22 Supinator muscle
23 Extensor carpi radialis muscle
24 Anconeus muscle
25 Extensor carpi radialis brevis muscle

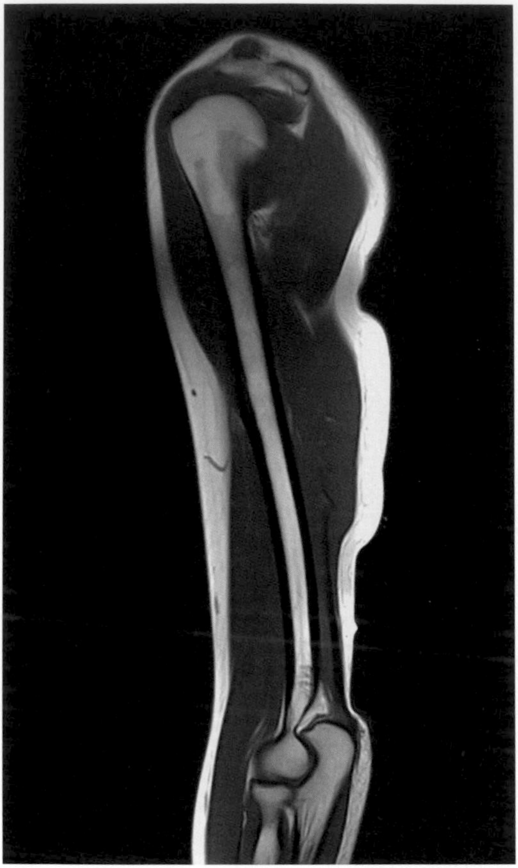

Proximal/
Cranial
Ventral
Dorsal
Distal

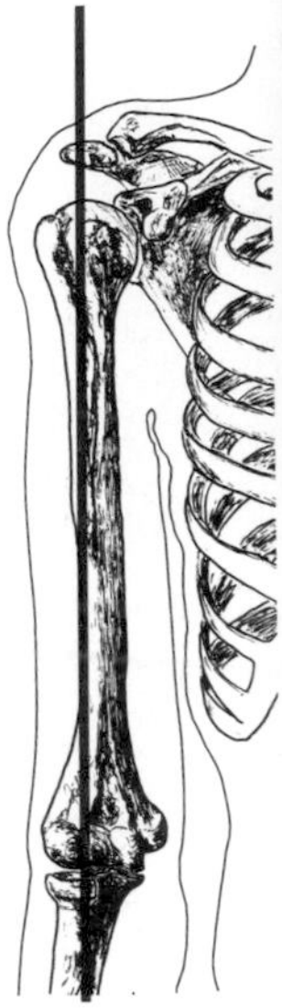

1 Clavicle
2 Acromioclavicular ligament
3 Acromion
4 Infraspinatus muscle
5 Supraspinatus muscle (tendon)
6 Humerus (head)
7 Humerus (greater tubercle)
8 Teres minor muscle
9 Humerus (neck)

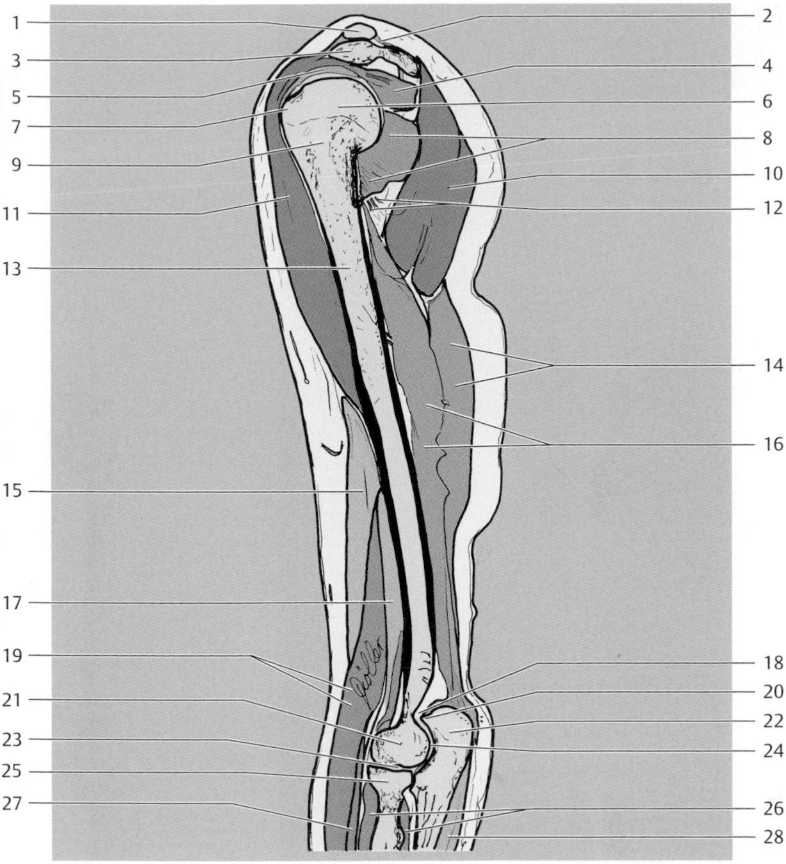

10 Deltoid muscle (acromial part)
11 Deltoid muscle
12 Posterior circumflex humeral artery and vein
13 Humerus (shaft)
14 Triceps brachii muscle (long head)
15 Biceps brachii muscle (long head)
16 Triceps brachii muscle (lateral head)
17 Brachialis muscle
18 Olecranon fossa
19 Brachioradialis muscle
20 Coronoid process
21 Humerus (capitulum)
22 Olecranon
23 Humeroradial joint
24 Humero-ulnar joint
25 Radius (head)
26 Supinator muscle
27 Extensor carpi radialis muscle
28 Flexor digitorum profundus muscle

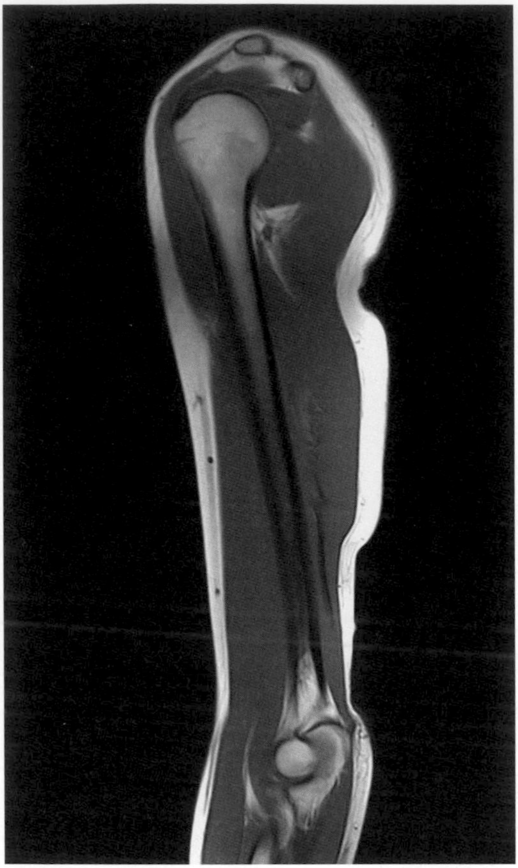

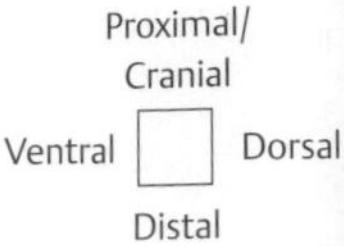

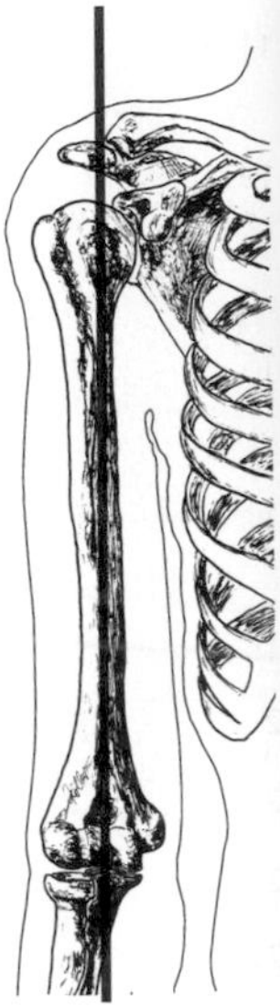

1 Clavicle
2 Acromioclavicular ligament
3 Supraspinatus muscle (+ tendon)
4 Acromion
5 Humerus (greater tubercle)
6 Infraspinatus muscle
7 Humerus (head)
8 Teres minor muscle
9 Deltoid muscle
10 Deltoid muscle (acromial part)
11 Humerus (shaft)

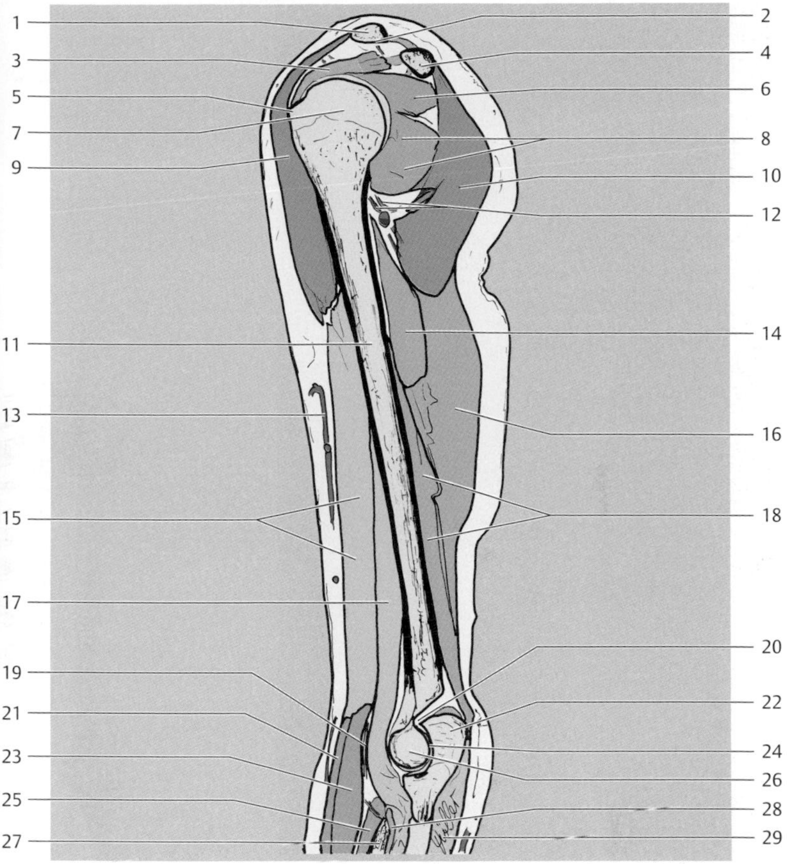

12 Posterior circumflex humeral artery and vein
13 Cephalic vein
14 Triceps brachii muscle (lateral head)
15 Biceps brachii muscle (long head)
16 Triceps brachii muscle (long head)
17 Brachialis muscle
18 Triceps brachii muscle (medial head)
19 Radial nerve
20 Olecranon fossa
21 Brachioradialis muscle
22 Olecranon
23 Extensor carpi radialis muscle
24 Humero-ulnar joint
25 Supinator muscle
26 Humerus (capitulum)
27 Radius (shaft)
28 Biceps brachii muscle (tendon)
29 Flexor digitorum profundus muscle

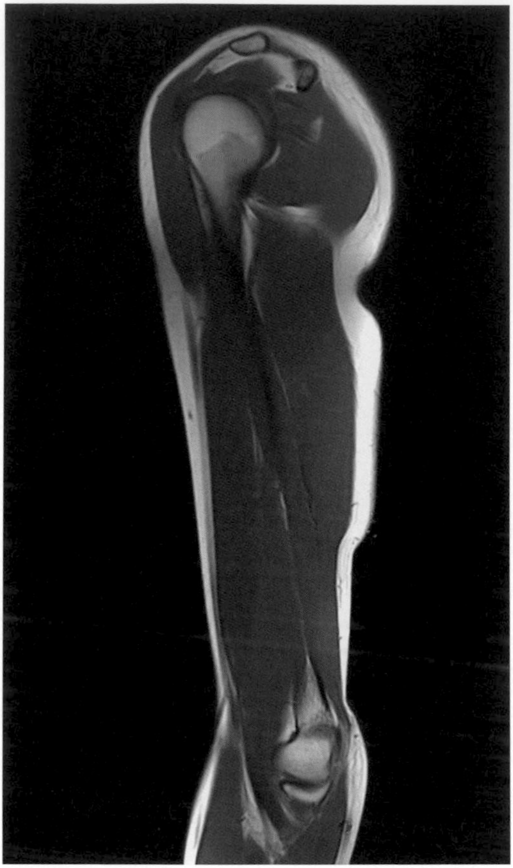

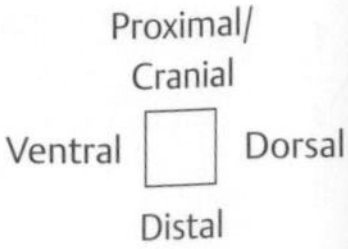
Proximal/
Cranial
Ventral
Dorsal
Distal

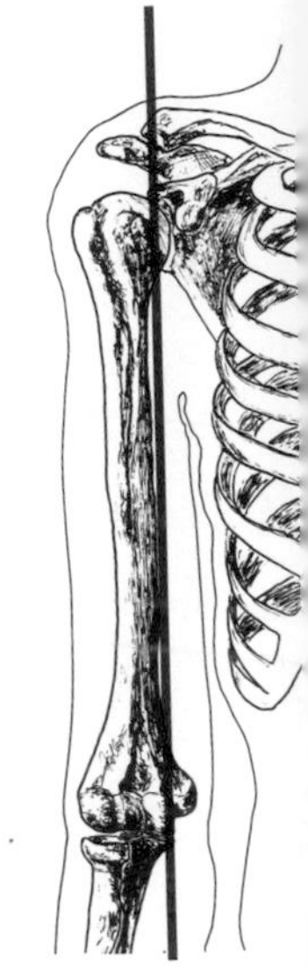

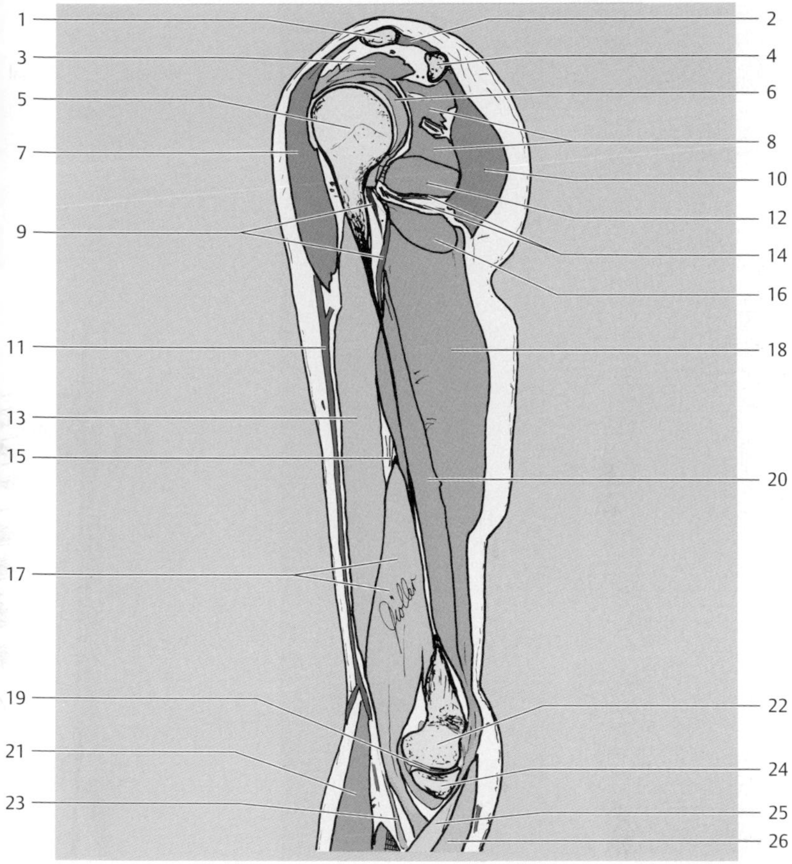

1 Clavicle
2 Trapezius muscle
3 Supraspinatus muscle (+ tendon)
4 Acromion
5 Humerus (head)
6 Joint capsule
7 Deltoid muscle
8 Infraspinatus muscle
9 Posterior circumflex humeral artery and vein
10 Deltoid muscle (acromial part)
11 Cephalic vein
12 Teres minor muscle
13 Biceps brachii muscle (long head)
14 Posterior circumflex humeral artery and vein, muscular branches
15 Median nerve
16 Teres major muscle
17 Brachialis muscle
18 Triceps brachii muscle (long head)
19 Humero-ulnar joint
20 Triceps brachii muscle (medial head)
21 Brachioradialis muscle
22 Humerus (trochlea)
23 Biceps brachii muscle (tendon)
24 Ulna
25 Flexor carpi ulnaris muscle
26 Flexor digitorum profundus muscle

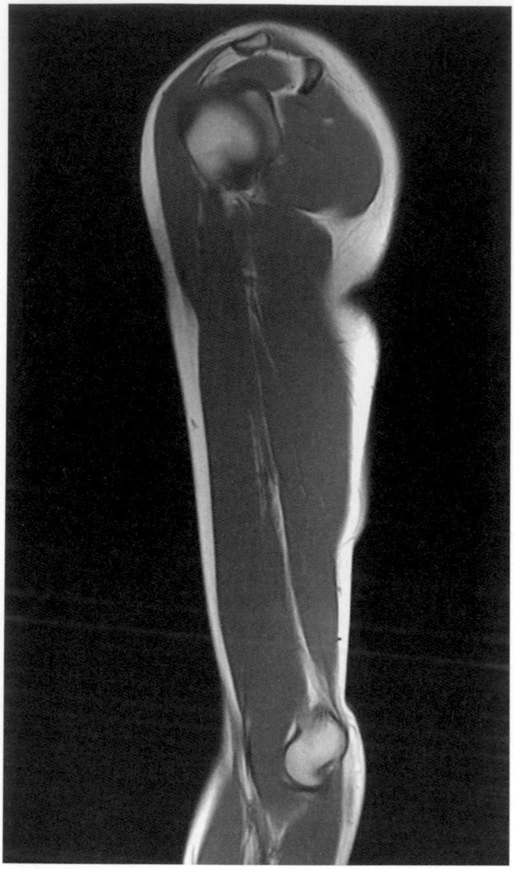

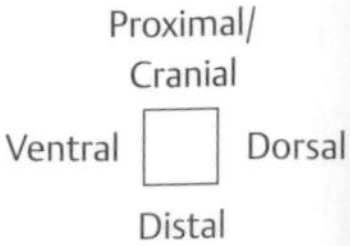

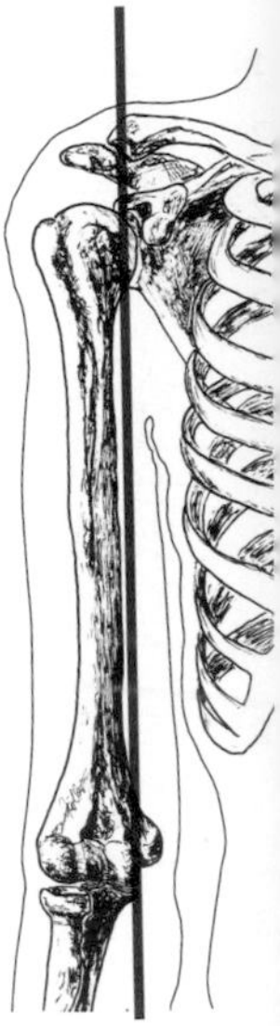

1 Clavicle
2 Trapezius muscle
3 Supraspinatus muscle (+ tendon)
4 Acromion
5 Joint capsule
6 Glenoid
7 Glenoid labrum
8 Infraspinatus muscle
9 Humerus (head)
10 Deltoid muscle (acromial part)

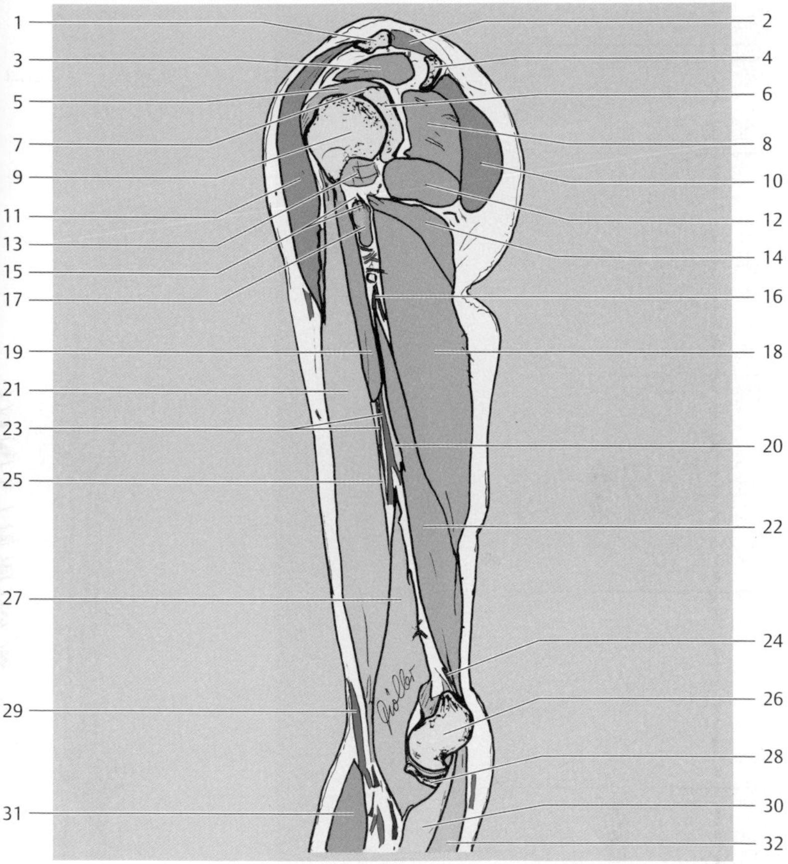

11 Deltoid muscle
12 Teres minor muscle
13 Glenohumeral ligament
14 Teres major muscle
15 Posterior circumflex humeral artery and vein
16 Posterior circumflex humeral artery and vein (muscular branch)
17 Latissimus dorsi muscle (insertion)
18 Triceps brachii muscle (long head)
19 Coracobrachialis muscle
20 Ulnar nerve
21 Biceps brachii muscle (long head)
22 Triceps brachii muscle (medial head)
23 Deep brachial artery and vein
24 Collateral ulnar artery and vein
25 Median nerve
26 Medial epicondyle
27 Brachialis muscle
28 Olecranon
29 Median cubital vein
30 Flexor carpi ulnaris muscle
31 Brachioradialis muscle
32 Flexor digitorum profundus muscle

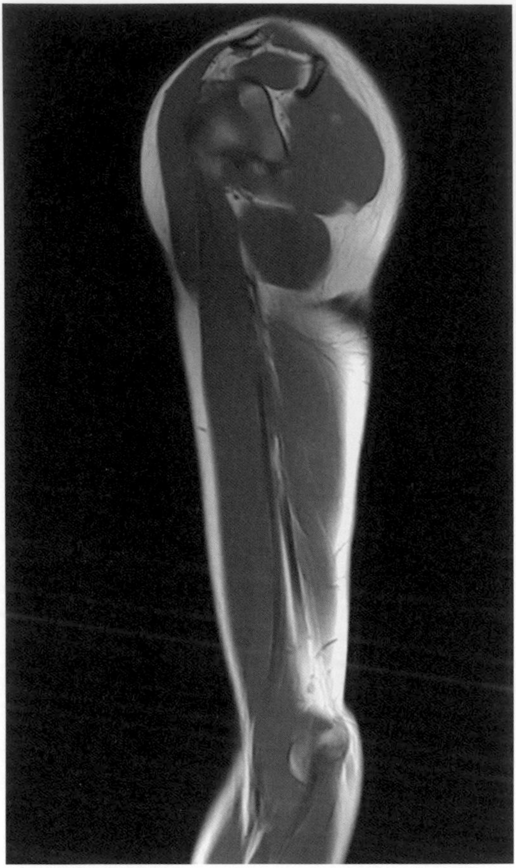

Proximal/
Cranial

Ventral Dorsal

Distal

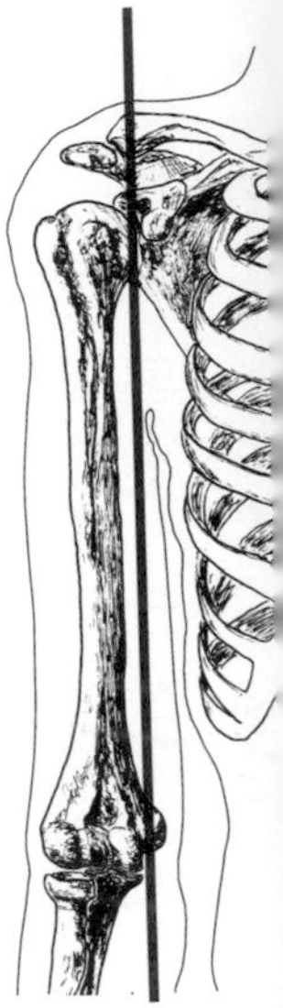

1 Clavicle
2 Trapezius muscle
3 Coracoclavicular ligament
4 Acromion
5 Supraspinatus muscle
6 Glenoid
7 Joint capsule
8 Deltoid muscle (acromial part)
9 Deltoid muscle
10 Infraspinatus muscle
11 Humerus (head)
12 Teres minor muscle

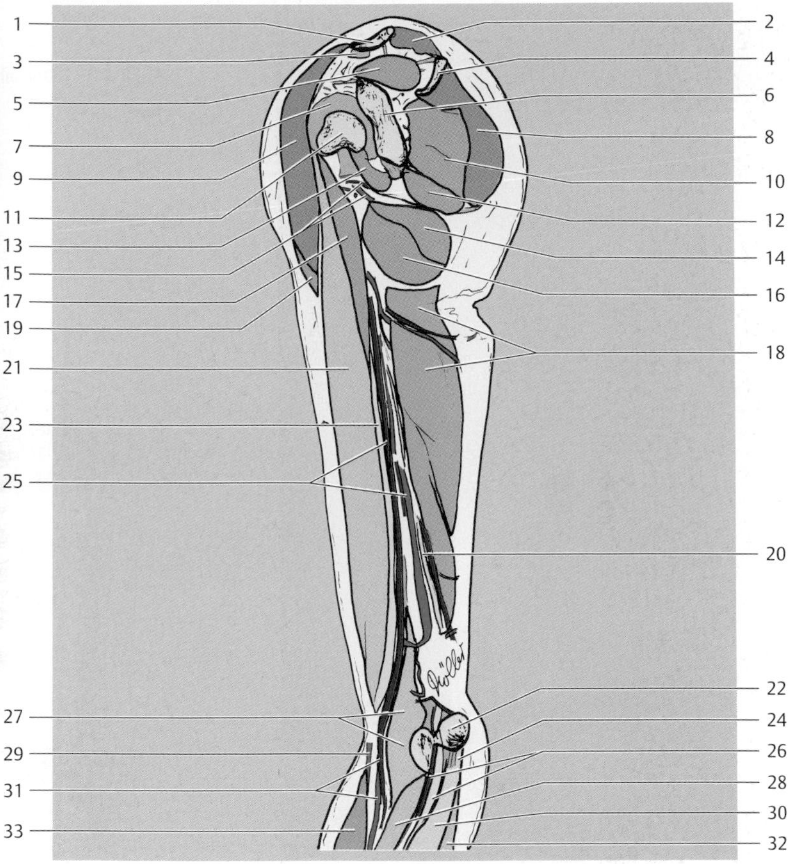

13 Subscapularis muscle
14 Teres major muscle
15 Posterior circumflex humeral artery and vein
16 Latissimus dorsi muscle
17 Coracobrachialis muscle
18 Triceps brachii muscle (long head)
19 Pectoralis major muscle
20 Ulnar nerve
21 Biceps brachii muscle (long head)
22 Humerus (trochlea)
23 Median nerve
24 Common head of flexor muscles
25 Brachial artery and vein
26 Ulnar nerve and collateral ulnar artery and vein
27 Brachialis muscle
28 Flexor digitorum superficialis muscle
29 Median cubital vein
30 Flexor carpi ulnaris muscle
31 Ulnar artery and vein
32 Flexor digitorum profundus muscle
33 Brachioradialis muscle

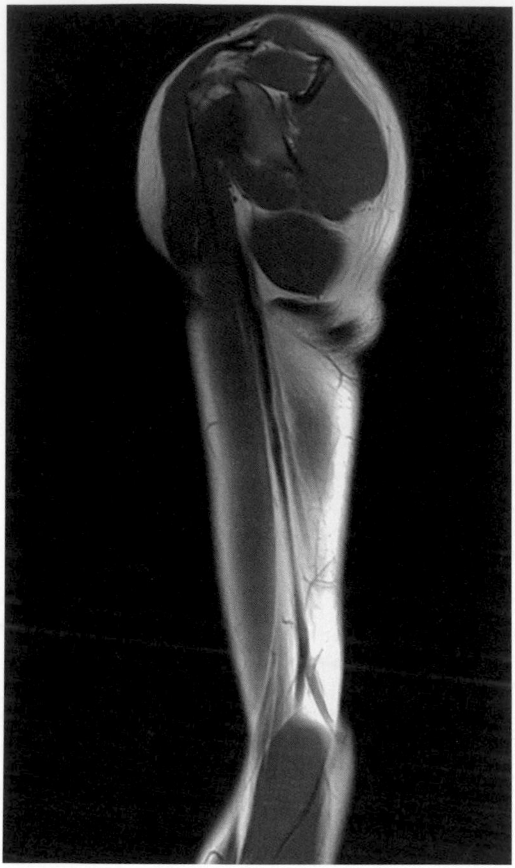

Proximal/
Cranial
Ventral Dorsal
Distal

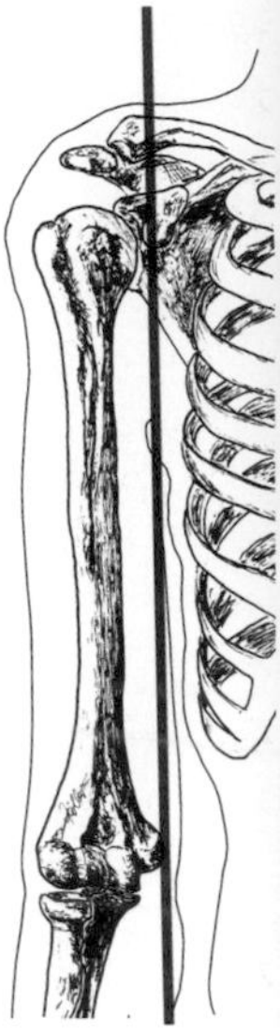

1 Clavicle
2 Trapezius muscle
3 Coracoid process
4 Supraspinatus muscle
5 Deltoid muscle
6 Acromion

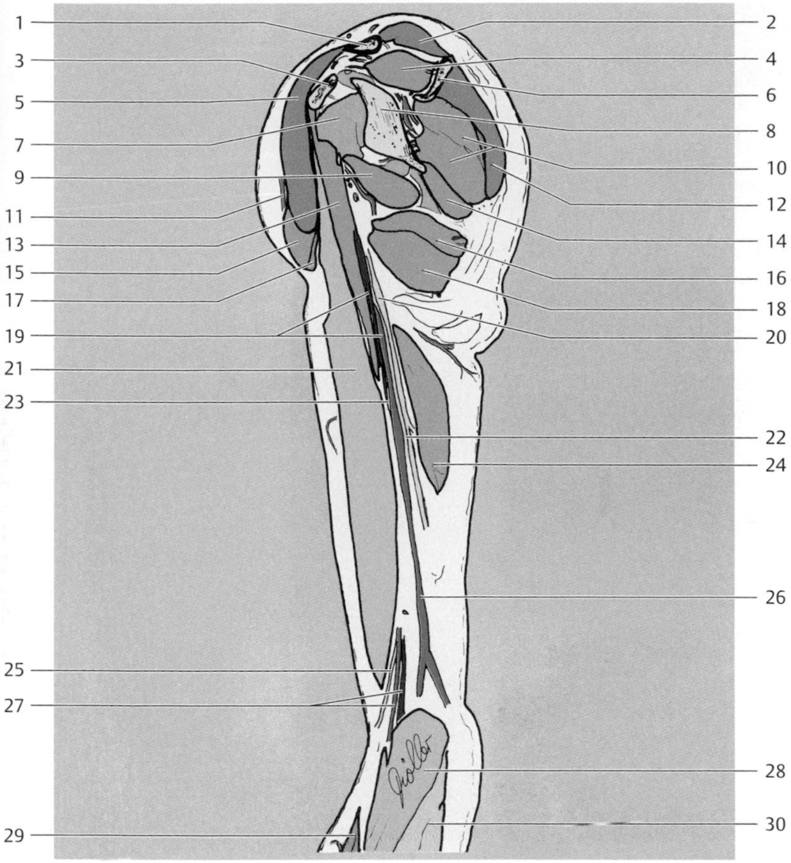

7 Joint capsule
8 Scapula (collum)
9 Subscapularis muscle
10 Infraspinatus muscle
11 Cephalic vein
12 Deltoid muscle (acromial part)
13 Coracobrachialis muscle
14 Teres minor muscle
15 Pectoralis major muscle
16 Teres major muscle
17 Pectoralis minor muscle
18 Latissimus dorsi muscle
19 Brachial artery and vein
20 Radial nerve
21 Biceps brachii muscle (long head)
22 Ulnar nerve
23 Median nerve
24 Triceps brachii muscle (long head)
25 Medial cutaneous nerve of arm
26 Basilic vein
27 Ulnar artery and vein
28 Brachialis muscle
29 Brachioradialis muscle
30 Flexor carpi ulnaris muscle

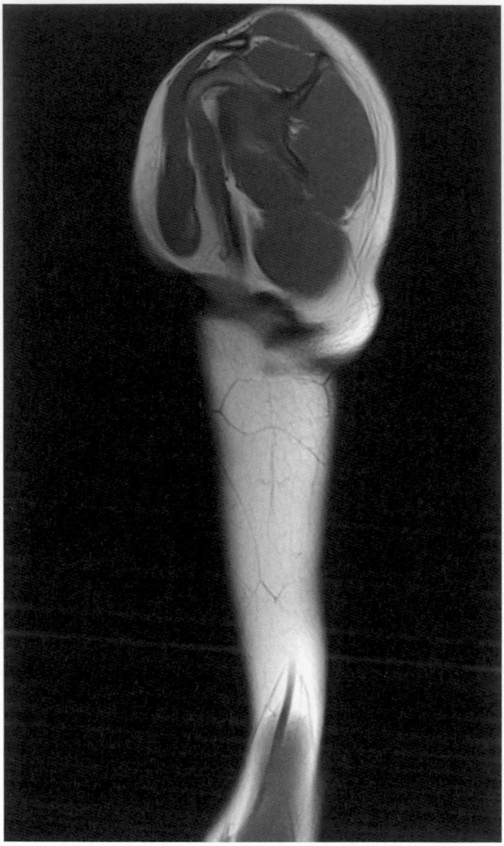

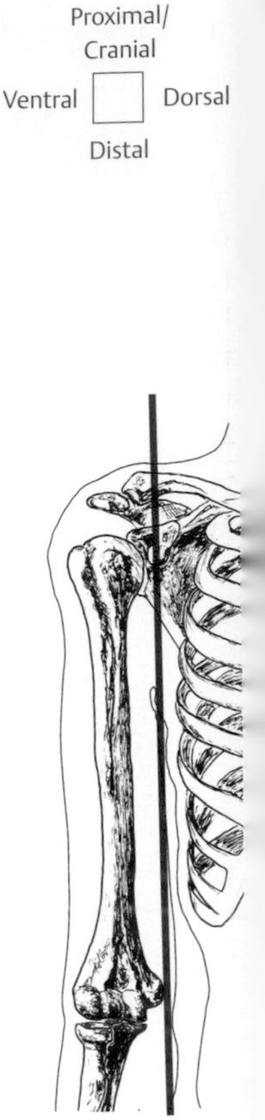
Proximal/
Cranial
Ventral
Dorsal
Distal

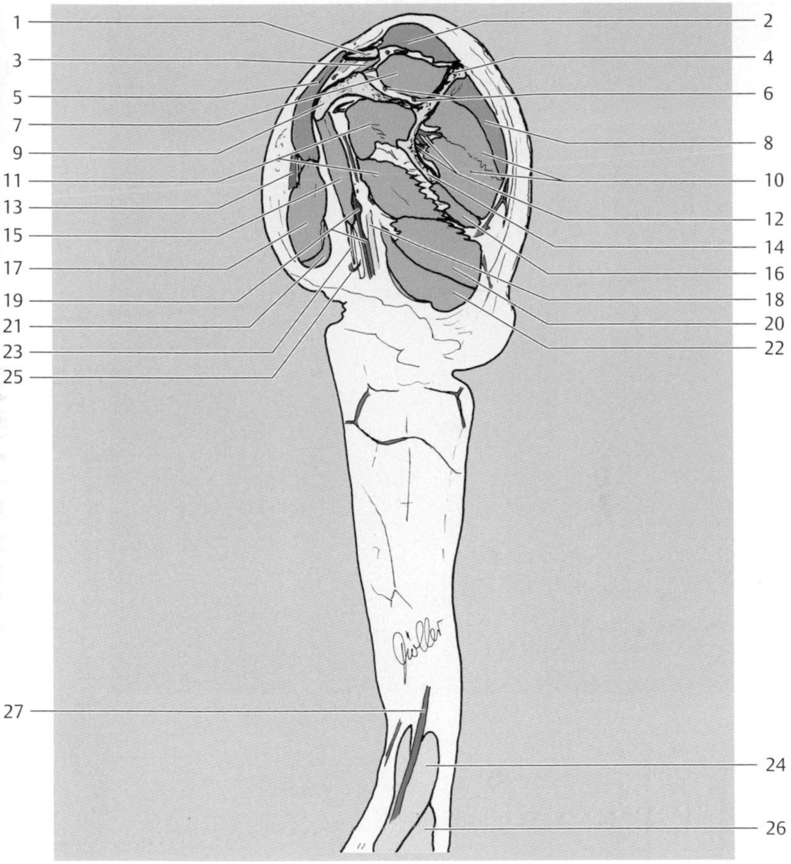

1 Clavicle
2 Trapezius muscle
3 Coracoclavicular ligament
4 Acromion
5 Deltoid muscle
6 Suprascapularis artery and vein
7 Supraspinatus muscle
8 Deltoid muscle (acromial part)
9 Coracoid process
10 Infraspinatus muscle
11 Subscapularis muscle
12 Circumflex scapulae artery and vein
13 Cephalic vein
14 Scapula
15 Coracobrachialis muscle
16 Teres minor muscle
17 Pectoralis major muscle
18 Radial nerve
19 Brachial artery and vein
20 Teres major muscle
21 Pectoralis minor muscle
22 Latissimus dorsi muscle
23 Median nerve
24 Pronator teres muscle
25 Ulnar nerve
26 Flexor carpi ulnaris muscle
27 Basilic vein

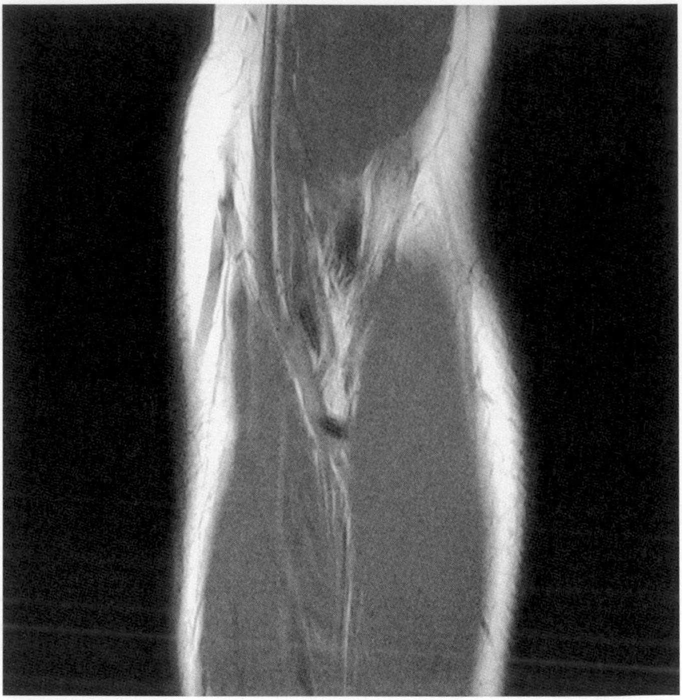

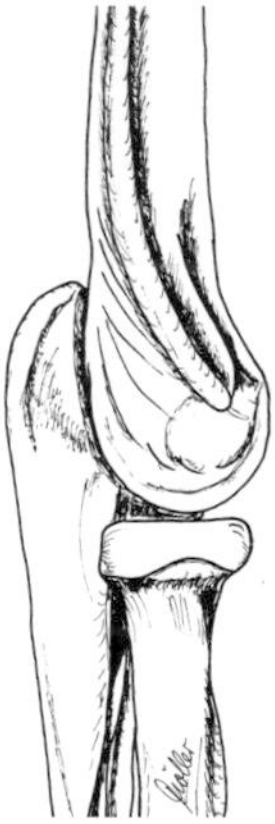

Proximal

Ulnar / Medial — Radial / Lateral

Distal

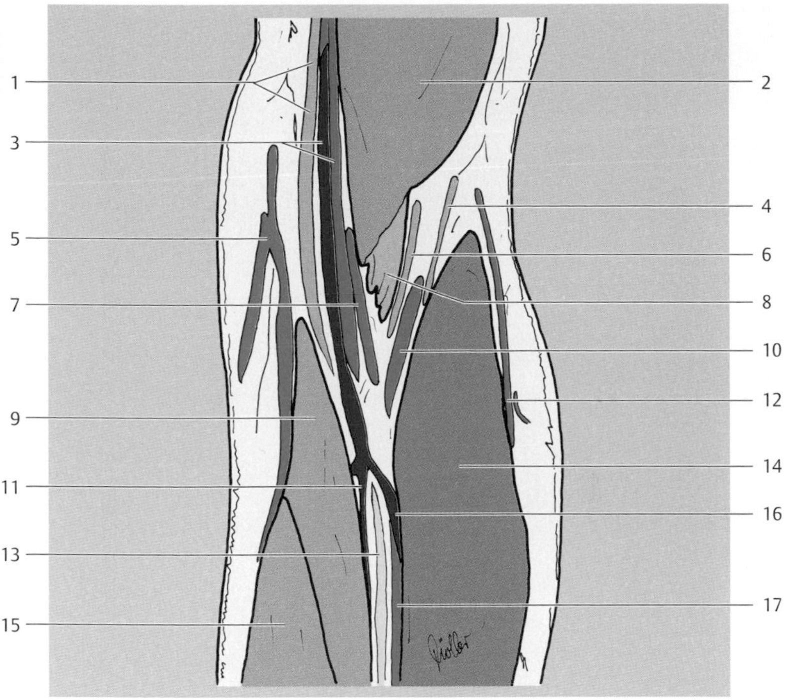

1 Median nerve
2 Brachialis muscle
3 Brachial artery and vein
4 Lateral cutaneous nerve of forearm
5 Basilic vein
6 Radial nerve (deep branch)
7 Median cubital vein
8 Biceps brachii muscle (tendon)
9 Pronator teres muscle
10 Median cephalic vein
11 Ulnar artery
12 Cephalic vein
13 Median nerve
14 Brachioradialis muscle
15 Flexor carpi radialis muscle
16 Radial artery
17 Median vein of forearm

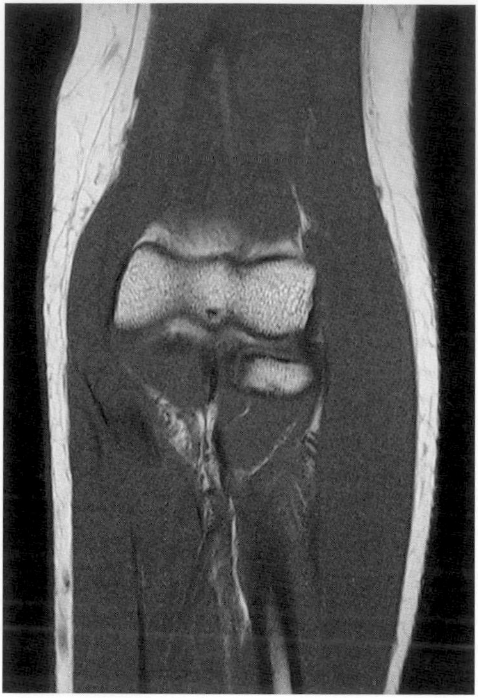

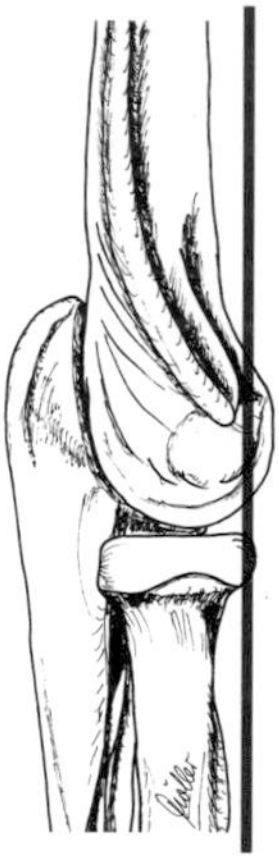

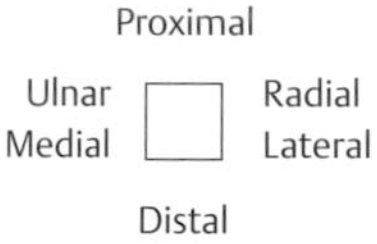
Proximal
Ulnar
Medial
Radial
Lateral
Distal

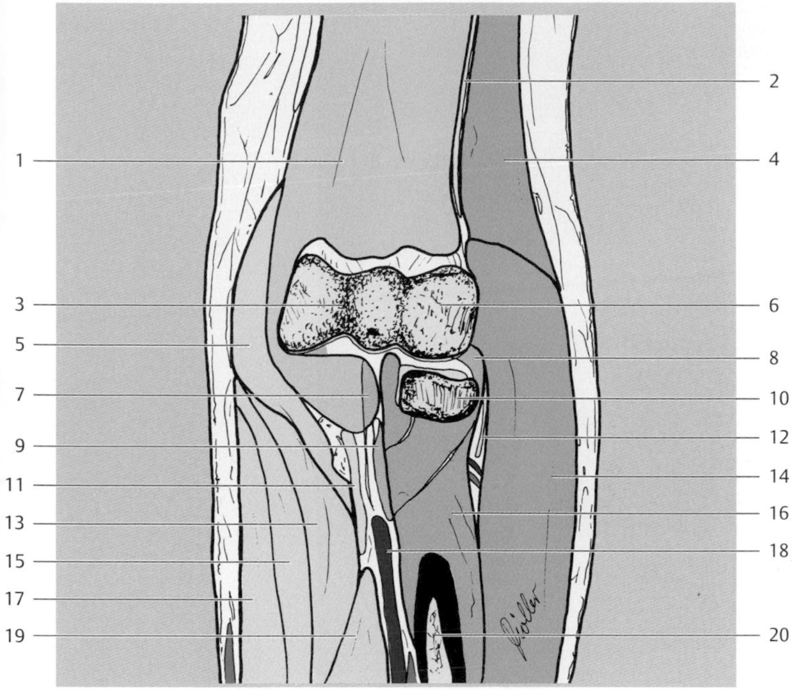

1 Brachialis muscle
2 Radial nerve
3 Humerus (trochlea)
4 Brachioradialis muscle
5 Pronator teres muscle
6 Humerus (capitulum)
7 Brachialis muscle (tendon)
8 Anular ligament and radial collateral ligament of wrist joint
9 Biceps brachii muscle (tendon)
10 Radius (head)
11 Median nerve
12 Radial nerve (deep branch)
13 Flexor carpi radialis muscle
14 Extensor carpi radialis longus and brevis muscles
15 Palmaris longus muscle
16 Supinator muscle
17 Flexor carpi ulnaris muscle
18 Interosseous artery and vein
19 Flexor digitorum profundus muscle
20 Radius (shaft)

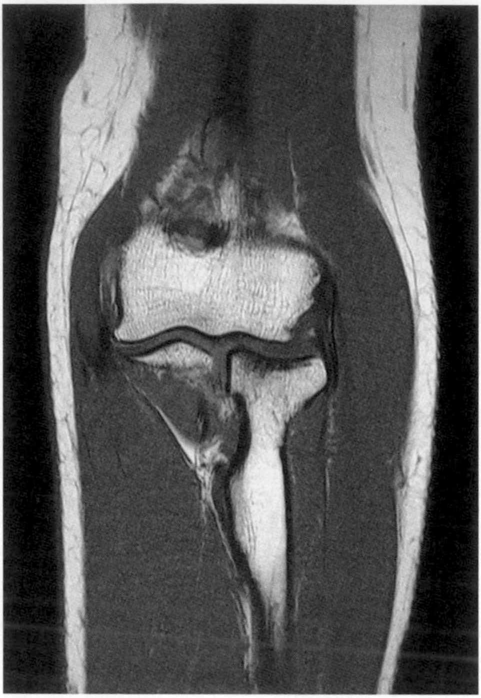

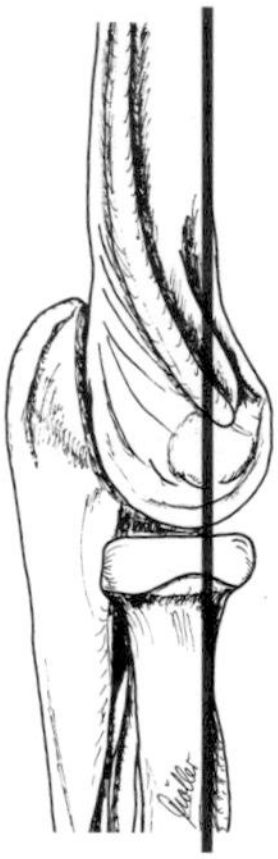

Proximal

Ulnar Medial | Radial Lateral

Distal

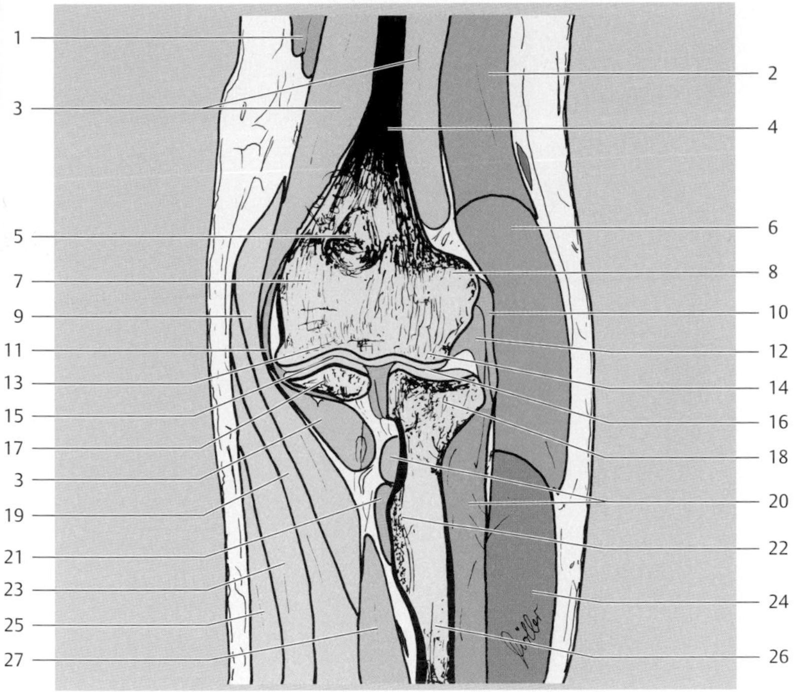

1 Triceps brachii muscle
2 Brachioradialis muscle
3 Brachialis muscle
4 Humerus (shaft)
5 Coronoid fossa
6 Extensor carpi radialis longus muscle
7 Medial epicondyle
8 Lateral epicondyle
9 Pronator teres muscle
10 Common extensor tendons (attachment)
11 Medial collateral ligament
12 Radial collateral ligament
13 Humerus (trochlea)
14 Humerus (capitulum)
15 Humero-ulnar joint
16 Humeroradial joint
17 Ulna (coronoid process)
18 Radius (head)
19 Flexor carpi radialis muscle
20 Supinator muscle
21 Biceps brachii muscle (tendon)
22 Radial tuberosity
23 Palmaris longus muscle
24 Extensor digitorum muscle
25 Flexor digitorum superficialis muscle
26 Radius (head)
27 Flexor digitorum profundus muscle

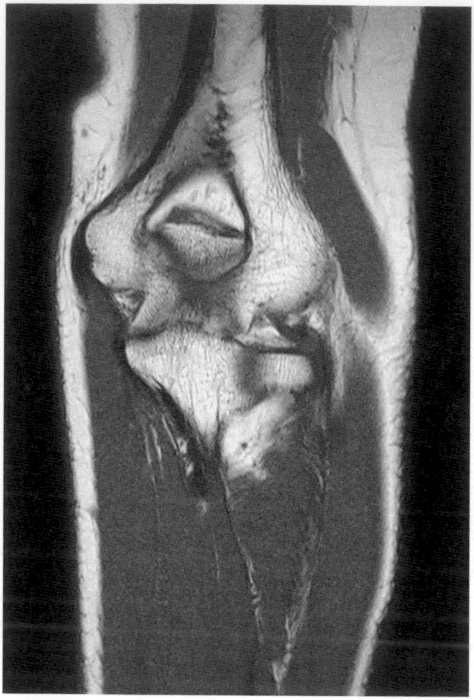

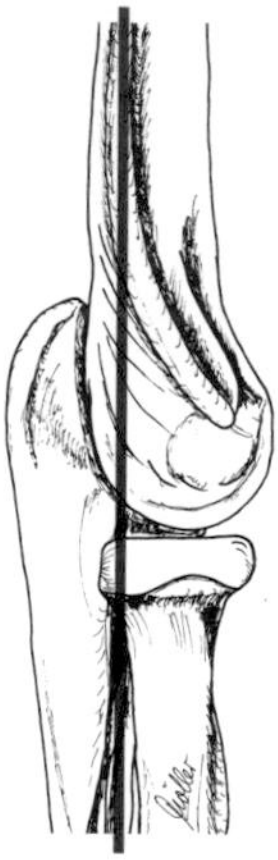

Proximal

Ulnar / Medial — Radial / Lateral

Distal

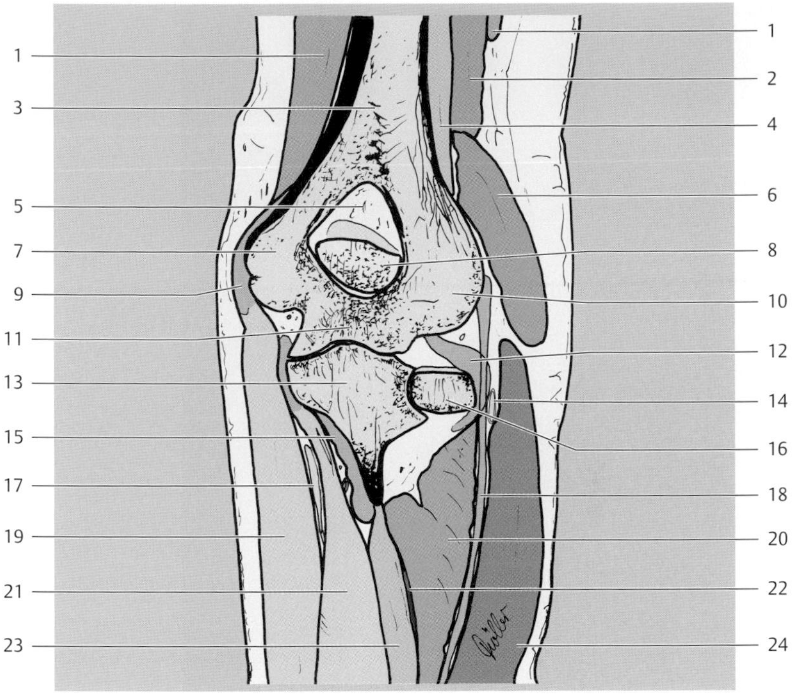

1 Triceps brachii muscle
2 Brachioradialis muscle
3 Humerus (shaft)
4 Brachialis muscle
5 Olecranon fossa (posterior fat body)
6 Extensor carpi radialis longus muscle
7 Medial epicondyle
8 Olecranon
9 Common flexor tendons (attachment)
10 Lateral epicondyle
11 Humerus (trochlea)
12 Anular ligament
13 Ulna (coronoid process)
14 Radial nerve (deep branch)
15 Brachialis muscle (tendon attachment)
16 Radius (head)
17 Ulnar nerve
18 Common extensor tendons
19 Flexor carpi ulnaris muscle
20 Supinator muscle
21 Flexor digitorum superficialis muscle
22 Common interosseous artery and vein
23 Flexor digitorum profundus muscle
24 Extensor digitorum muscle

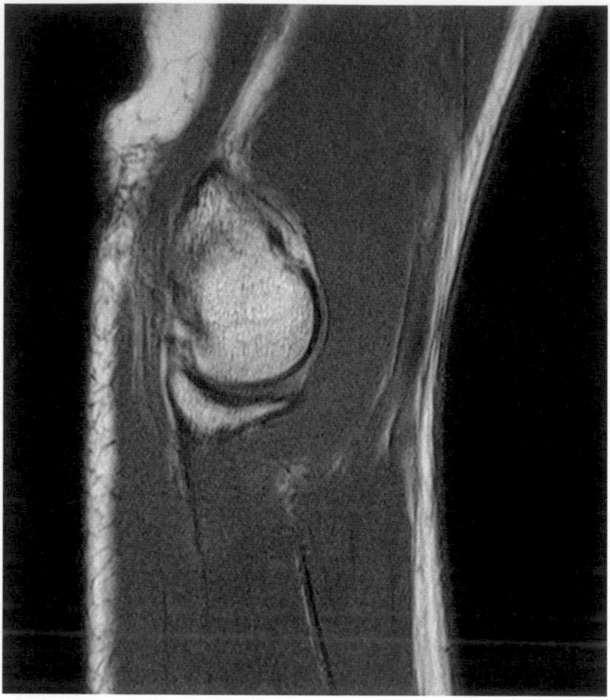

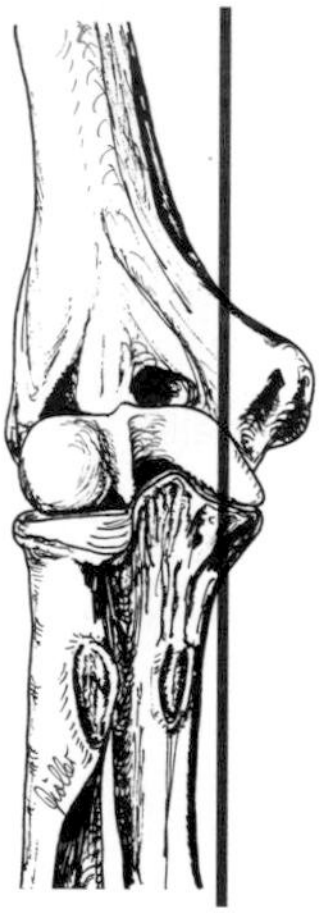

Proximal

Dorsal ☐ Ventral

Distal

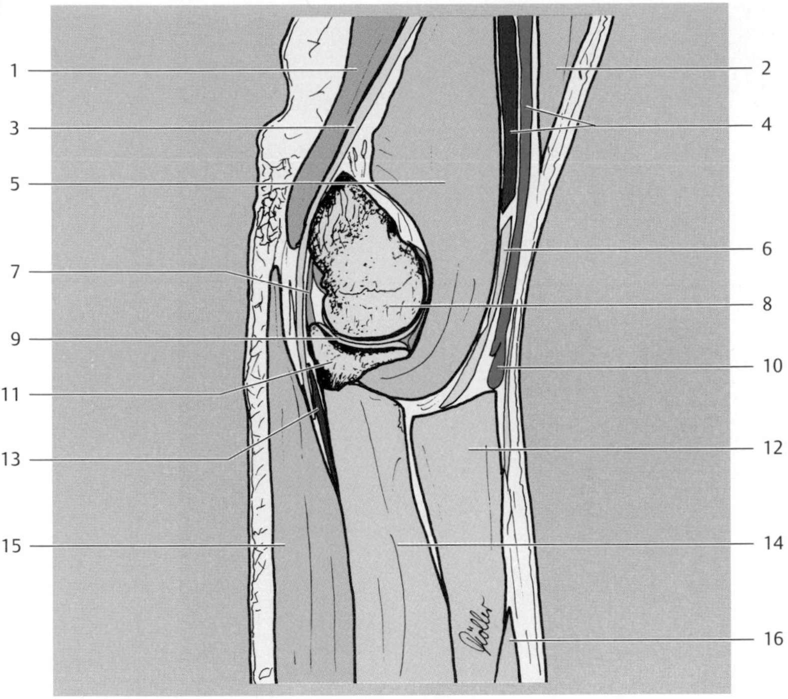

1 Triceps brachii muscle
2 Biceps brachii muscle
3 Ulnar nerve
4 Brachial artery and vein
5 Brachialis muscle
6 Median nerve
7 Collateral ulnar ligament, posterior part (+ posterior capsule of the elbow joint)
8 Humerus (trochlea)
9 Humero-ulnar joint
10 Median cubital vein
11 Olecranon
12 Pronator teres muscle
13 Ulnar recurrent artery
14 Flexor digitorum superficialis muscle
15 Flexor digitorum profundus muscle
16 Flexor carpi radialis muscle

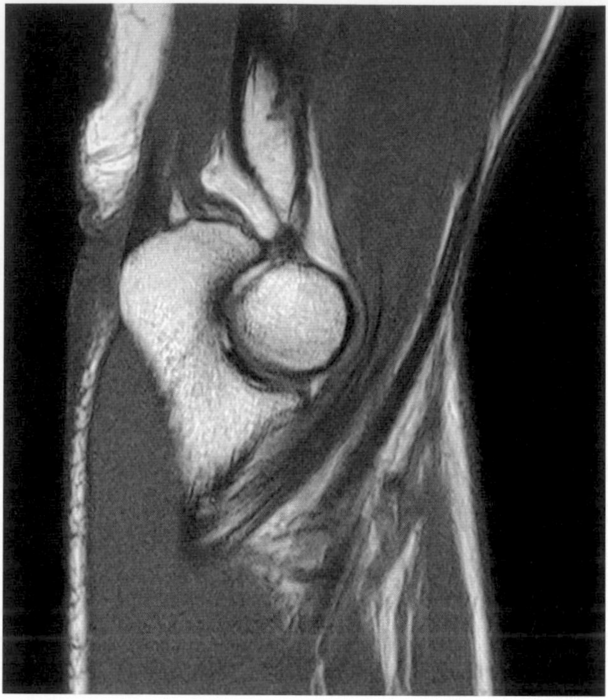

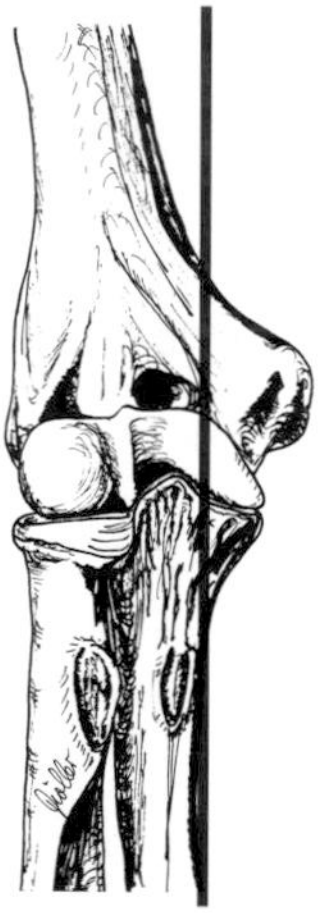

Proximal

Dorsal ☐ Ventral

Distal

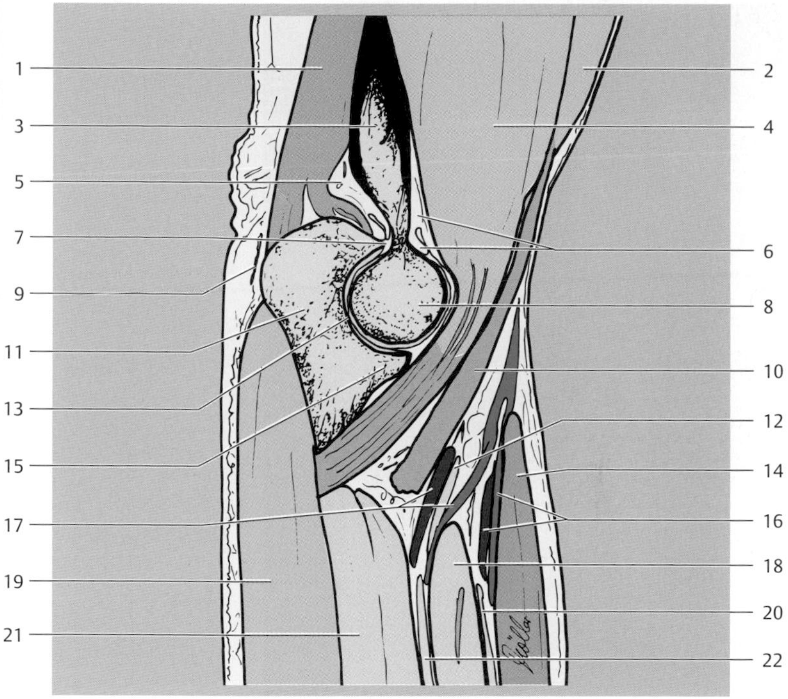

1 Triceps brachii muscle
2 Biceps brachii muscle
3 Humerus
4 Brachialis muscle
5 Posterior fat body of elbow
6 Anterior fat body and coronoid fossa
7 Olecranon fossa
8 Humerus (trochlea)
9 Olecranon bursa
10 Biceps muscle (tendon)
11 Olecranon
12 Ulnar nerve
13 Trochlear notch
14 Brachioradialis muscle
15 Coronoid process
16 Radial artery and vein
17 Ulnar artery and vein
18 Pronator teres muscle
19 Flexor digitorum profundus muscle
20 Radial nerve
21 Flexor digitorum superficialis muscle
22 Median nerve

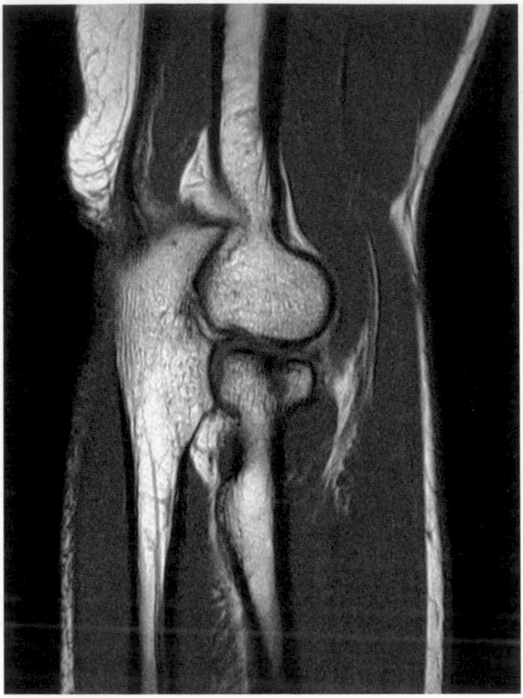

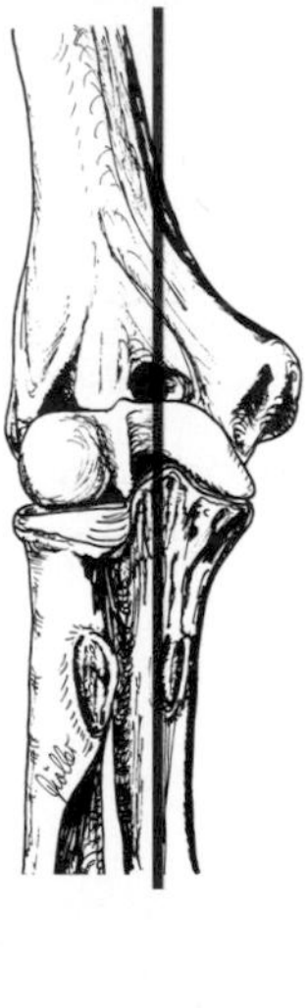

Proximal

Dorsal ☐ Ventral

Distal

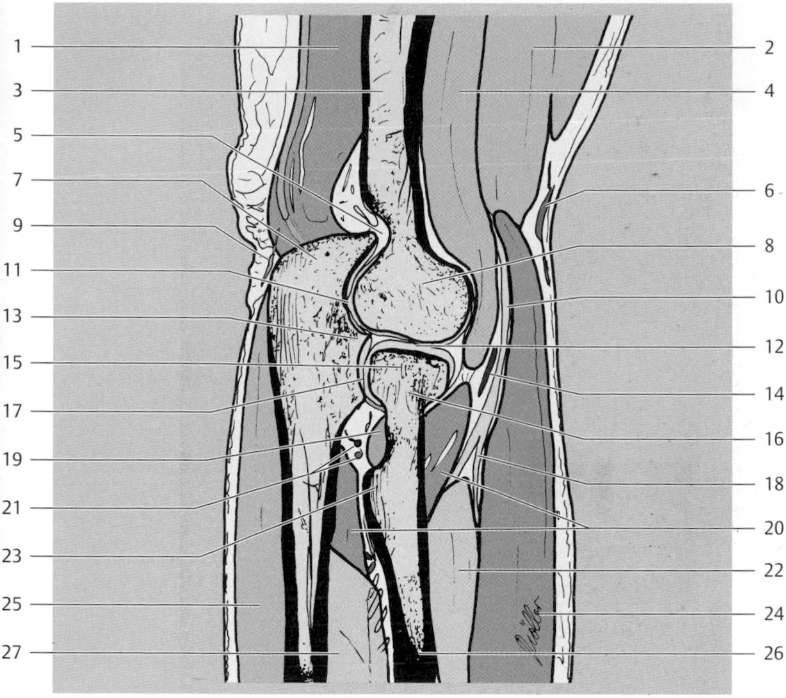

1 Triceps brachii muscle
2 Biceps brachii muscle
3 Humerus (shaft)
4 Brachialis muscle
5 Olecranon fossa
6 Cephalic vein
7 Olecranon
8 Humerus (capitulum)
9 Olecranon bursa
10 Radial nerve
11 Trochlear notch
12 Humeroradial joint
13 Coronoid process
14 Profunda brachii artery
15 Radius (head)
16 Radius (neck)
17 Proximal radioulnar joint
18 Radial nerve (superficial branch)
19 Biceps muscle (tendon attachment)
20 Supinator muscle
21 Interosseous artery and vein
22 Flexor digitorum superficialis muscle
23 Radial tuberosity
24 Brachioradialis muscle
25 Flexor digitorum profundus muscle
26 Radius (shaft)
27 Pronator teres muscle (ulnar head)

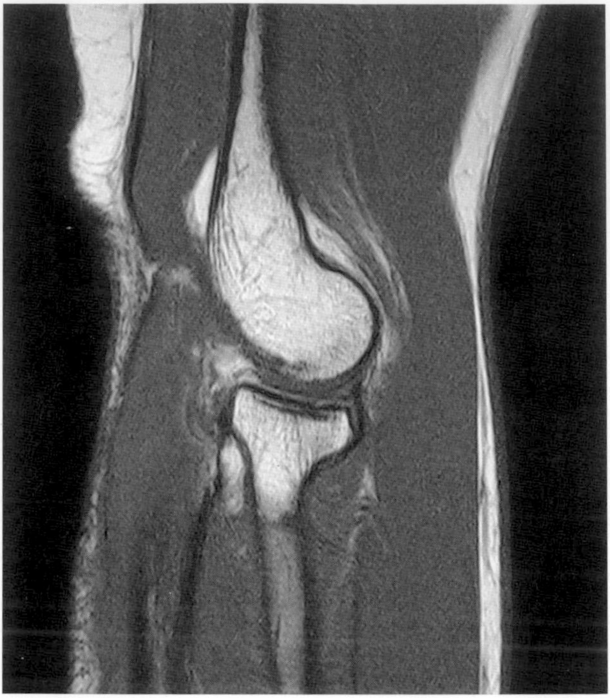

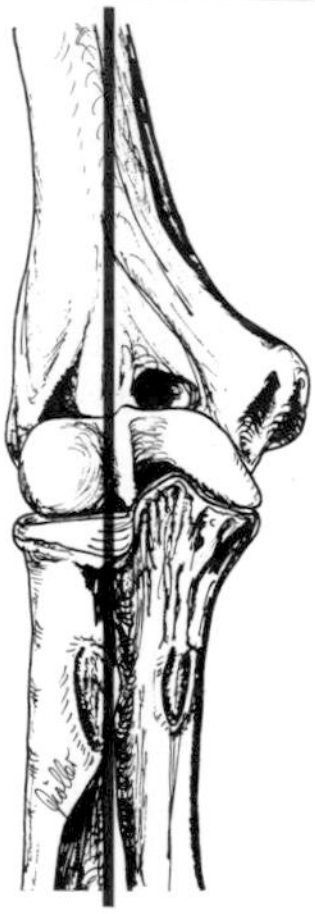

Proximal

Dorsal Ventral

Distal

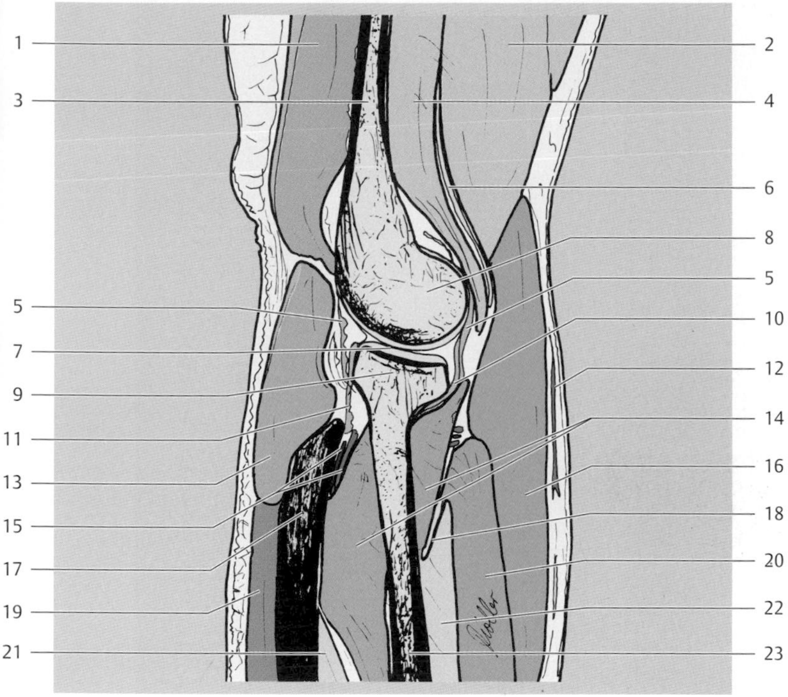

1 Triceps brachii muscle
2 Biceps brachii muscle
3 Humerus (shaft)
4 Brachialis muscle
5 Joint capsule
6 Radial nerve
7 Humeroradial joint
8 Humerus (capitulum)
9 Radius (head)
10 Anular ligament of radius
11 Radial collateral ligament
12 Cephalic vein
13 Anconeus muscle
14 Supinator muscle
15 Interosseous artery and vein
16 Brachioradialis muscle
17 Ulna (shaft)
18 Radial nerve (deep branch)
19 Extensor carpi ulnaris muscle
20 Extensor carpi radialis longus muscle
21 Pronator teres muscle (ulnar head)
22 Flexor digitorum superficialis muscle (radial head)
23 Radius (shaft)

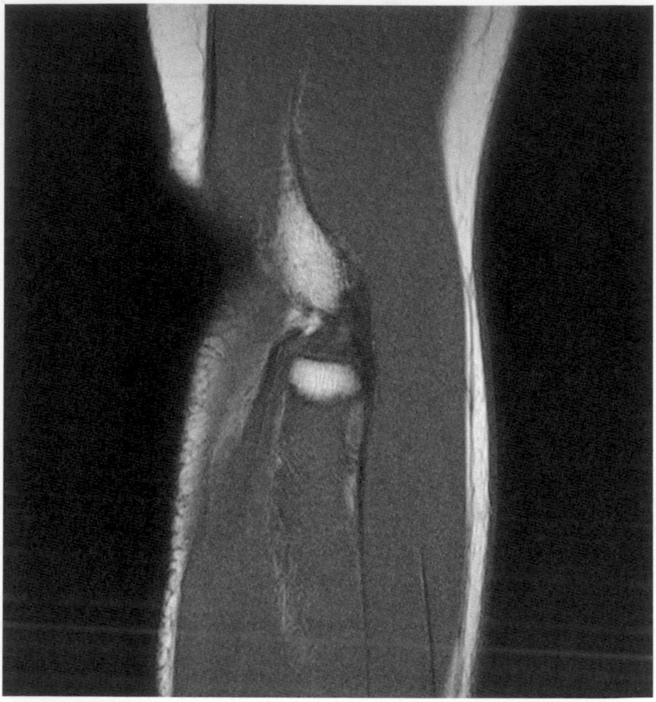

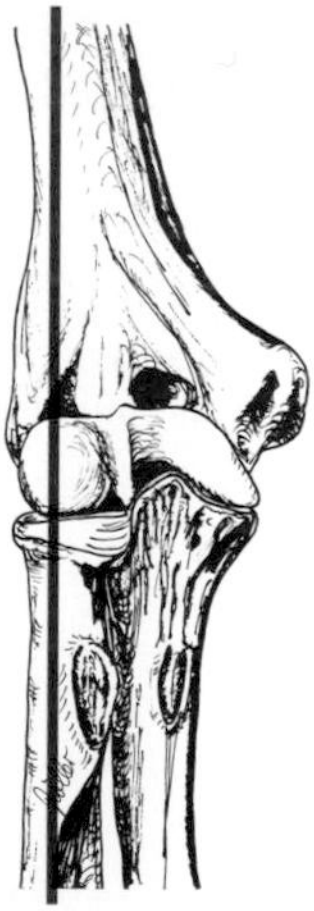

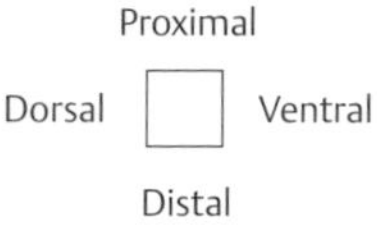
Proximal
Dorsal
Ventral
Distal

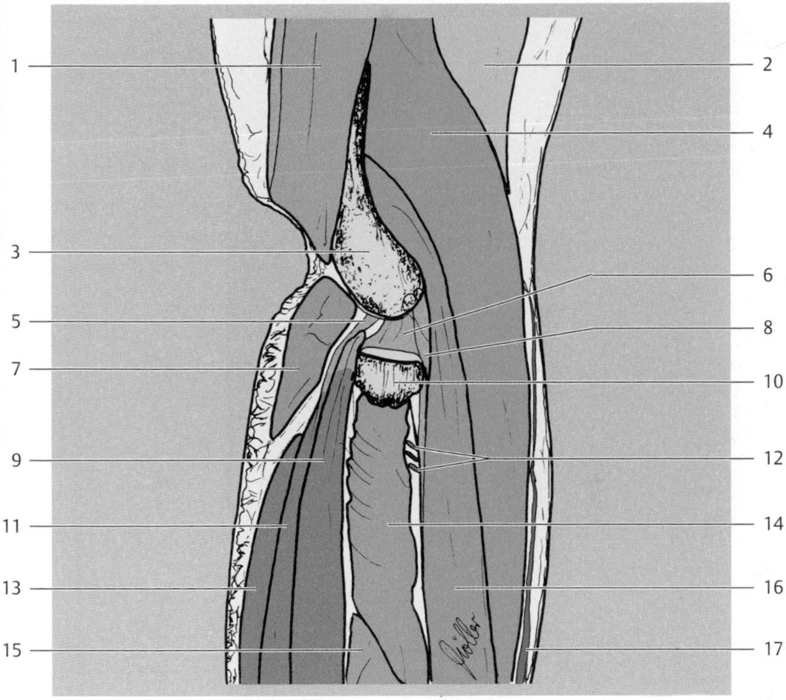

1 Triceps brachii muscle
2 Brachialis muscle
3 Humerus (capitulum)
4 Brachioradialis muscle
5 Joint capsule
6 Radial collateral ligament
7 Anconeus muscle
8 Anular ligament of radius
9 Extensor digitorum muscle
10 Radius (head)
11 Extensor digiti minimi muscle
12 Anterior interosseous artery and veins
13 Extensor carpi ulnaris muscle
14 Supinator muscle
15 Abductor pollicis longus muscle
16 Extensor carpi radialis longus muscle
17 Cephalic vein

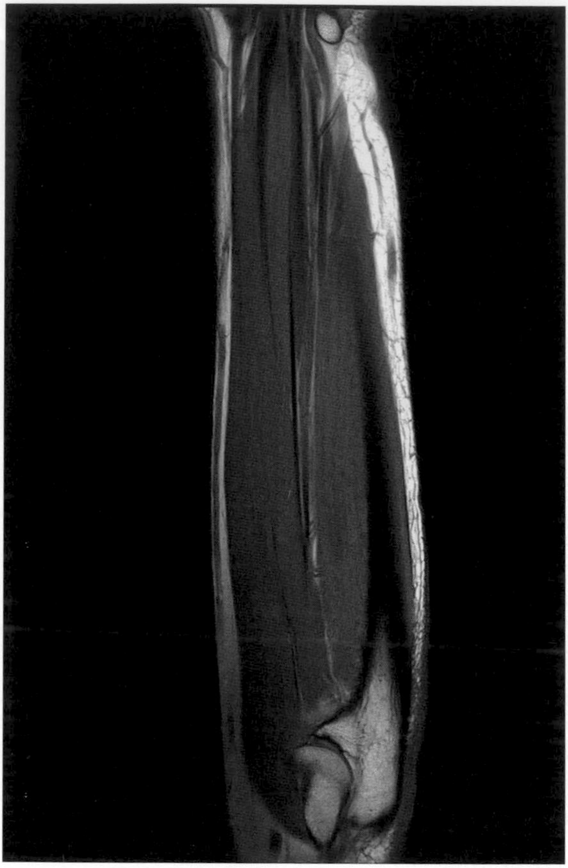

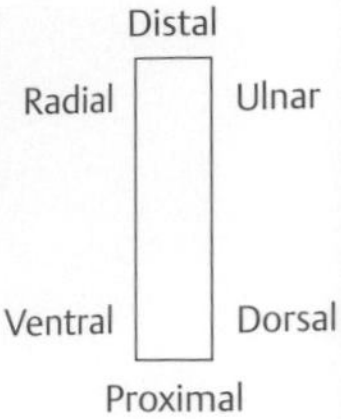
Distal
Radial
Ulnar
Ventral
Dorsal
Proximal

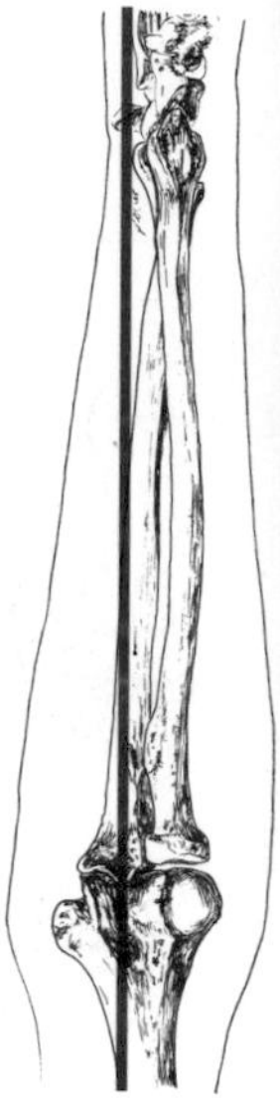

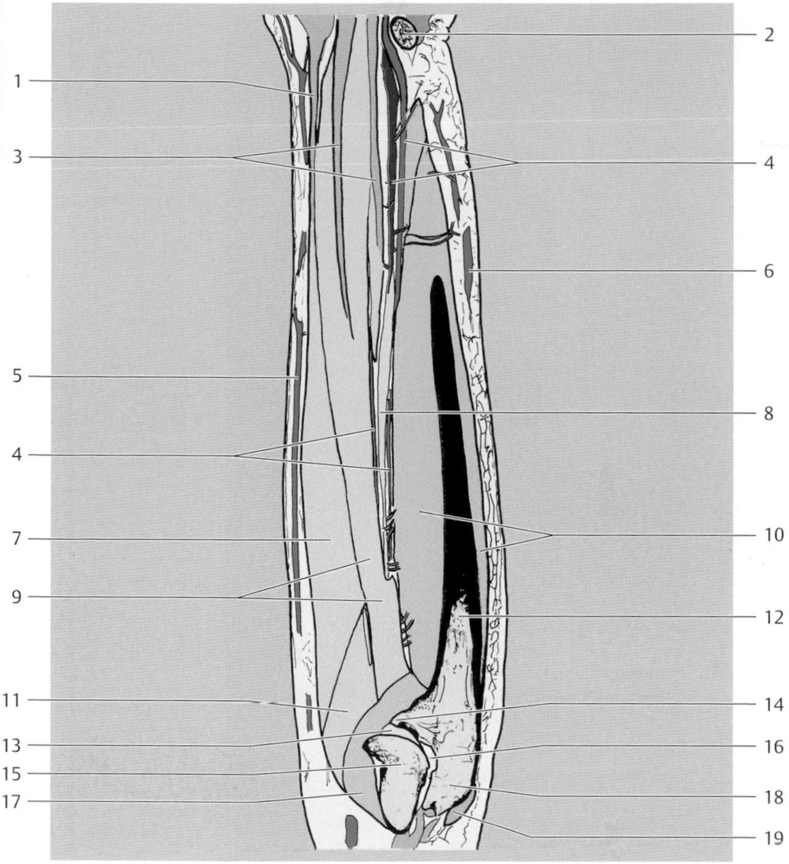

1 Flexor carpi radialis muscle (tendon)
2 Pisiform
3 Flexor digitorum superficialis muscle and tendon
4 Ulnar artery and vein
5 Cephalic vein
6 Basilic vein
7 Flexor carpi radialis muscle
8 Ulnar nerve
9 Flexor digitorum superficialis muscle
10 Flexor digitorum profundus muscle
11 Pronator teres muscle
12 Ulna (shaft)
13 Humero-ulnar joint
14 Coronoid process
15 Humerus (Trochlea)
16 Trochlear notch
17 Brachialis muscle
18 Olecranon
19 Triceps brachii muscle (tendon attachment)

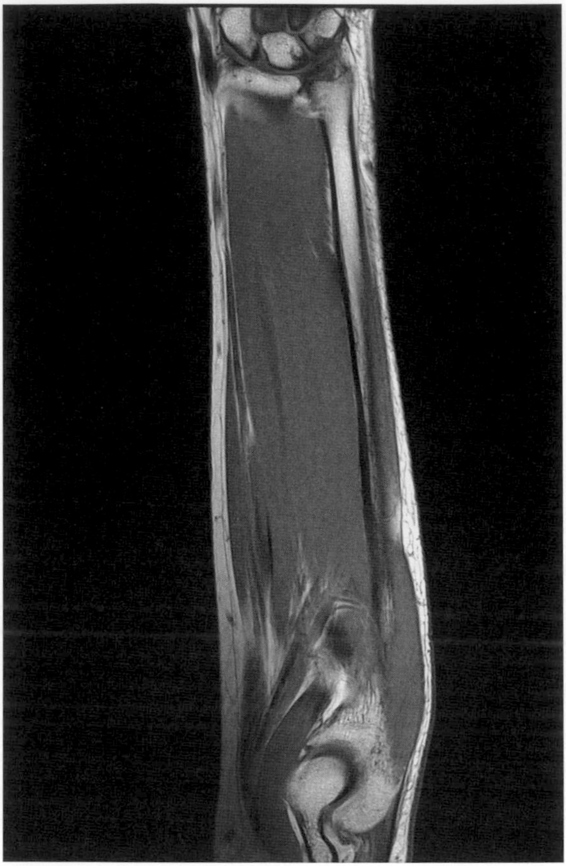

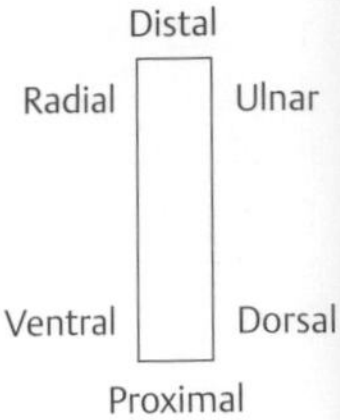

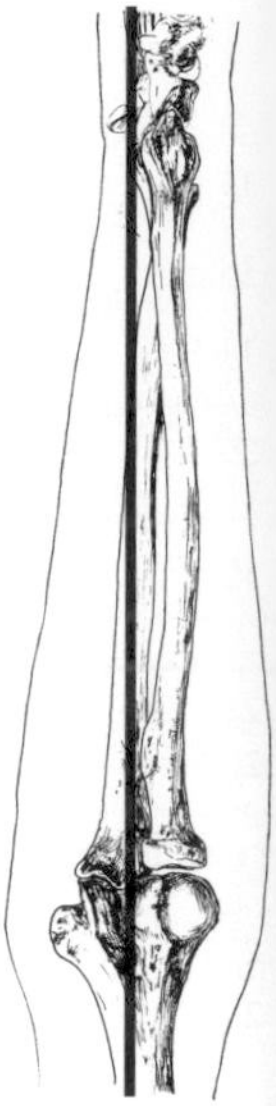

1 Capitate
2 Hamate
3 Scaphoid
4 Triquetrum
5 Lunate
6 Triangular fibrocartilage
7 Radius
8 Ulna

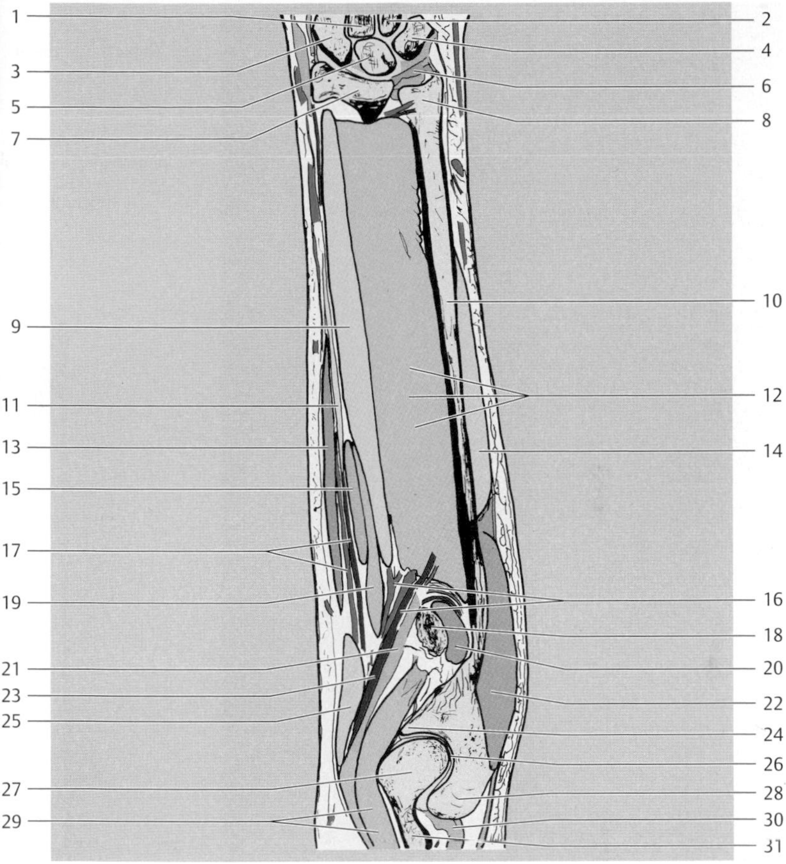

9 Flexor digitorum superficialis muscle
10 Ulna (shaft)
11 Median nerve
12 Flexor digitorum profundus muscle
13 Brachioradialis muscle
14 Flexor carpi ulnaris muscle
15 Pronator teres muscle (tendon)
16 Ulnar artery and vein
17 Radial artery and vein
18 Radial tuberosity
19 Flexor pollicis muscle
20 Supinator muscle
21 Biceps brachii muscle (tendon)
22 Anconeus muscle
23 Brachialis artery
24 Coronoid process
25 Pronator teres muscle
26 Humero-ulnar joint
27 Humerus (Trochlea)
28 Olecranon
29 Brachialis muscle
30 Triceps brachii muscle (tendon)
31 Humerus (shaft)

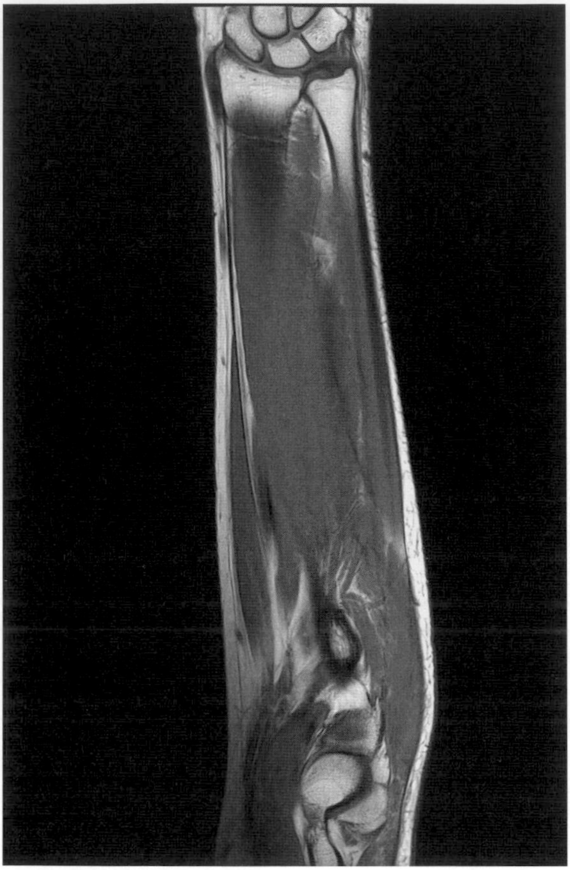

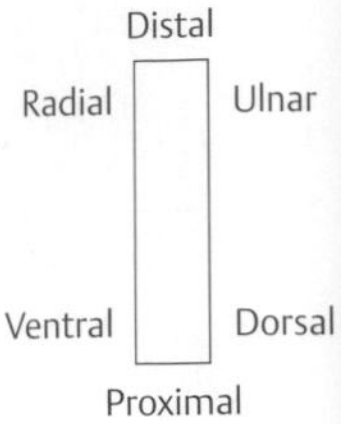

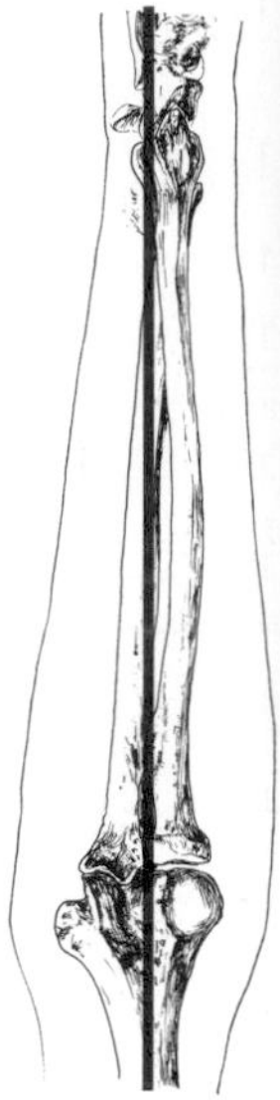

1 Capitate
2 Hamate
3 Scaphoid
4 Triquetrum
5 Lunate
6 Disk equivalent
7 Abductor pollicis longus + brachioradialis muscle (tendons)
8 Ulnar collateral ligament of wrist joint
9 Radius
10 Triangular fibrocartilage
11 Cephalic vein
12 Ulna
13 Extensor carpi ulnaris muscle
14 Pronator quadratus muscle

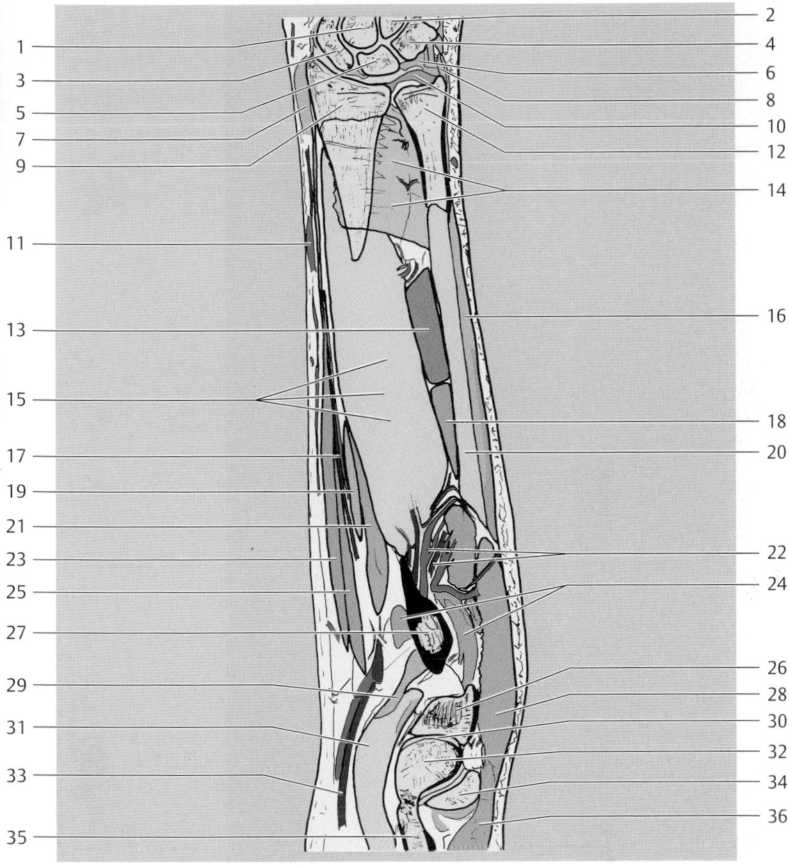

15 Flexor digitorum superficialis muscle
16 Extensor indicis muscle (+ tendon)
17 Radial artery and vein
18 Extensor pollicis longus muscle
19 Pronator teres muscle (tendon)
20 Flexor carpi ulnaris muscle
21 Flexor pollicis longus muscle
22 Ulnar artery and vein
23 Brachioradialis muscle
24 Supinator muscle
25 Extensor carpi radialis longus muscle
26 Radioulnar joint
27 Radial tuberosity
28 Anconeus muscle
29 Biceps brachii muscle (tendon)
30 Humero-ulnar joint
31 Brachialis muscle
32 Humerus (Trochlea)
33 Brachialis artery
34 Olecranon
35 Humerus (shaft)
36 Triceps brachii muscle (+ tendon)

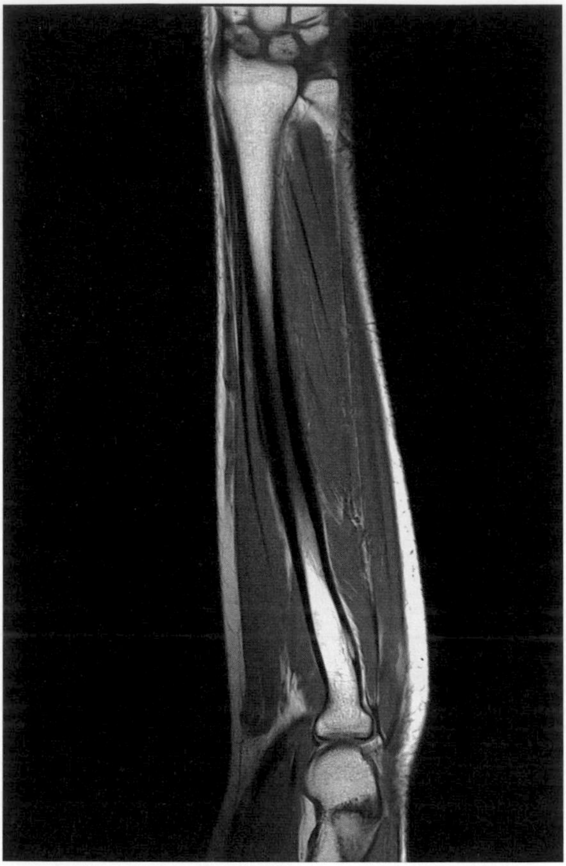

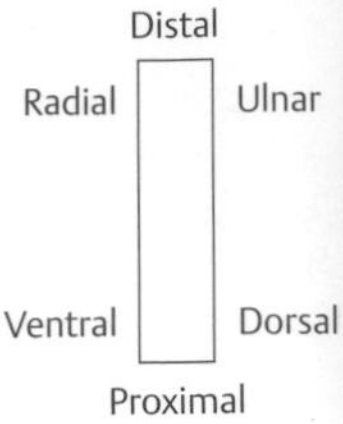

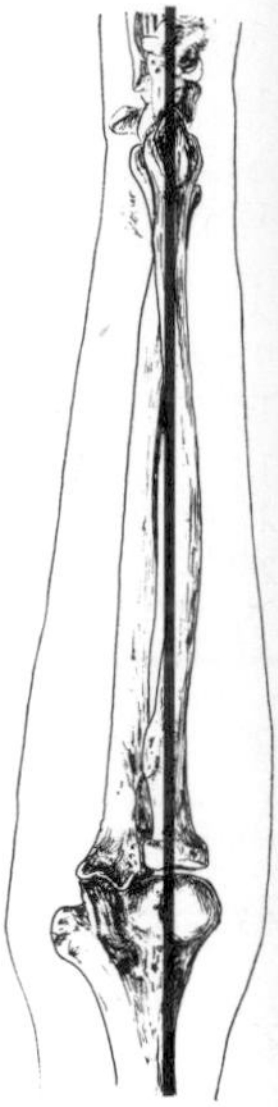

1 Trapezoid
2 Hamate
3 Capitate
4 Triquetrum
5 Scaphoid
6 Ulna

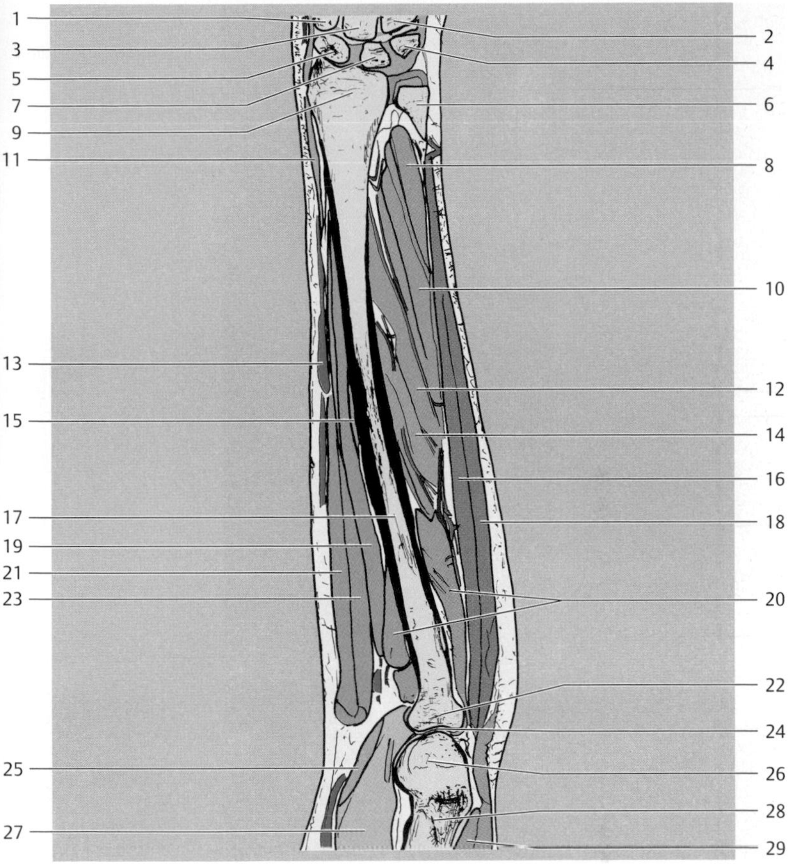

7 Lunate
8 Extensor indicis muscle
9 Radius
10 Extensor pollicis brevis muscle
11 Flexor pollicis longus muscle (tendon)
12 Extensor pollicis longus muscle
13 Cephalic vein
14 Abductor pollicis longus muscle
15 Pronator teres muscle (tendon)
16 Extensor digiti minimi muscle
17 Radius (shaft)
18 Extensor carpi ulnaris muscle
19 Extensor carpi radialis brevis muscle
20 Supinator muscle
21 Brachioradialis muscle
22 Radius (head)
23 Extensor carpi radialis longus muscle
24 Humeroradial joint
25 Biceps brachii muscle (tendon)
26 Humerus (capitulum)
27 Brachialis muscle
28 Humerus (shaft)
29 Triceps brachii muscle

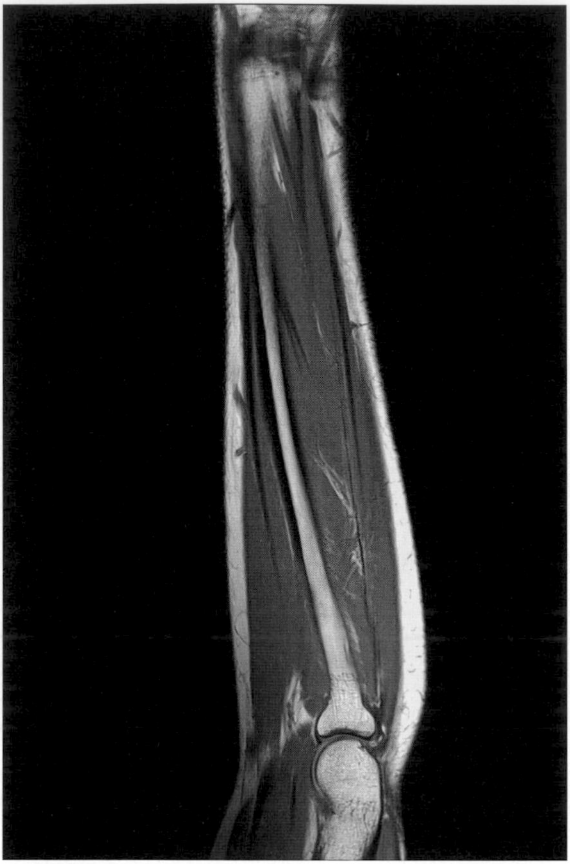

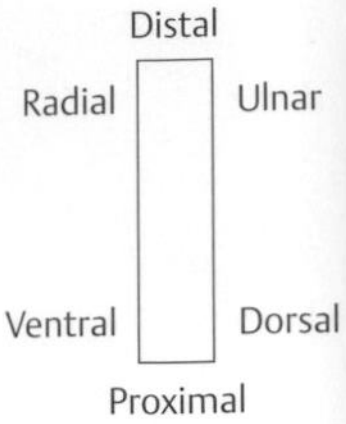

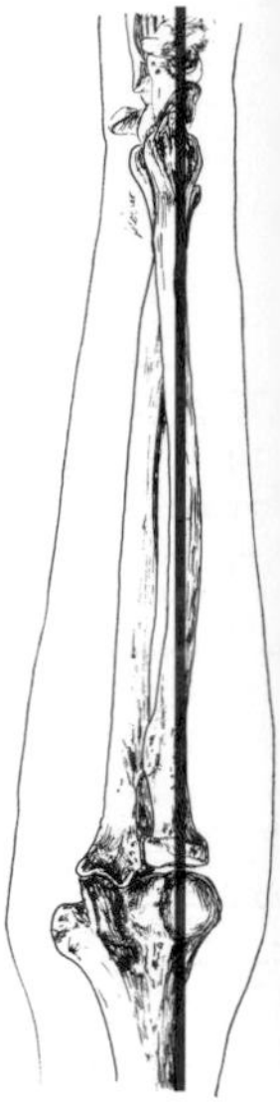

1 Joint capsule + dorsal radiocarpal ligament
2 Extensor digiti minimi muscle (tendon)
3 Radius
4 Ulna
5 Extensor pollicis longus muscle (+ tendon)
6 Extensor indicis muscle (+ tendon)

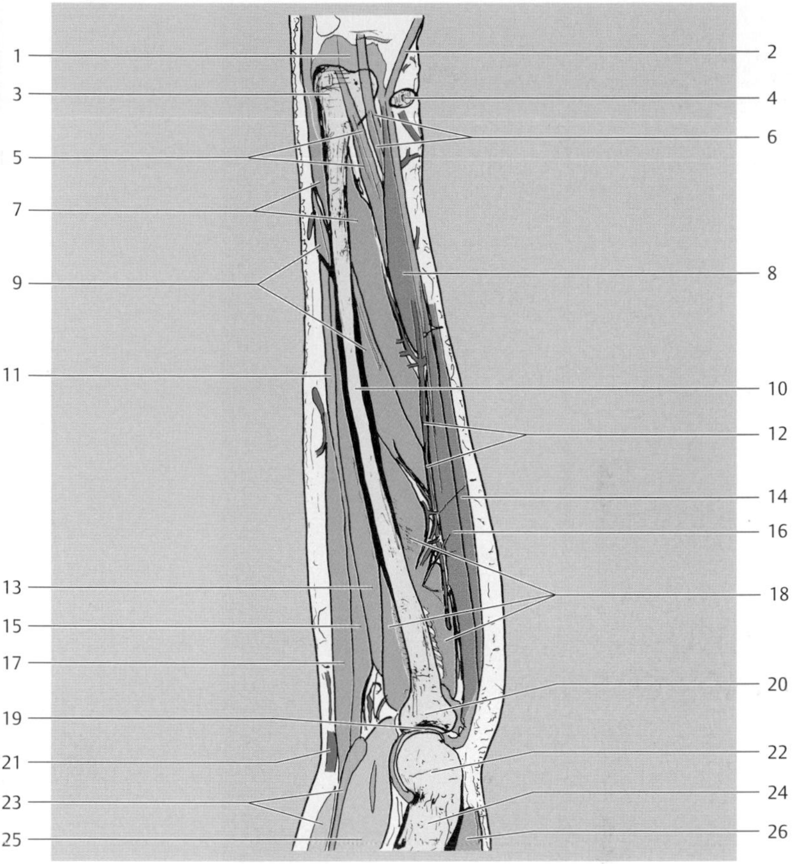

7 Extensor pollicis brevis muscle
8 Extensor digitorum muscle
9 Abductor pollicis longus muscle
10 Radius (shaft)
11 Extensor carpi radialis longus muscle (tendon)
12 Posterior interosseous artery and vein
13 Extensor carpi radialis brevis muscle
14 Extensor carpi ulnaris muscle
15 Extensor carpi radialis longus muscle
16 Extensor digiti minimi muscle
17 Brachioradialis muscle
18 Supinator muscle
19 Humeroradial joint
20 Radius (head)
21 Median cubital vein
22 Humerus (capitulum)
23 Biceps brachii muscle (+ tendon)
24 Humerus (shaft)
25 Brachialis muscle
26 Triceps brachii muscle (+ tendon)

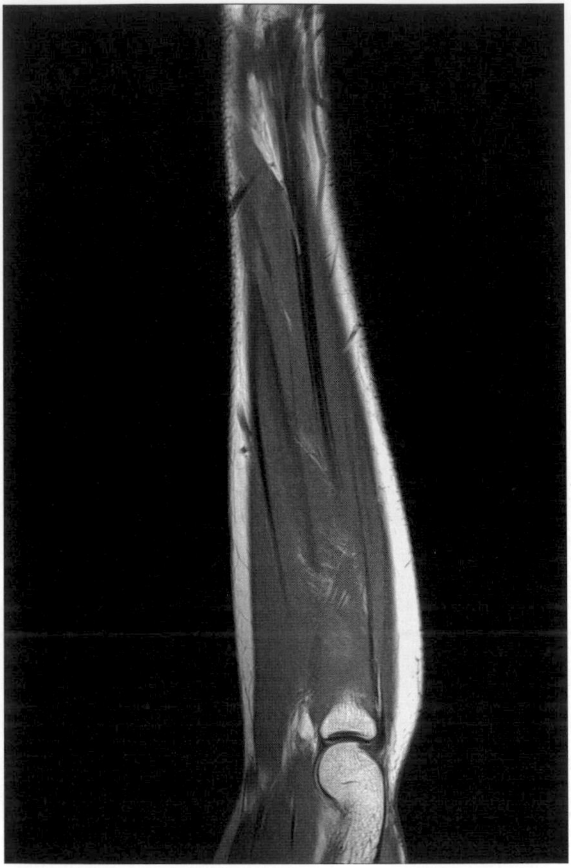

Distal

Radial Ulnar

Ventral Dorsal

Proximal

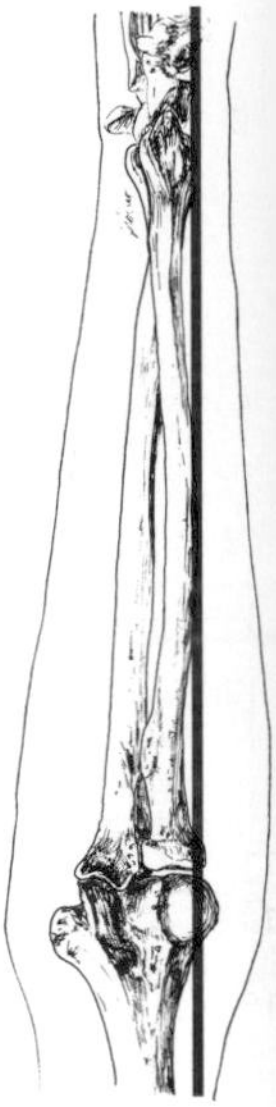

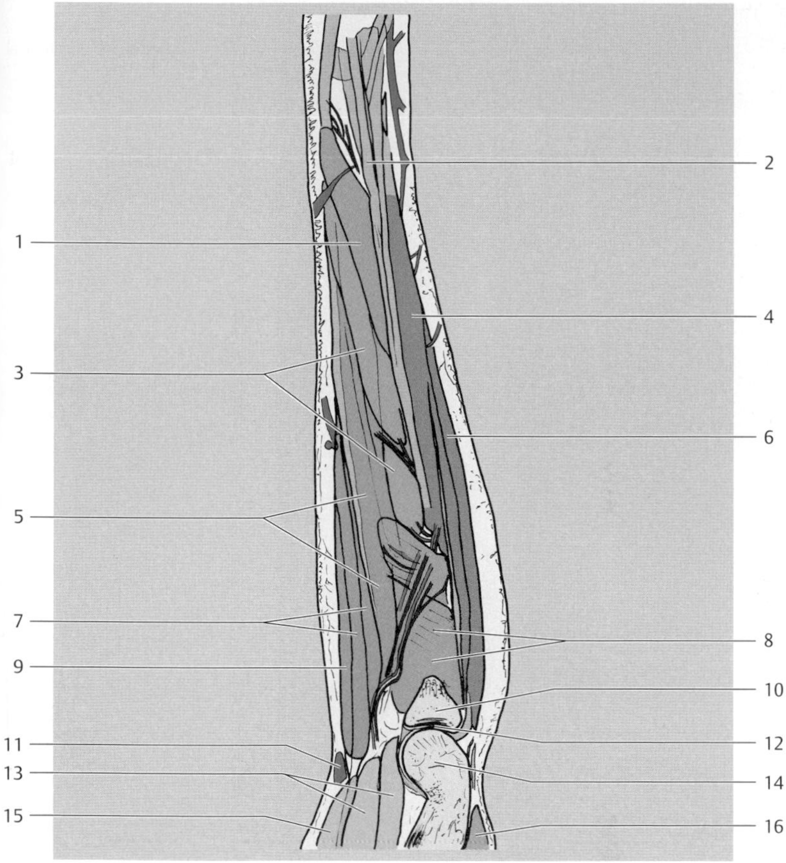

1 Extensor pollicis brevis muscle
2 Extensor digitorum muscle (tendon)
3 Abductor pollicis longus muscle
4 Extensor digitorum muscle (+ tendon)
5 Extensor carpi radialis brevis muscle
6 Extensor digiti minimi muscle
7 Extensor carpi radialis longus muscle
8 Supinator muscle
9 Brachioradialis muscle
10 Radius (head)
11 Median cubital vein
12 Humeroradial joint
13 Brachialis muscle
14 Humerus (capitulum)
15 Biceps brachii muscle (+ tendon)
16 Triceps brachii muscle

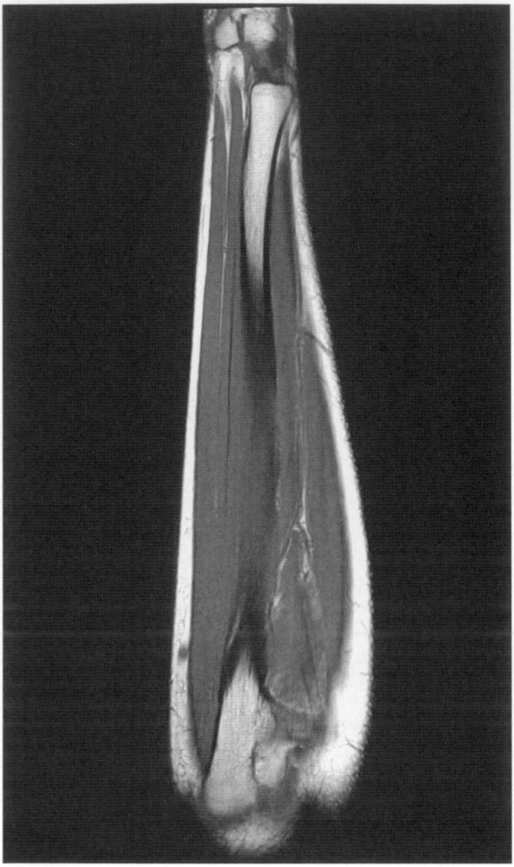

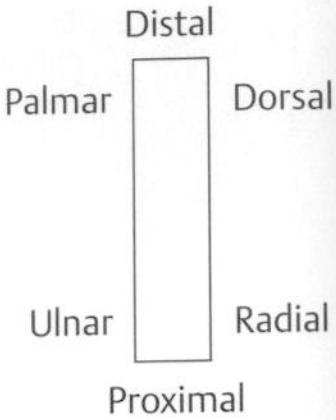

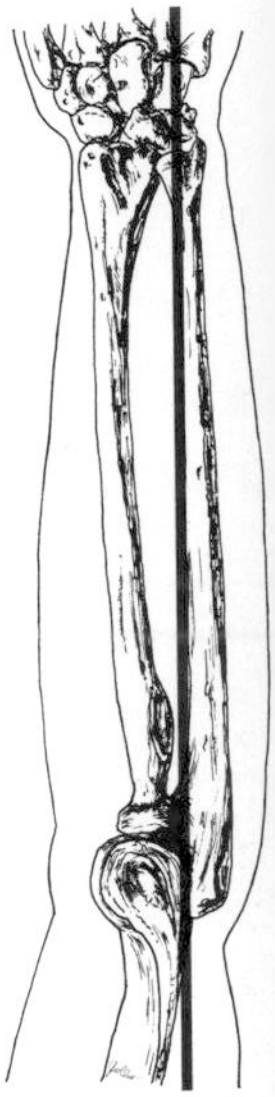

1 Abductor digiti minimi muscle
2 Triquetrum
3 Pisiform
4 Ulnar styloid process
5 Palmar ulnocarpal ligament
6 Ulna
7 Ulnar nerve

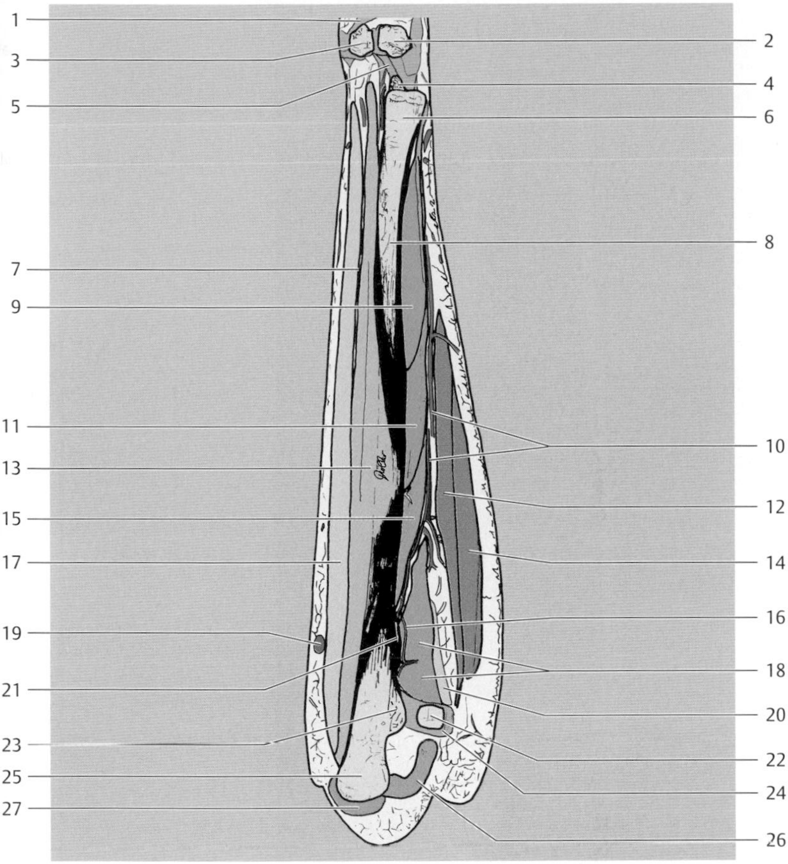

8 Ulna (shaft)
9 Extensor indicis muscle
10 Posterior interosseous artery and vein
11 Extensor pollicis brevis muscle
12 Extensor digiti minimi muscle
13 Flexor digitorum profundus muscle
14 Extensor digitorum muscle
15 Abductor pollicis longus muscle
16 Recurrent interosseous artery and vein
17 Flexor carpi ulnaris muscle
18 Supinator muscle
19 Basilic vein
20 Extensor carpi ulnaris muscle
21 Brachialis muscle (attachment)
22 Radius (head)
23 Radial tuberosity
24 Anular ligament
25 Olecranon
26 Anconeus muscle
27 Triceps brachii muscle

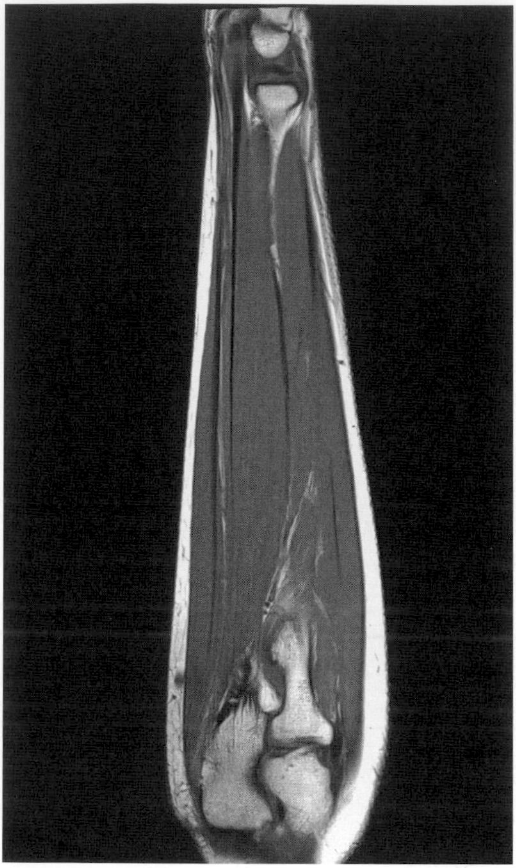

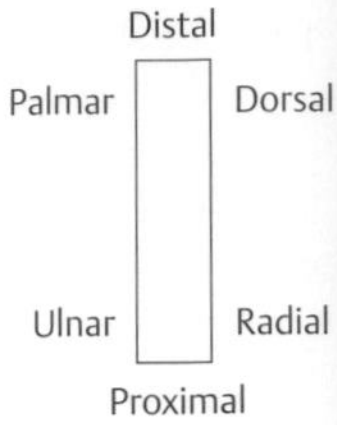

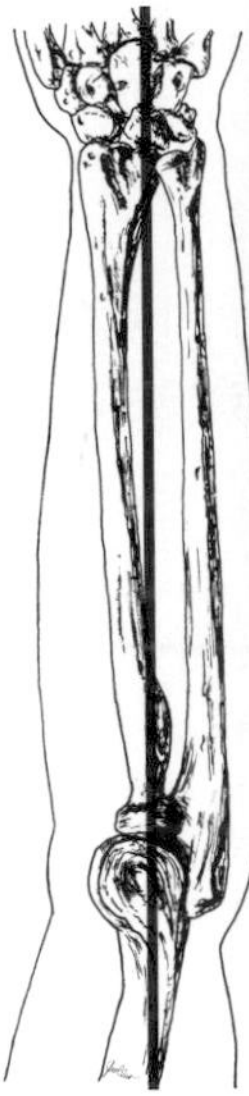

1 Ulnar vein
2 Hamate
3 Flexor digitorum profundus muscle (tendon)
4 Triquetrum
5 Ulnar nerve
6 Extensor digiti minimi muscle (tendon)
7 Pronator quadratus muscle
8 Ulna
9 Anterior interosseous artery and vein
10 Extensor digiti minimi muscle
11 Extensor indicis muscle

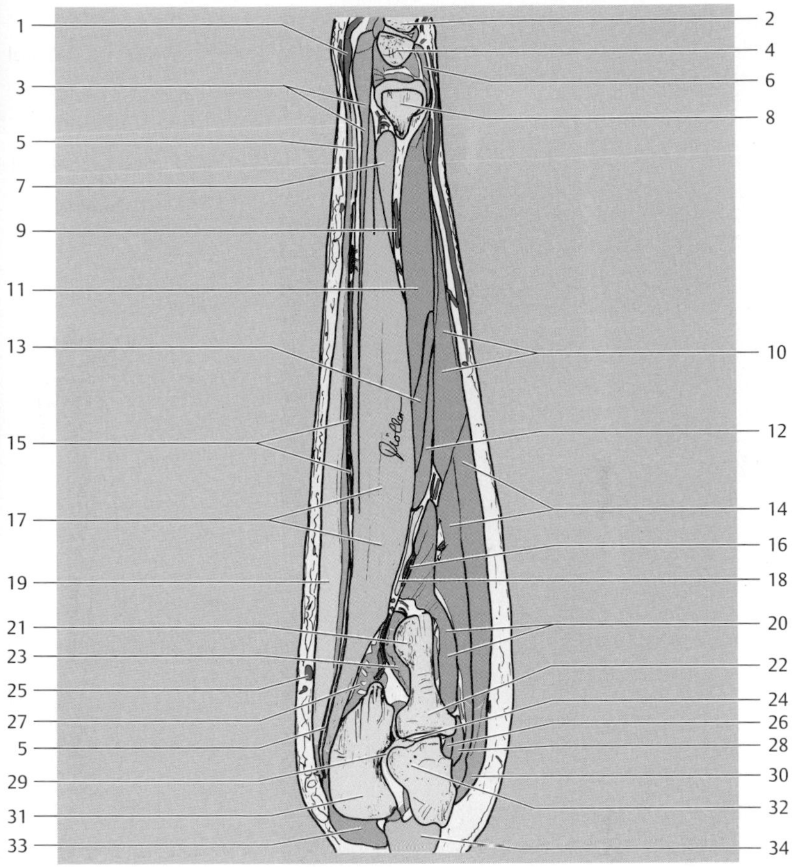

12 Abductor pollicis longus muscle
13 Extensor pollicis brevis muscle
14 Extensor digitorum muscle (+ tendon)
15 Ulnar artery and vein
16 Interosseous artery and vein
17 Flexor digitorum profundus muscle
18 Median nerve
19 Flexor carpi ulnaris muscle
20 Supinator muscle
21 Radial tuberosity
22 Radius (head)
23 Biceps brachii muscle (+ tendon)
24 Humeroradial joint
25 Basilic vein
26 Anular ligament
27 Brachialis muscle (attachment)
28 Radial collateral ligament
29 Humero-ulnar joint
30 Common extensor tendon (attachment)
31 Olecranon
32 Humerus (capitulum)
33 Triceps brachii muscle (+ tendon)
34 Brachialis muscle

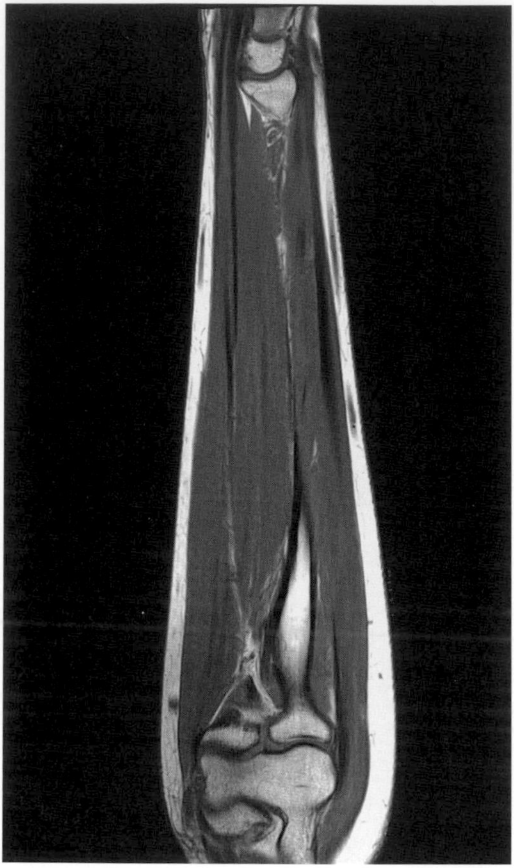

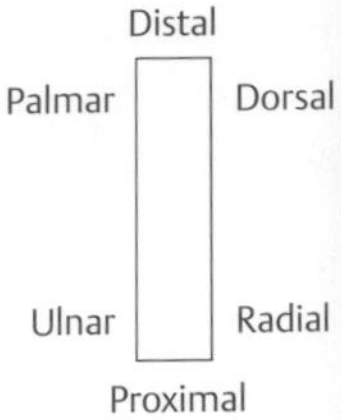

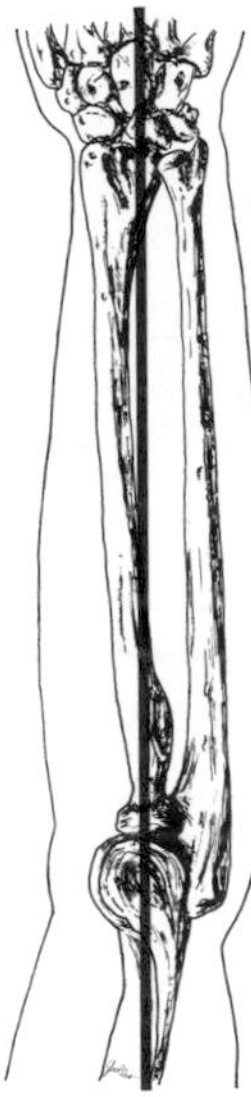

1 Median nerve
2 Capitate
3 Wrist joint
4 Lunate
5 Flexor digitorum profundus muscle (tendon)
6 Radius
7 Flexor digitorum superficialis muscle (tendon)
8 Extensor indicis muscle
9 Pronator quadratus muscle
10 Posterior interosseous artery and vein

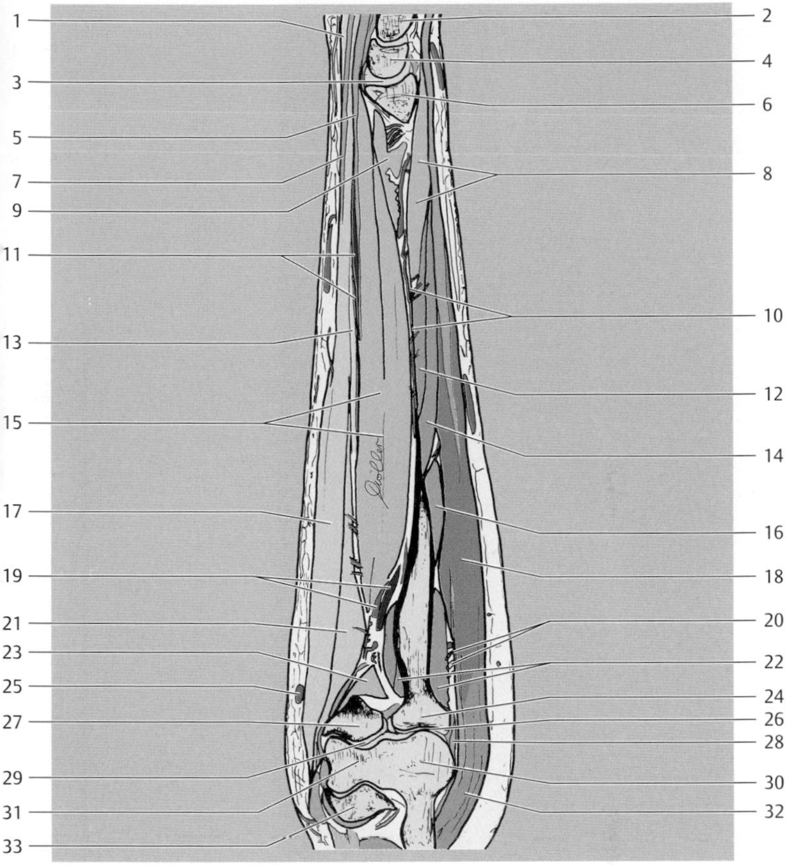

11 Ulnar artery and vein
12 Extensor pollicis brevis muscle
13 Ulnar nerve
14 Extensor pollicis longus muscle
15 Flexor digitorum profundus muscle
16 Abductor pollicis longus muscle
17 Flexor carpi ulnaris muscle
18 Extensor digitorum muscle
19 Anterior interosseous artery and vein
20 Radial nerve (deep branch) and radial recurrent artery
21 Flexor digitorum superficialis muscle
22 Supinator muscle
23 Brachialis muscle
24 Radius (head)
25 Basilic vein
26 Humeroradial joint
27 Olecranon
28 Radial collateral ligament
29 Humero-ulnar joint
30 Humerus (capitulum)
31 Humerus (trochlea)
32 Extensor carpi radialis brevis muscle
33 Coronoid process

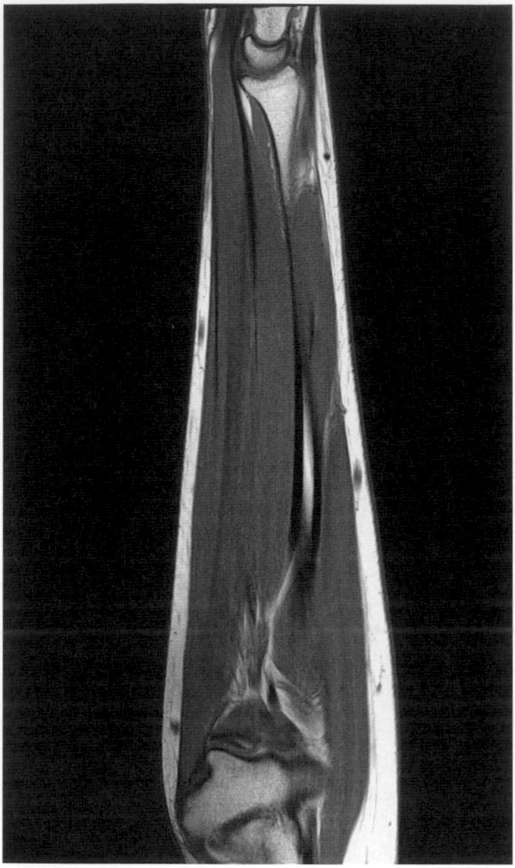

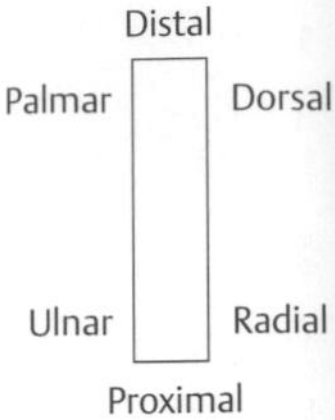

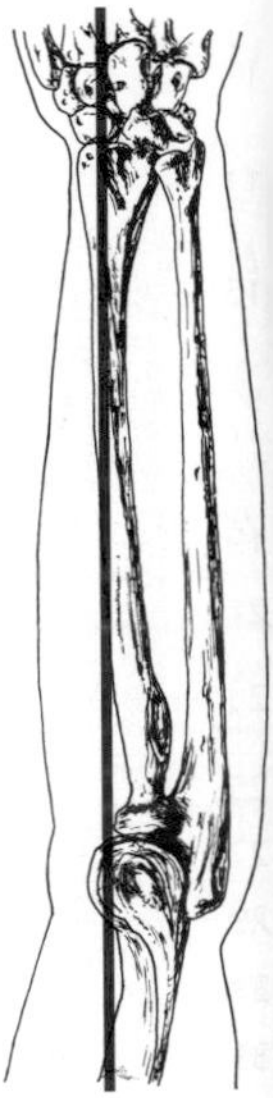

1 Capitate
2 Extensor digitorum muscle (tendon)
3 Flexor digitorum superficialis muscle (tendon)
4 Lunate
5 Wrist joint
6 Radius
7 Flexor digitorum profundus muscle (tendon)
8 Anterior interosseous artery and vein
9 Pronator quadratus muscle
10 Extensor pollicis brevis muscle

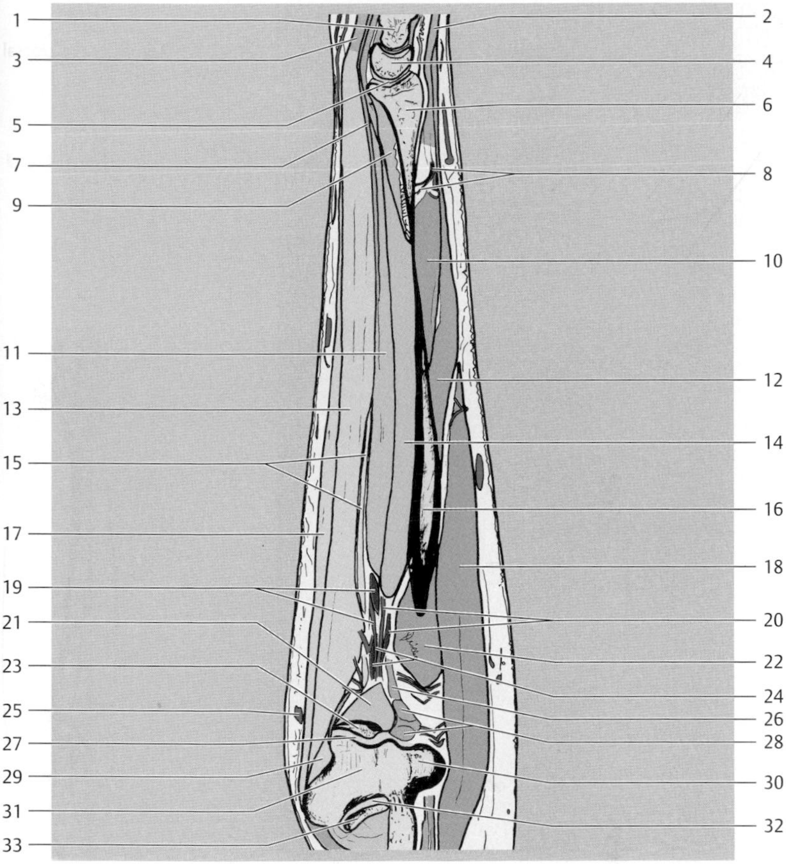

11 Flexor digitorum profundus muscle
12 Abductor pollicis muscle
13 Flexor digitorum superficialis muscle
14 Flexor pollicis longus muscle
15 Median nerve
16 Radius (shaft)
17 Palmaris longus muscle
18 Extensor carpi radialis longus and brevis muscle
19 Ulnar artery and vein
20 Posterior interosseous artery and vein
21 Brachialis muscle
22 Supinator muscle
23 Olecranon
24 Radial artery and vein
25 Basilic vein
26 Biceps brachii muscle (tendon)
27 Humero-ulnar joint
28 Anular ligament
29 Pronator teres muscle
30 Humerus (capitulum)
31 Humerus (trochlea)
32 Olecranon fossa
33 Coronoid process

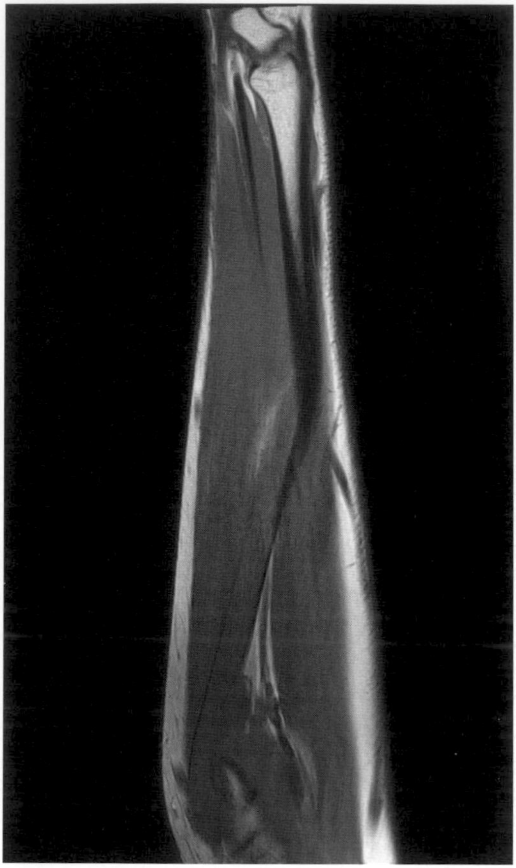

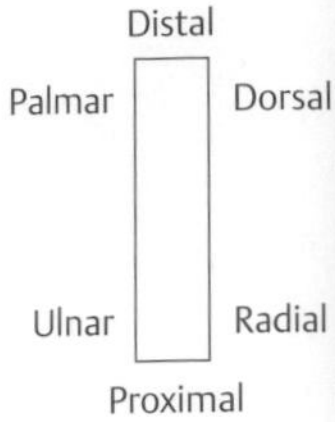
Distal
Palmar
Dorsal
Ulnar
Radial
Proximal

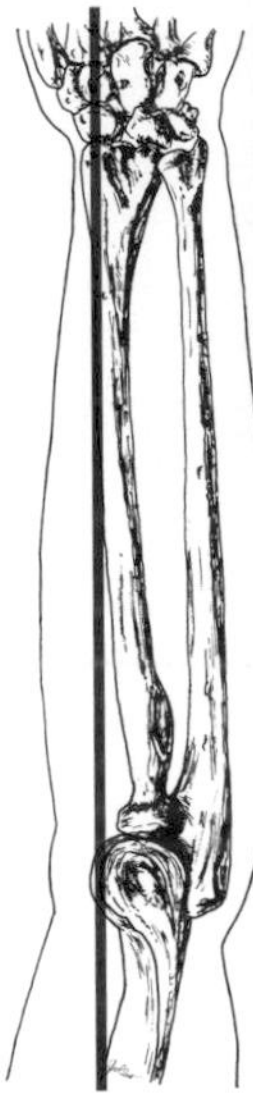

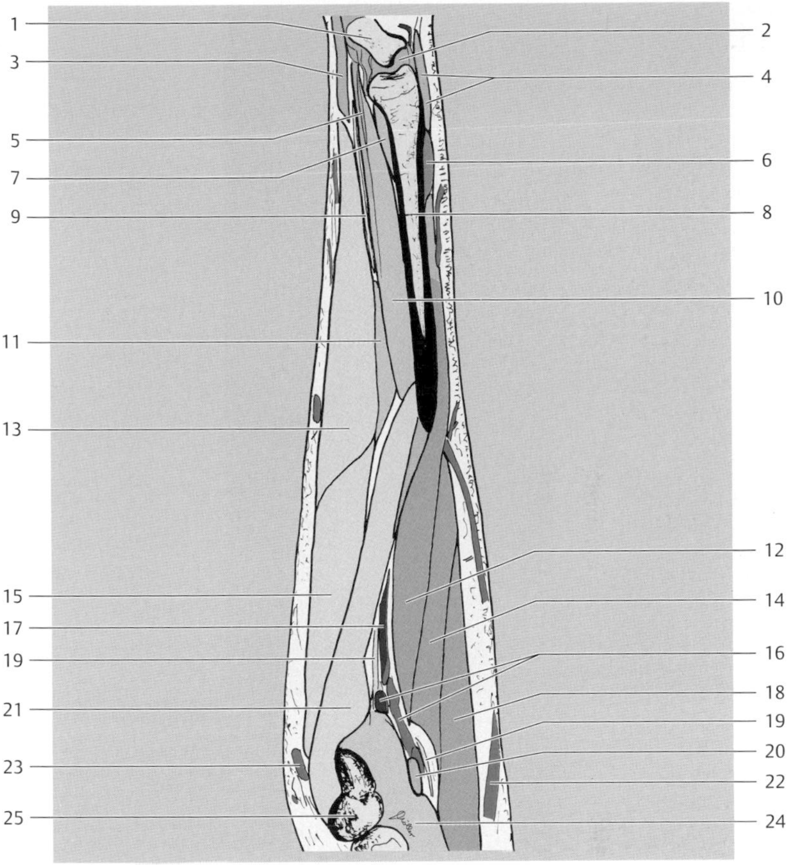

1 Scaphoid
2 Wrist joint
3 Flexor carpi radialis muscle (tendon)
4 Extensor carpi radialis brevis muscle (tendon)
5 Flexor pollicis longus muscle (tendon)
6 Extensor digitorum muscle
7 Pronator quadratus muscle
8 Radius (shaft)
9 Median nerve
10 Flexor pollicis longus muscle
11 Flexor digitorum profundus muscle
12 Extensor carpi radialis brevis muscle
13 Flexor digitorum superficialis muscle
14 Extensor carpi radialis longus muscle
15 Flexor carpi radialis muscle
16 Brachial artery and vein
17 Radial artery and vein
18 Brachioradialis muscle
19 Radial nerve
20 Biceps brachii muscle (tendon)
21 Pronator teres muscle
22 Cephalic vein
23 Basilic vein
24 Brachialis muscle
25 Medial epicondyle

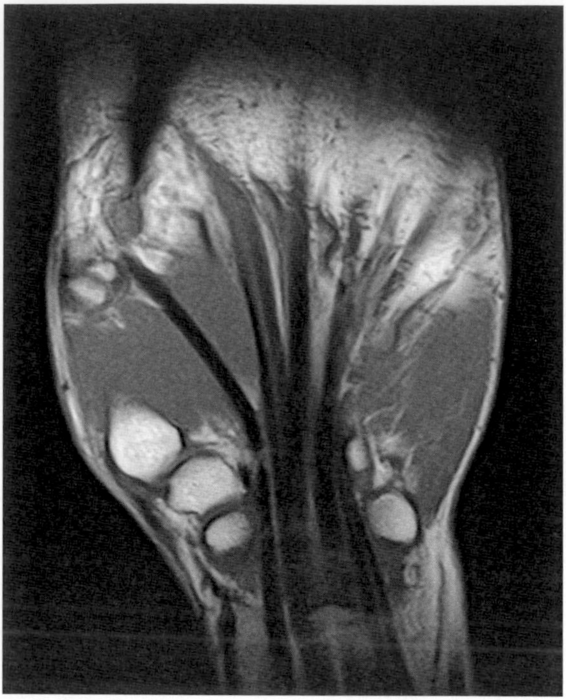

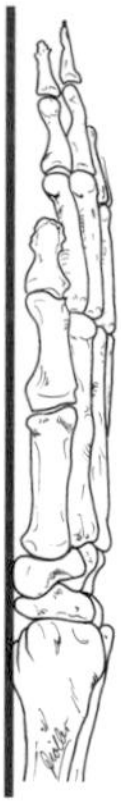

Distal

Radial Ulnar

Proximal

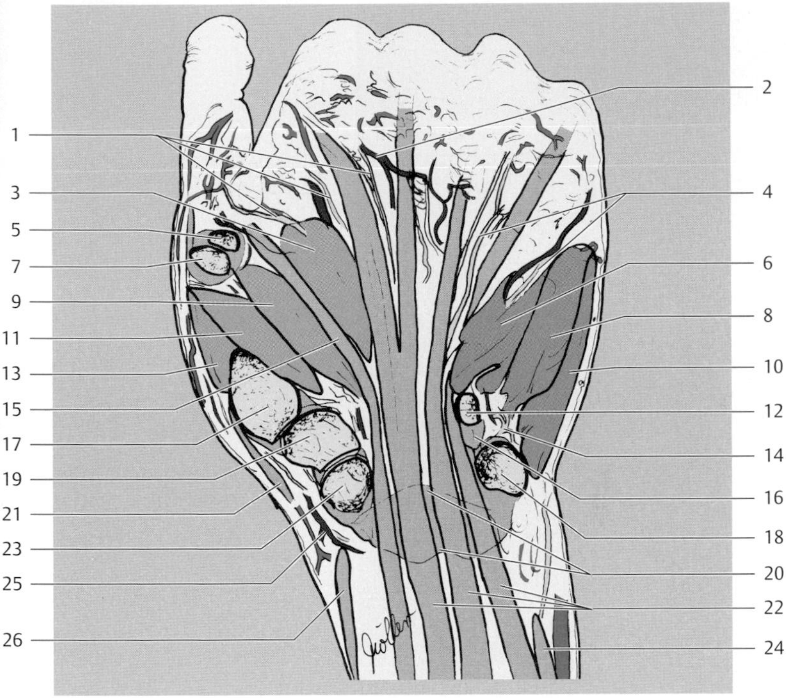

1 Proper palmar digital nerves (of median nerve)
2 Proper palmar digital arteries
3 Adductor pollicis muscle (transverse head)
4 Proper palmar digital nerves (of ulnar nerve)
5 Proximal phalanx I (base)
6 Opponens digiti minimi muscle
7 Metacarpal I (head)
8 Flexor digiti minimi muscle
9 Flexor pollicis brevis muscle (deep head)
10 Abductor digiti minimi muscle
11 Abductor pollicis muscle
12 Hamate (hook)
13 Opponens pollicis muscle
14 Ulnar nerve (deep branch)
15 Flexor pollicis longus muscle (tendon)
16 Pisohamate ligament
17 Metacarpal I (base)
18 Pisiform
19 Trapezium
20 Palmar radiocarpal ligament
21 Abductor pollicis longus muscle (tendon attachment)
22 Flexor digitorum profundus muscle (tendons)
23 Scaphoid
24 Flexor carpi ulnaris muscle (tendon)
25 Radial artery (superficial palmar branch)
26 Brachioradialis muscle (tendon)

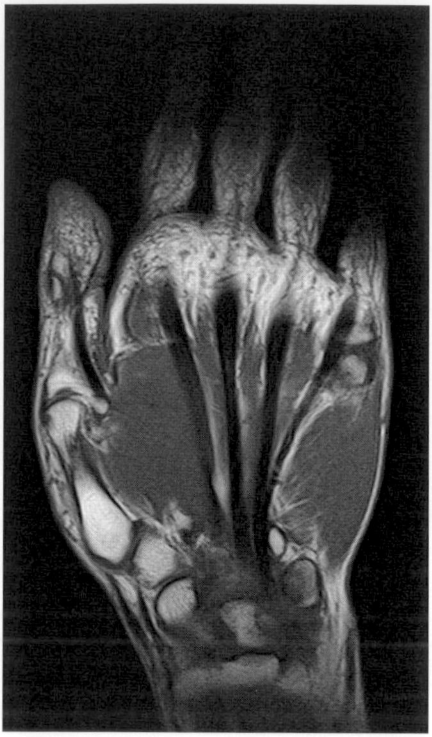

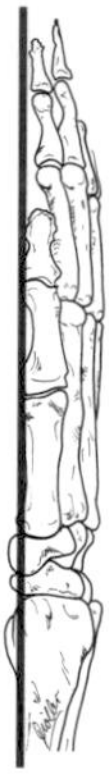

Distal

Radial ☐ Ulnar

Proximal

1 Distal phalanx I
2 Proper palmar digital arteries and nerves
3 Proximal phalanx I (head)
4 Lumbrical muscles
5 Flexor pollicis longus muscle (tendon)

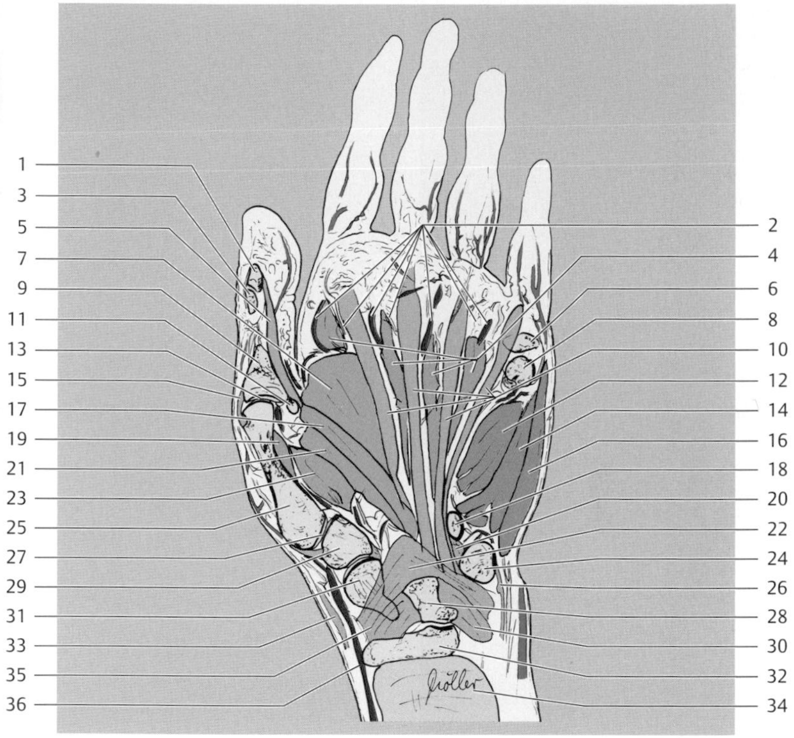

6 Proximal phalanx V (base)
7 Adductor pollicis muscle (transverse head)
8 Metacarpal V (head)
9 Proximal phalanx I (base)
10 Flexor digitorum profundus muscle (tendons)
11 Sesamoid bone
12 Opponens digiti minimi muscle
13 Metacarpophalangeal joint I
14 Flexor digiti minimi muscle
15 Joint capsule
16 Abductor digiti minimi muscle
17 Adductor pollicis muscle (oblique head)
18 Hamate (hook)
19 Interosseous muscle
20 Pisohamate ligament
21 Flexor pollicis brevis muscle
22 Radiate carpal ligament
23 Opponens pollicis muscle
24 Pisiform
25 Metacarpal I
26 Ulnar collateral ligament of wrist joint
27 Carpometacarpal joint I
28 Lunate
29 Trapezium
30 Palmar ulnocarpal ligament
31 Scaphoid
32 Radius
33 Extensor pollicis brevis muscle (tendon)
34 Pronator quadratus muscle
35 Palmar radiocarpal ligament
36 Radial artery

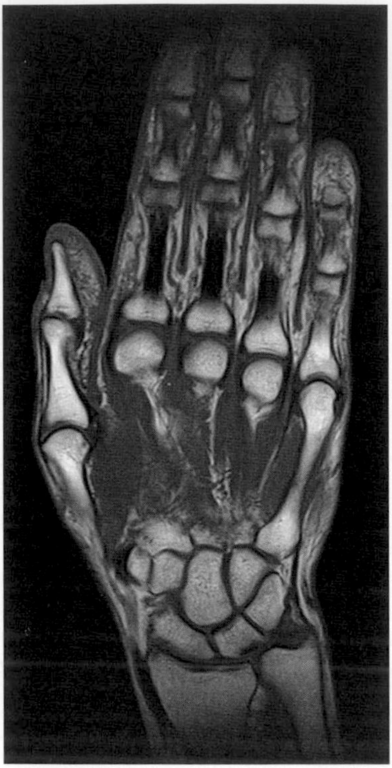

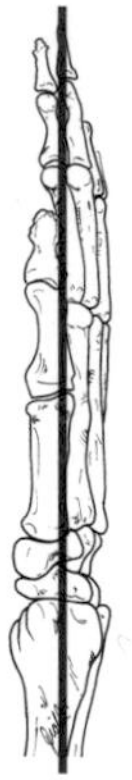

Distal

Radial Ulnar

Proximal

1 Distal phalanx II
2 Distal interphalangeal joint
3 Middle phalanx (base)
4 Proper palmar digital nerves and arteries
5 Proximal phalanx (head)
6 Flexor digitorum muscle (tendon)
7 Distal phalanx I
8 Proximal interphalangeal joint
9 Metacarpal II (head)
10 Collateral ligament

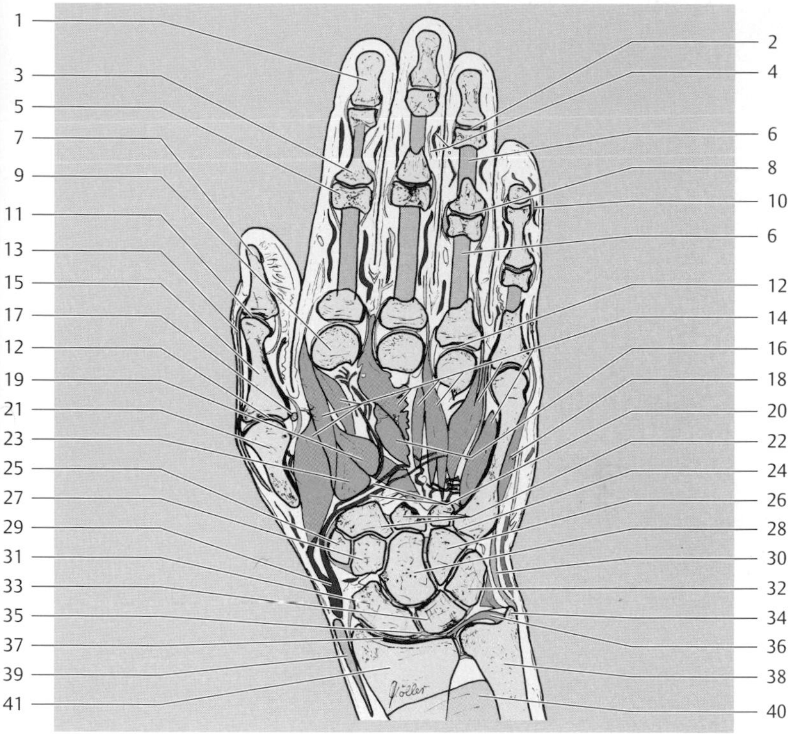

11 Interphalangeal joint I
12 Metacarpophalangeal joint
13 Extensor pollicis longus muscle (tendon)
14 Interosseous muscles
15 Proximal phalanx I
16 Adductor pollicis muscle (transverse head)
17 Sesamoid bone
18 Abductor digiti minimi muscle
19 Adductor pollicis muscle (oblique head)
20 Deep palmar arch and palmar carpal arch
21 Metacarpal I (head)
22 Metacarpals (bases)
23 Flexor pollicis brevis muscle
24 Carpometacarpal joint
25 Trapezium
26 Hamate
27 Trapezoid
28 Capitate
29 Radial artery
30 Ulnar collateral ligament of wrist joint
31 Scaphoid
32 Triquetrum
33 Lunate
34 Ulnar styloid process
35 Interosseous ligament (scapholunate)
36 Triangular fibrocartilage complex (TFC)
37 Wrist joint
38 Ulna
39 Brachioradialis muscle (tendon)
40 Pronator quadratus muscle
41 Radius

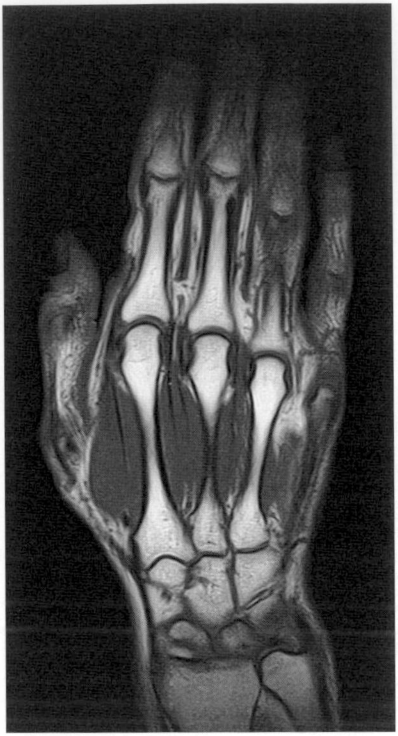

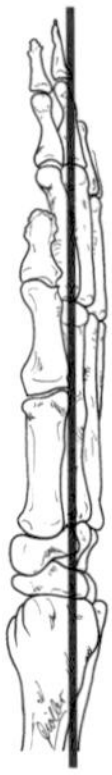

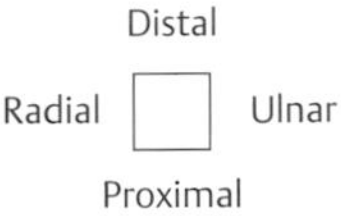

1 Middle phalanx (base)
2 Dorsal digital arteries and nerves
3 Collateral ligament
4 Proximal interphalangeal joint
5 Proximal phalanx (head)
6 Metacarpophalangeal joint
7 Proximal phalanx (shaft)
8 Interosseous muscles
9 Proximal phalanx (base)
10 Dorsal metacarpal vein
11 Metacarpal (head)
12 Joint capsule

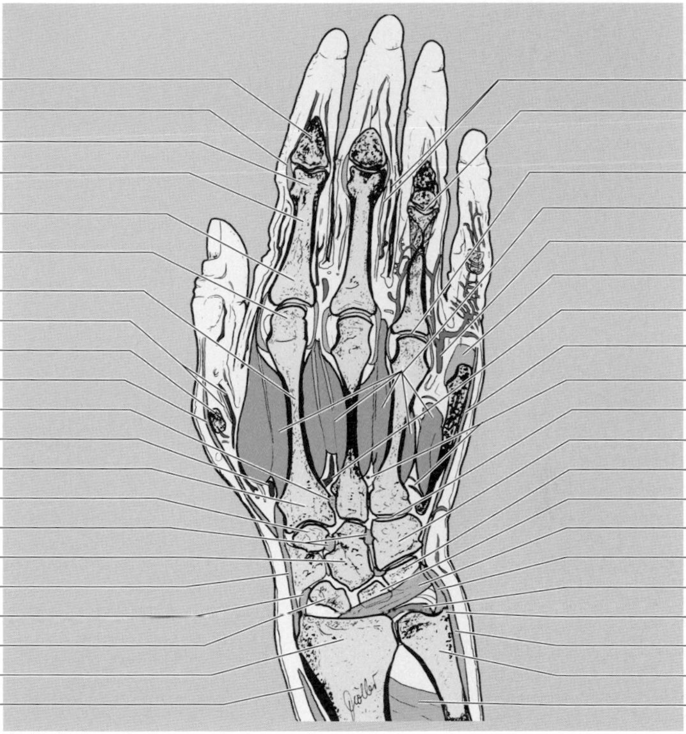

13 Metacarpal (shaft)
14 Dorsal metacarpal arteries
15 Dorsal metacarpal artery and nerve of thumb
16 Extensor digitorum muscle (tendon)
17 Metacarpal I (head)
18 Dorsal metacarpal arteries (perforating branches)
19 Extensor pollicis longus muscle (tendon)
20 Carpometacarpal joint
21 Interosseous metacarpal ligaments
22 Hamate
23 Radial artery (dorsal carpal branch)
24 Triquetrum
25 Metacarpal II (base)
26 Lunate
27 Trapezoid
28 Dorsal radiocarpal ligament
29 Interosseous intercarpal ligament
30 Ulnar collateral ligament of wrist joint
31 Capitate
32 Ulnar articular disk
33 Extensor carpi radialis longus muscle (tendon)
34 Ulnar styloid process
35 Radial collateral ligament of wrist joint
36 Extensor carpi ulnaris muscle (tendon)
37 Scaphoid
38 Ulna
39 Radius
40 Interosseous membrane
41 Brachioradialis muscle (tendon)

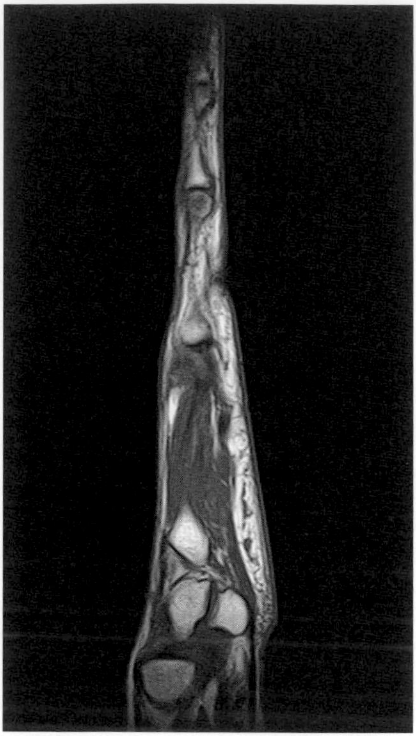

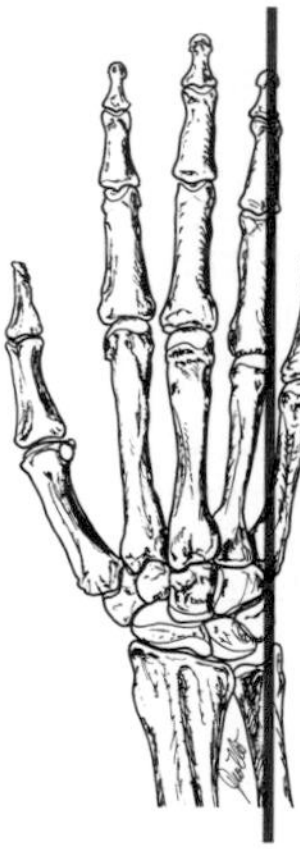

Distal

Dorsal ☐ Palmar

Proximal

1 Distal phalanx
2 Distal interphalangeal joint
3 Joint capsule
4 Middle phalanx (head)
5 Middle phalanx (base)
6 Palmar collateral ligament
7 Proximal interphalangeal joint
8 Flexor digitorum muscle (tendon)
9 Proximal phalanx (head)

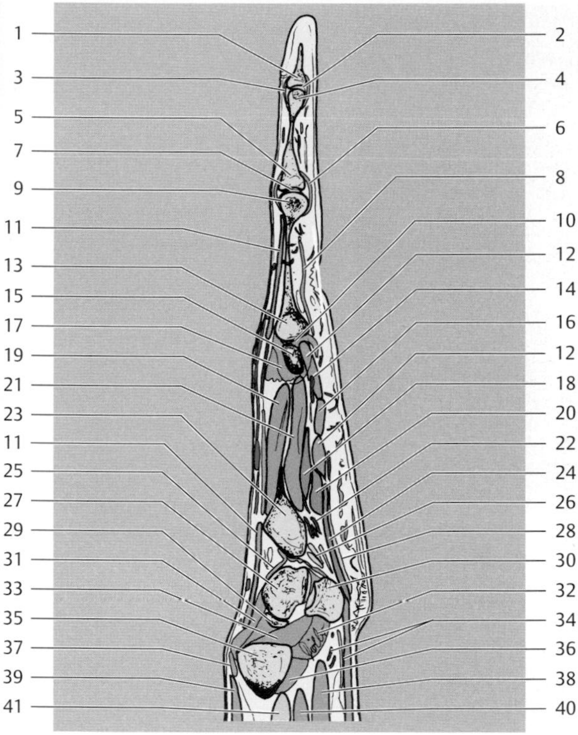

10 Metacarpophalangeal joint
11 Extensor digitorum muscle (tendon)
12 Lumbrical muscles
13 Proximal phalanx (base)
14 Palmar metacarpal artery
15 Metacarpal (head)
16 Flexor digiti minimi muscle (tendon)
17 Collateral ligament and attachment of interosseous muscles
18 Opponens digiti minimi muscle
19 Dorsal interosseous muscle
20 Flexor digiti minimi brevis muscle
21 Palmar interosseous muscle
22 Deep palmar arch
23 Metacarpal V (base)
24 Abductor digiti minimi muscle
25 Dorsal carpometacarpal ligament
26 Ulnar nerve (deep branch)
27 Triquetrum
28 Palmaris brevis muscle
29 Lunate
30 Pisiform
31 Dorsal radiocarpal ligament
32 Palmar ulnocarpal ligament
33 Triangular fibrocartilage complex (+ disk equivalent)
34 Ulnar artery and nerve
35 Ulna
36 Palmar radioulnar ligament
37 Dorsal radioulnar ligament
38 Flexor digitorum profundus muscle (tendon)
39 Extensor carpi ulnaris muscle (tendon)
40 Extensor digitorum superficialis muscle (tendon)
41 Pronator quadratus muscle

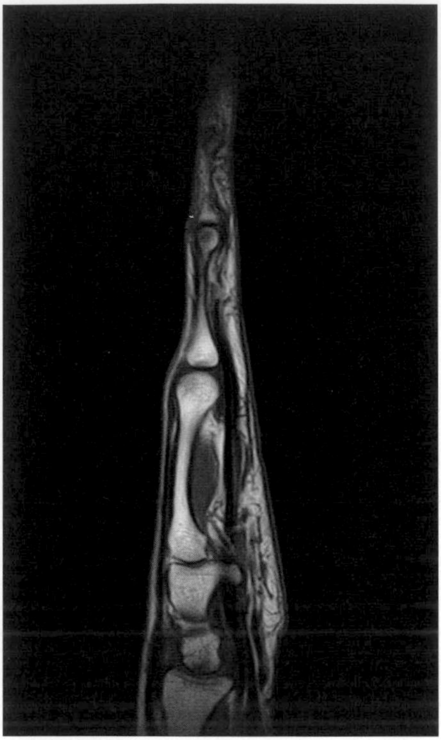

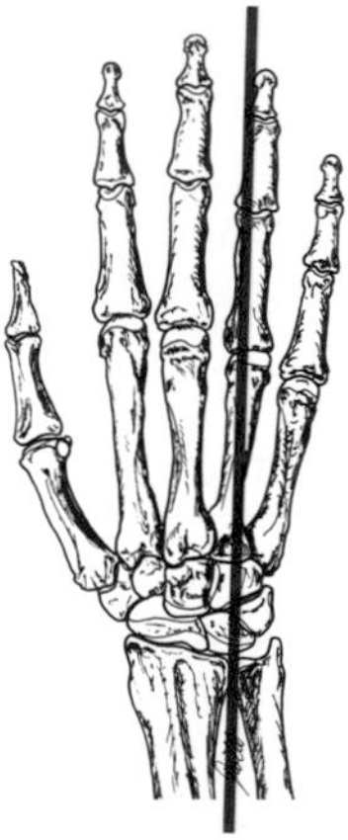

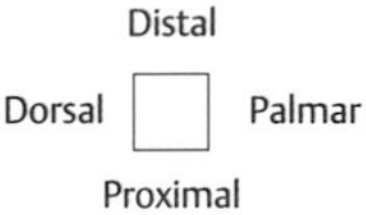

1 Collateral ligament
2 Middle phalanx (head)
3 Dorsal digital vein
4 Palmar digital vein
5 Middle phalanx (base)
6 Palmar (collateral) ligament
7 Proximal interphalangeal joint
8 Palmar digital artery and nerve
9 Proximal phalanx (head)
10 Flexor digitorum superficialis muscle (tendon)

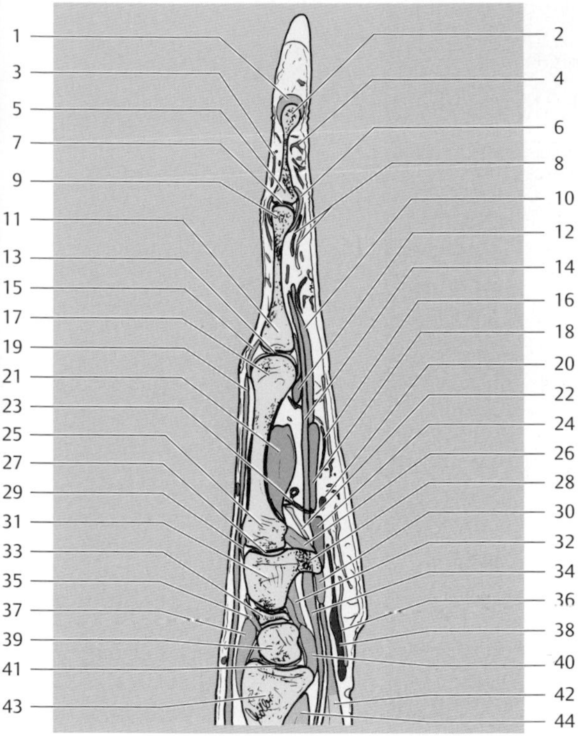

11 Proximal phalanx (base)
12 Palmar interosseous muscle
13 Metacarpophalangeal joint
14 Flexor digitorum profundus muscle (tendon)
15 Joint capsule
16 Palmar digital artery
17 Metacarpal (head)
18 Lumbrical muscle
19 Extensor digitorum muscle (tendon)
20 Superficial palmar arch
21 Palmar interosseous muscle
22 Ulnar nerve (deep branch)
23 Deep palmar arch
24 Flexor digiti minimi brevis muscle
25 Metacarpal (base)
26 Palmar carpometacarpal ligament
27 Carpometacarpal joint
28 Hamate (hook)
29 Dorsal carpometacarpal ligament
30 Flexor retinaculum
31 Hamate
32 Palmar intercarpal ligament
33 Triquetrum
34 Flexor digitorum muscle (tendon)
35 Dorsal intercarpal ligament
36 Palmar carpal ligament
37 Dorsal radiocarpal ligament
38 Ulnar artery
39 Lunate
40 Palmar ulnocarpal ligament
41 Radiocarpal joint
42 Flexor carpi ulnaris muscle
43 Radius
44 Pronator quadratus muscle

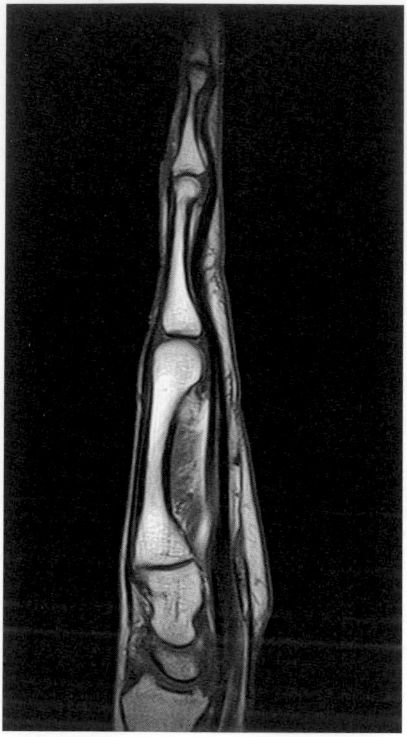

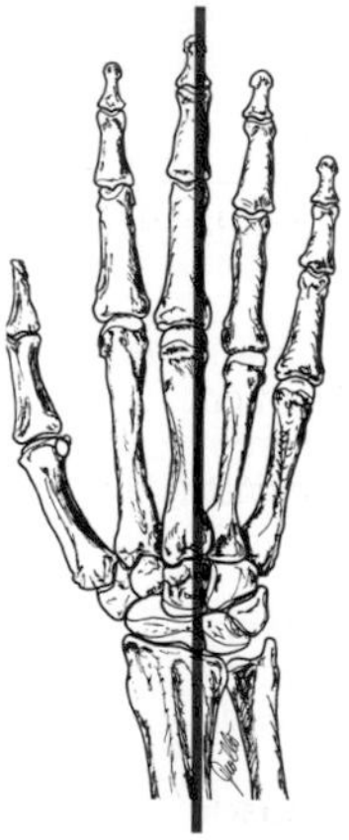

Distal

Dorsal ☐ Palmar

Proximal

1 Distal phalanx
2 Middle phalanx (head)
3 Distal interphalangeal joint
4 Palmar ligament
5 Joint capsule
6 Palmar digital artery
7 Middle phalanx (base)
8 Flexor digitorum muscle (tendon)

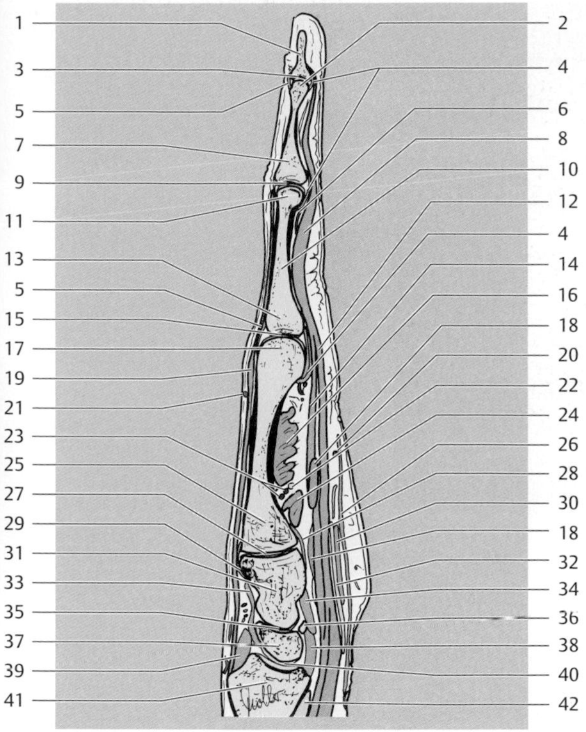

9 Proximal interphalangeal joint
10 Proximal phalanx (shaft)
11 Proximal phalanx (head)
12 Flexor digitorum superficialis muscle (tendon)
13 Proximal phalanx (base)
14 Flexor digitorum profundus muscle (tendon)
15 Metacarpophalangeal joint
16 Adductor pollicis muscle (transverse head)
17 Metacarpal (head)
18 Lumbrical muscles
19 Extensor digitorum muscle (tendon)
20 Superficial palmar arch
21 Palmar digital vein
22 Ulnar nerve (deep branch)
23 Deep palmar arch
24 Adductor pollicis muscle (deep head)
25 Metacarpal (base)
26 Palmar aponeurosis
27 Carpometacarpal joint
28 Palmar carpometacarpal ligament
29 Dorsal carpometacarpal ligament
30 Flexor retinaculum
31 Capitate
32 Median nerve
33 Dorsal intercarpal ligament
34 Palmar intercarpal ligament
35 Intercarpal (scaphocapitate) joint
36 Lunate
37 Scaphoid
38 Palmar radiocarpal ligament
39 Dorsal radiocarpal ligament
40 Wrist joint
41 Radius
42 Pronator quadratus muscle

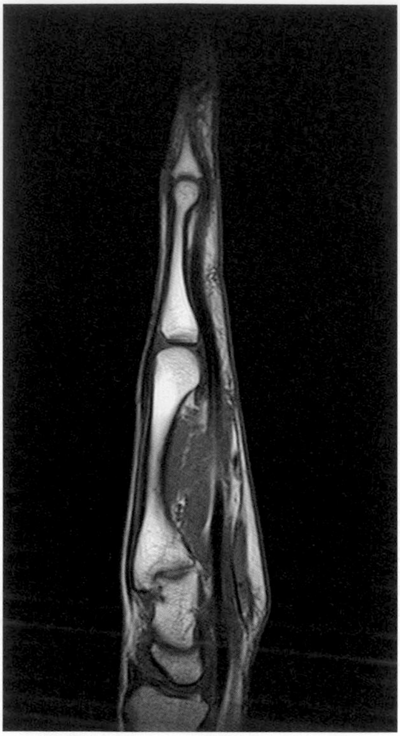

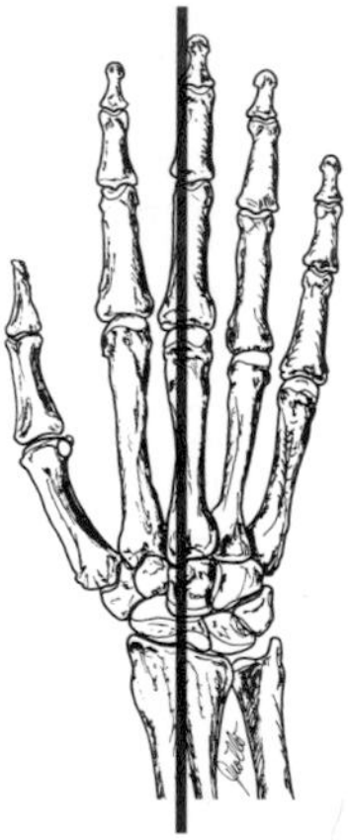

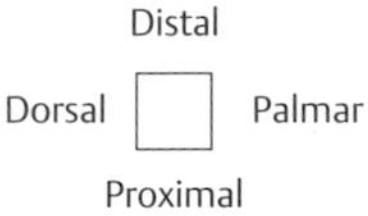

1 Collateral ligament (distal interphalangeal joint)
2 Proximal interphalangeal joint
3 Middle phalanx (base)
4 Palmar ligament
5 Proximal phalanx (head)
6 Flexor digitorum muscle (tendon)
7 Joint capsule

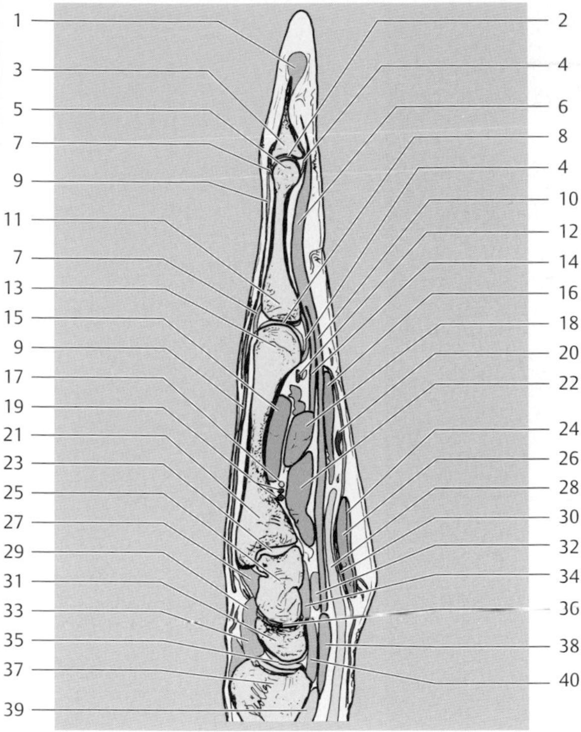

8 Metacarpophalangeal joint
9 Extensor digitorum muscle (tendon)
10 Flexor digitorum superficialis muscle (tendon)
11 Proximal phalanx (base)
12 Common palmar arteries
13 Metacarpal (head)
14 Flexor digitorum profundus muscle (tendon)
15 Interosseous muscle
16 Lumbrical muscles
17 Ulnar nerve (deep branch)
18 Adductor pollicis muscle (transverse head)
19 Deep palmar arch
20 Superficial palmar arch
21 Metacarpal (base)
22 Adductor pollicis muscle (oblique head)
23 Carpometacarpal joint
24 Palmar aponeurosis
25 Capitate
26 Abductor pollicis brevis muscle
27 Dorsal carpometacarpal ligament
28 Median nerve
29 Dorsal intercarpal ligament
30 Flexor retinaculum
31 Scaphoid
32 Flexor pollicis muscle (deep head)
33 Dorsal radiocarpal ligament
34 Palmar intercarpal ligament
35 Radiocarpal joint
36 Intercarpal (scaphocapitate) joint
37 Radius
38 Flexor pollicis longus muscle (tendon)
39 Pronator quadratus muscle
40 Palmar radiocarpal ligament

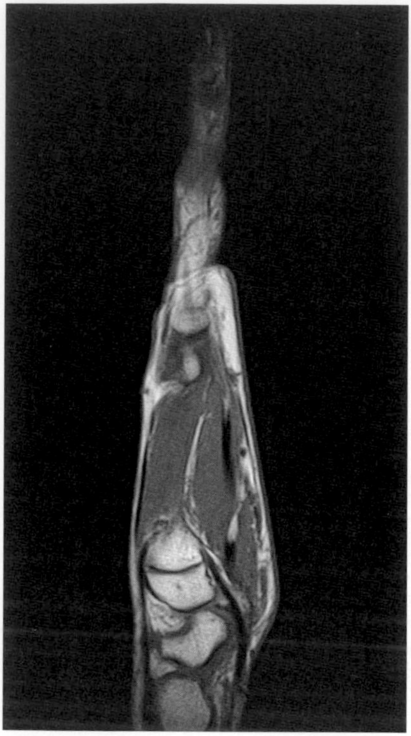

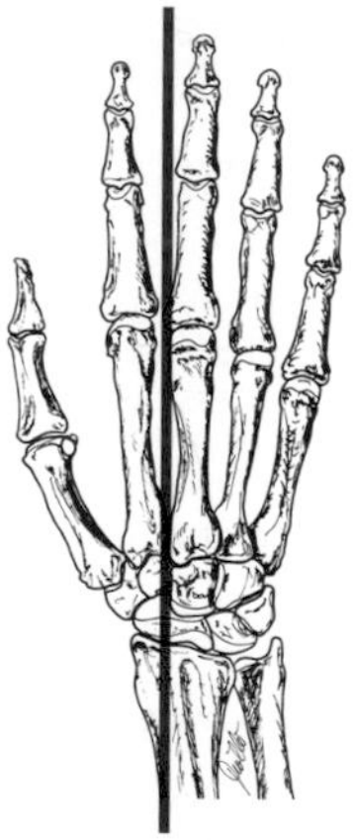

Distal

Dorsal ☐ Palmar

Proximal

1 Dorsal digital vein
2 Common palmar digital artery
3 Proximal phalanx (base)
4 Lumbrical muscles
5 Collateral ligament (metacarpophalangeal joint)
6 Adductor pollicis muscle (transverse head)

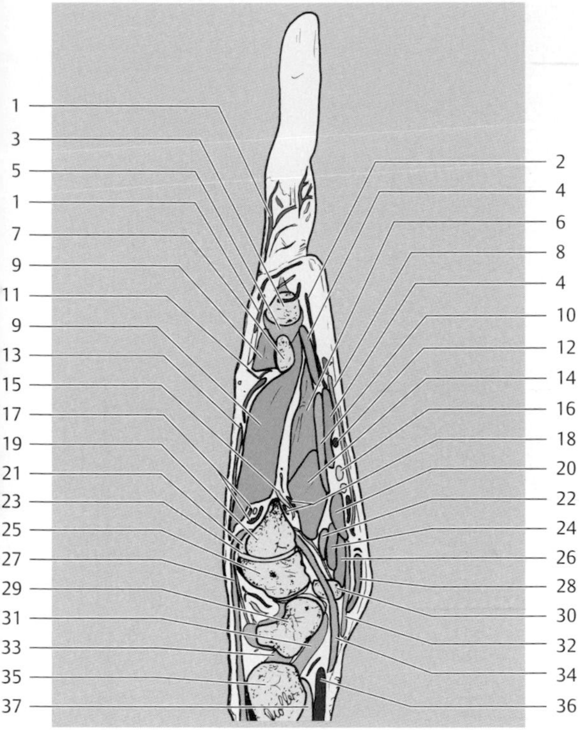

7 Metacarpal (head)
8 Palmar aponeurosis
9 Interosseous muscle
10 Flexor digitorum muscle (tendon)
11 Dorsal digital artery
12 Superficial palmar arch
13 Extensor digitorum muscle (tendon)
14 Adductor pollicis muscle (oblique head)
15 Ulnar nerve (deep branch)
16 Common palmar digital nerve (of median nerve)
17 Dorsal digital arteries and nerves
18 Deep palmar arch
19 Metacarpal II (base)
20 Flexor pollicis brevis muscle (superficial head)
21 Metacarpal III (base)
22 Flexor pollicis longus muscle (tendon)
23 Carpometacarpal joint
24 Flexor pollicis brevis muscle (deep head)
25 Trapezoid
26 Opponens pollicis muscle
27 Extensor carpi radialis brevis muscle
28 Abductor pollicis brevis muscle
29 Scaphoid
30 Hamate (hook)
31 Palmar radiocarpal ligament
32 Flexor retinaculum
33 Radial collateral ligament of wrist joint
34 Flexor carpi radialis muscle (tendon)
35 Radius
36 Radial artery
37 Pronator quadratus muscle

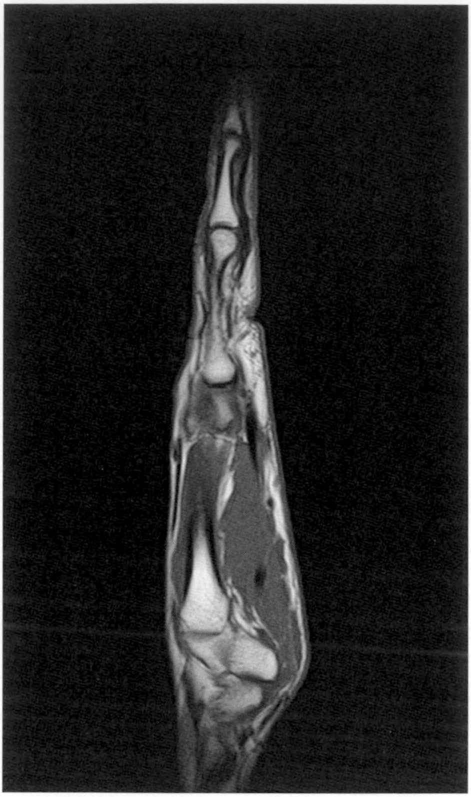

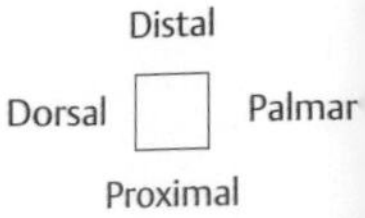

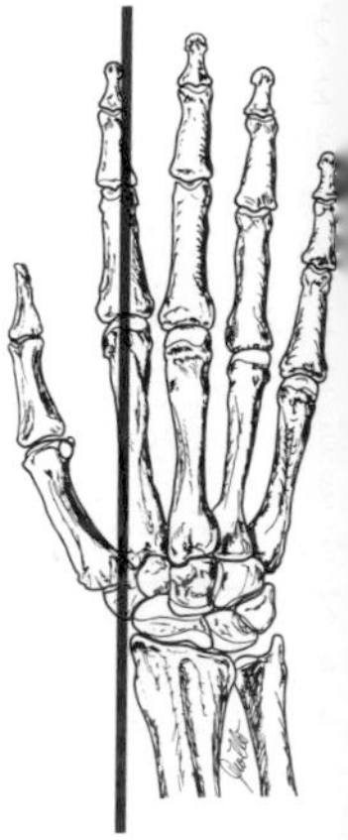

1 Distal phalanx
2 Palmar (collateral) ligament
3 Distal interphalangeal joint
4 Flexor digitorum muscle (tendon)
5 Middle phalanx (head)
6 Proper palmar digital artery
7 Extensor digitorum muscle (tendon)
8 Proper palmar digital nerve
9 Middle phalanx (base)
10 Flexor digitorum muscle (tendon)
11 Collateral ligament
12 Lumbrical muscle
13 Proximal phalanx (head)
14 Adductor pollicis muscle (transverse head)
15 Proper dorsal digital artery
16 Common palmar digital nerve
17 Proximal phalanx (base)
18 Superficial palmar arch
19 Metacarpal (head)
20 Median nerve
21 Collateral ligament
22 Adductor pollicis muscle (oblique head)
23 Digital artery (perforating branch)
24 Common metacarpal artery
25 Dorsal digital vein

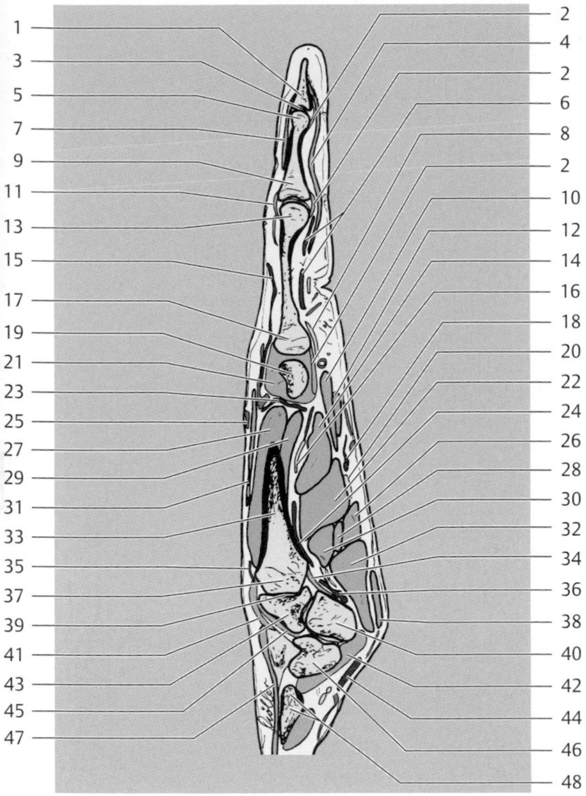

26 Flexor pollicis brevis muscle (superficial head)
27 Dorsal interosseous muscle
28 Flexor pollicis longus muscle (tendon)
29 Palmar interosseous muscle
30 Flexor pollicis brevis muscle (deep head)
31 Extensor digitorum II muscle (tendon)
32 Opponens pollicis muscle
33 Metacarpal II (shaft)
34 Palmar carpometacarpal ligament
35 Dorsal metacarpal artery
36 Deep palmar arch
37 Metacarpal II (base)
38 Abductor pollicis brevis muscle
39 Carpometacarpal joint
40 Trapezium (tubercle)
41 Dorsal carpometacarpal ligament
42 Radial collateral ligament of wrist joint
43 Trapezoid
44 Radial artery (superficial branch)
45 Dorsal intercarpal ligament
46 Scaphoid
47 Extensor carpi radialis longus muscle (tendon)
48 Radius with styloid process

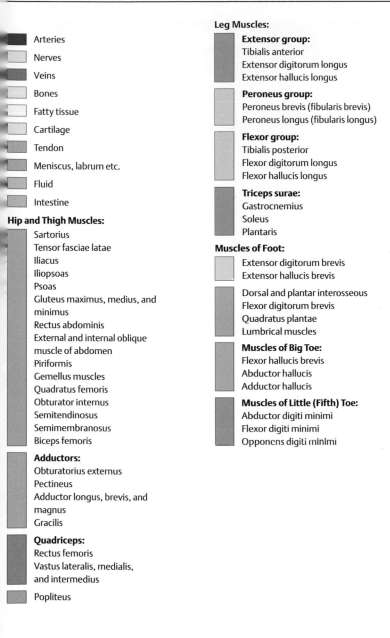

- Arteries
- Nerves
- Veins
- Bones
- Fatty tissue
- Cartilage
- Tendon
- Meniscus, labrum etc.
- Fluid
- Intestine

Hip and Thigh Muscles:

Sartorius
Tensor fasciae latae
Iliacus
Iliopsoas
Psoas
Gluteus maximus, medius, and minimus
Rectus abdominis
External and internal oblique muscle of abdomen
Piriformis
Gemellus muscles
Quadratus femoris
Obturator internus
Semitendinosus
Semimembranosus
Biceps femoris

Adductors:
Obturatorius externus
Pectineus
Adductor longus, brevis, and magnus
Gracilis

Quadriceps:
Rectus femoris
Vastus lateralis, medialis, and intermedius

Popliteus

Leg Muscles:

Extensor group:
Tibialis anterior
Extensor digitorum longus
Extensor hallucis longus

Peroneus group:
Peroneus brevis (fibularis brevis)
Peroneus longus (fibularis longus)

Flexor group:
Tibialis posterior
Flexor digitorum longus
Flexor hallucis longus

Triceps surae:
Gastrocnemius
Soleus
Plantaris

Muscles of Foot:

Extensor digitorum brevis
Extensor hallucis brevis

Dorsal and plantar interosseous
Flexor digitorum brevis
Quadratus plantae
Lumbrical muscles

Muscles of Big Toe:
Flexor hallucis brevis
Abductor hallucis
Adductor hallucis

Muscles of Little (Fifth) Toe:
Abductor digiti minimi
Flexor digiti minimi
Opponens digiti minimi

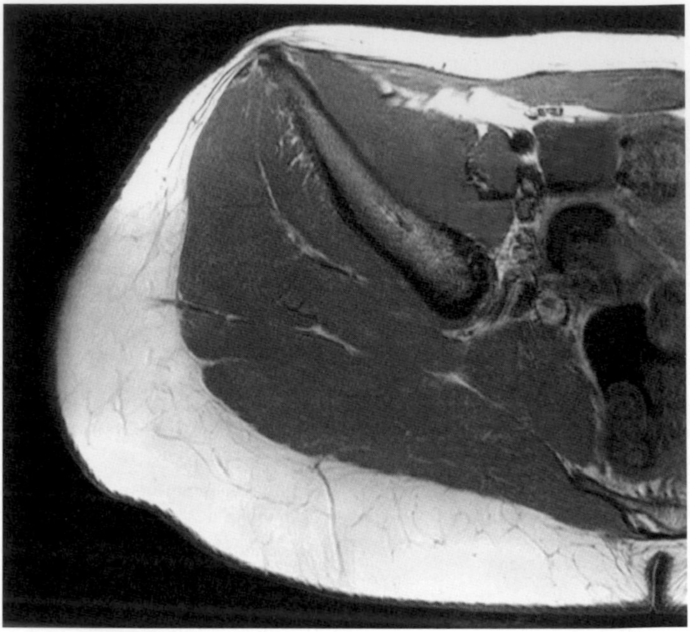

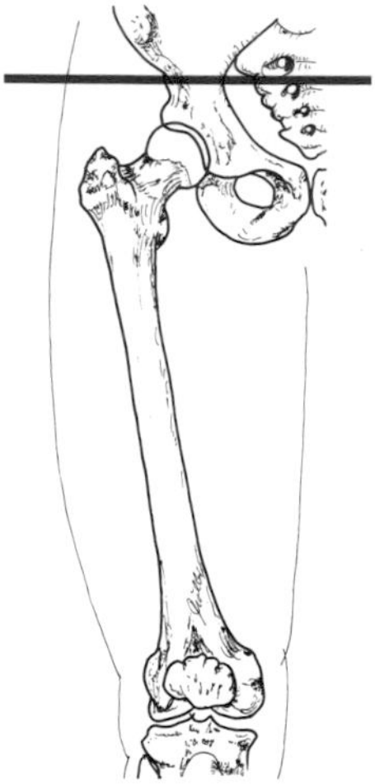

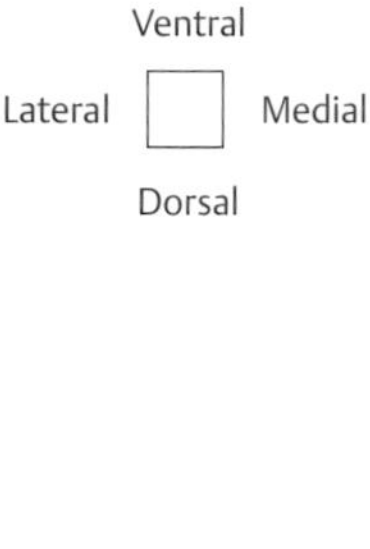
Ventral
Lateral
Medial
Dorsal

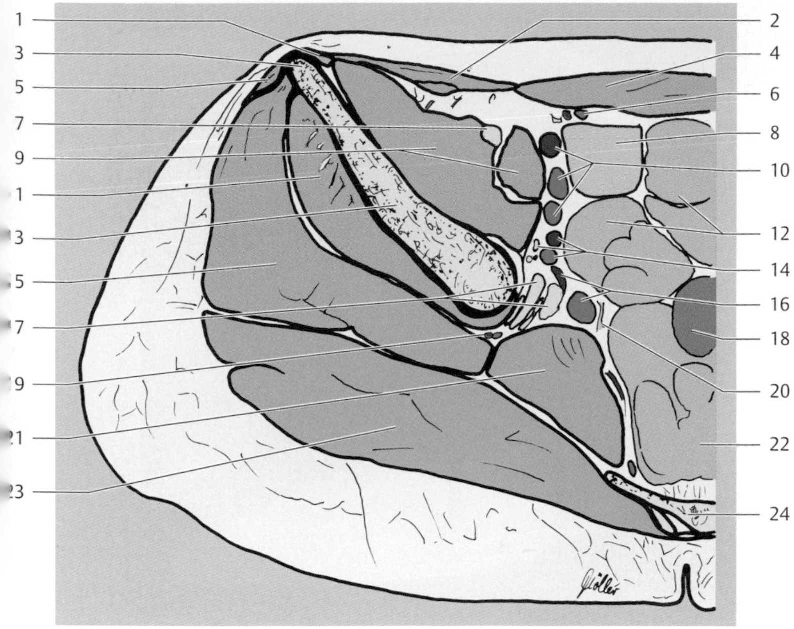

1 Inguinal ligament
2 Internal oblique abdominal muscle and transversus abdominis muscle
3 Anterior superior iliac spine
4 Rectus abdominis muscle
5 Tensor fasciae latae muscle
6 Inferior epigastric artery and vein
7 Femoral nerve
8 Urinary bladder
9 Iliopsoas muscle
10 External iliac artery and veins
11 Gluteus minimus muscle
12 Small intestine
13 Ilium
14 Obturator artery, vein, and nerve
15 Gluteus medius muscle
16 Internal iliac artery and vein
17 Sacral plexus
18 Uterus
19 Superior gluteal artery and vein
20 Ureter
21 Piriformis muscle
22 Sigmoid colon
23 Gluteus maximus muscle
24 Sacrum

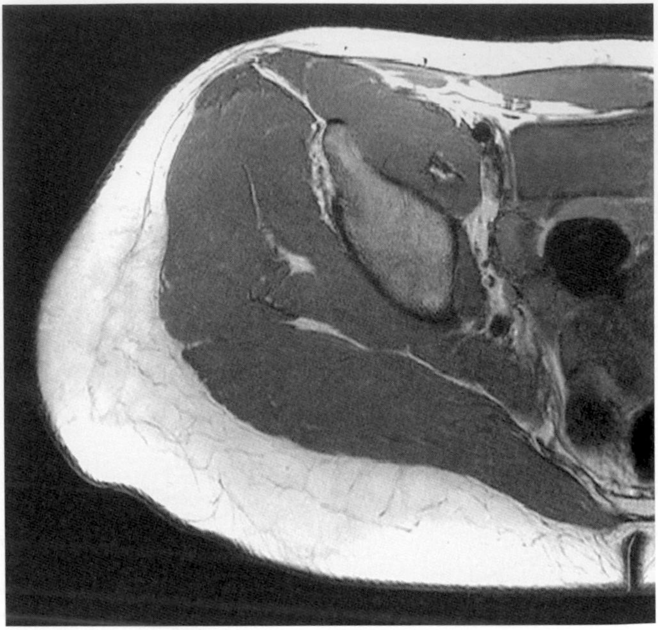

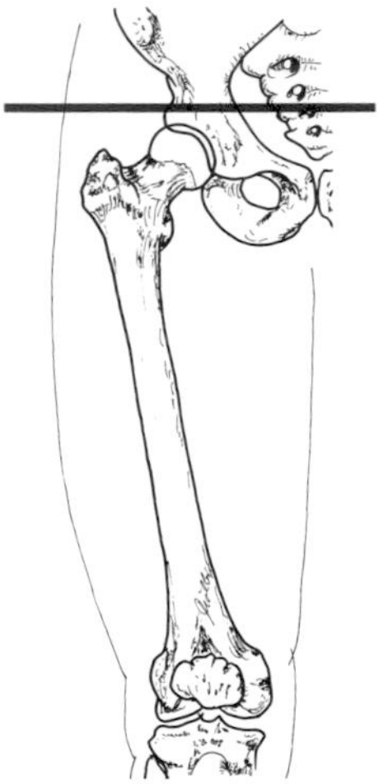

Ventral
Lateral
Medial
Dorsal

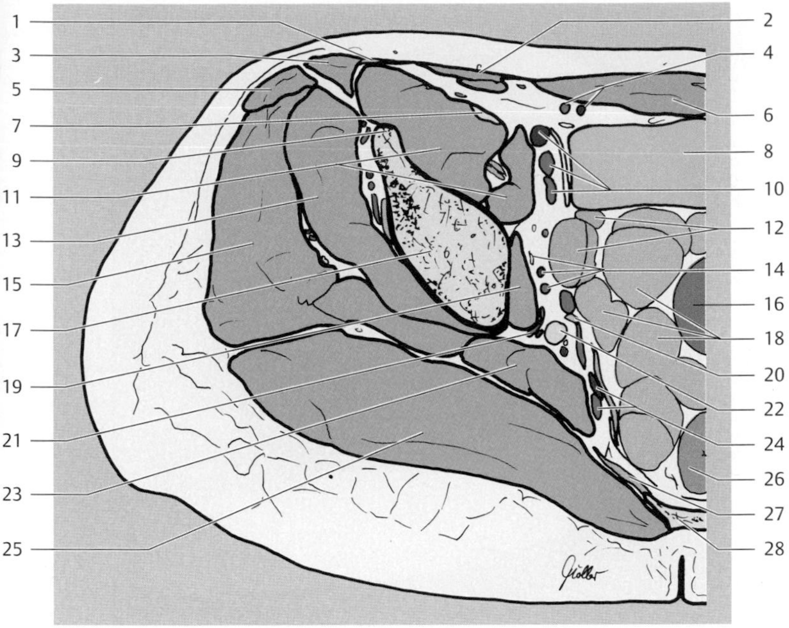

1 Inguinal ligament
2 Internal oblique abdominal muscle + transverse abdominal muscle
3 Sartorius muscle
4 Inferior epigastric artery and vein
5 Tensor fasciae latae muscle
6 Rectus abdominis muscle
7 Femoral nerve
8 Urinary bladder
9 Inferior anterior iliac spine
10 External iliac artery and veins
11 Iliopsoas muscle
12 Ovary and uterine tube
13 Gluteus minimus muscle
14 Obturator artery, vein, and nerve
15 Gluteus medius muscle
16 Uterus
17 Ilium
18 Small intestine
19 Obturator internus muscle
20 Ureter
21 Superior gluteal artery and vein
22 Lumbosacral plexus
23 Piriformis muscle
24 Internal iliac artery and vein
25 Gluteus maximus muscle
26 Rectum
27 Sacrotuberous ligament
28 Sacrum

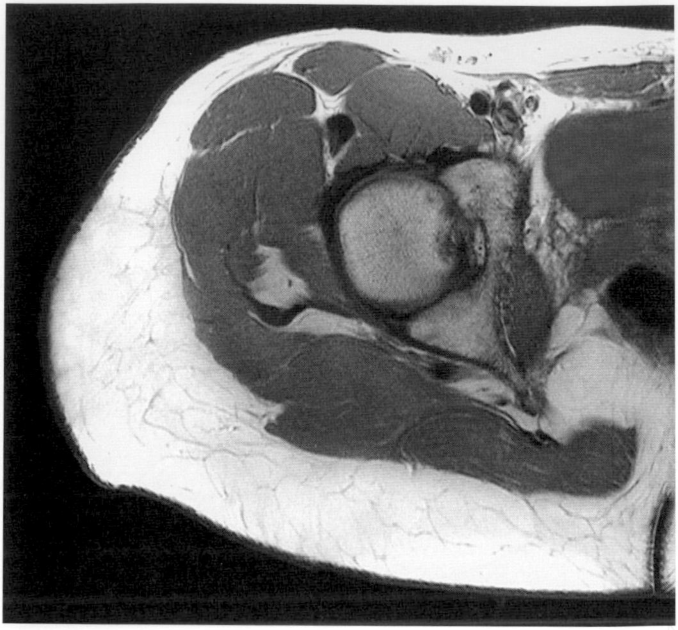

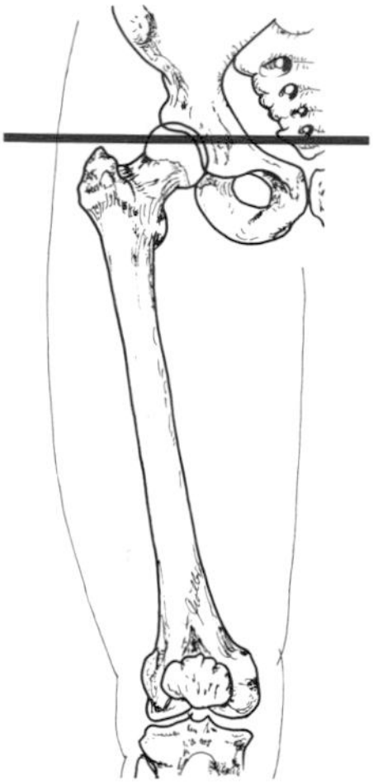

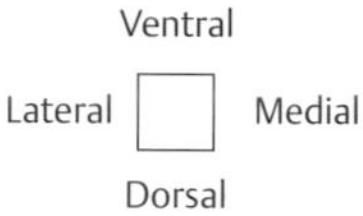
Ventral
Lateral
Medial
Dorsal

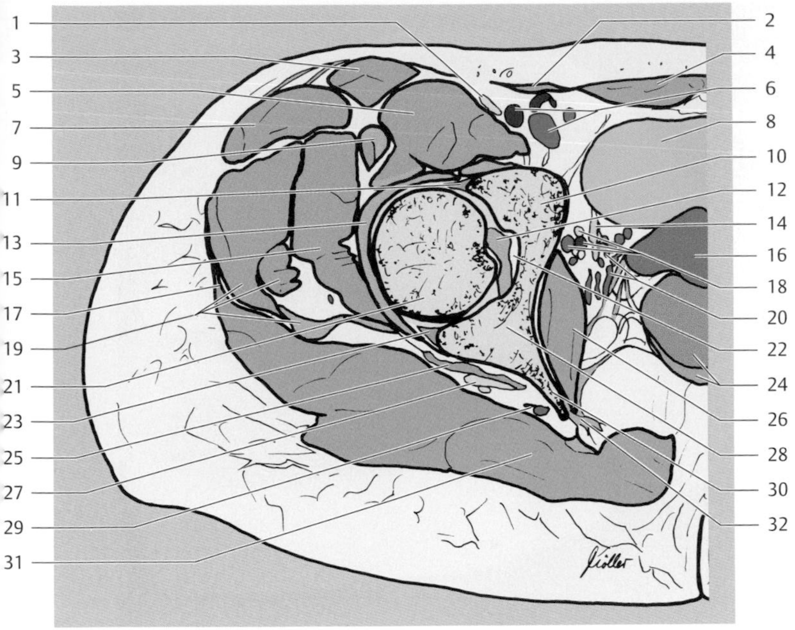

1 Femoral nerve
2 Internal oblique abdominal muscle + transverse abdominal muscle
3 Sartorius muscle
4 Rectus abdominis muscle
5 Iliopsoas muscle
6 External iliac artery and vein
7 Tensor fasciae latae muscle
8 Urinary bladder
9 Rectus femoris muscle (tendon)
10 Pubis (superior ramus)
11 Anterior glenoid labrum
12 Ligament of head of femur
13 Iliofemoral ligament
14 Ureter
15 Gluteus minimus muscle
16 Uterus
17 Iliotibial tract
18 Obturator artery, vein, and nerve
19 Gluteus medius muscle (+ tendon)
20 Uterine venous plexus
21 Head of femur
22 Acetabular fossa
23 Posterior glenoid labrum
24 Rectum and levator ani muscle
25 Piriformis muscle
26 Obturator internus muscle
27 Sciatic nerve
28 Ischium
29 Superior gluteal artery and vein
30 Ischial spine
31 Gluteus maximus muscle
32 Sacrotuberal ligament

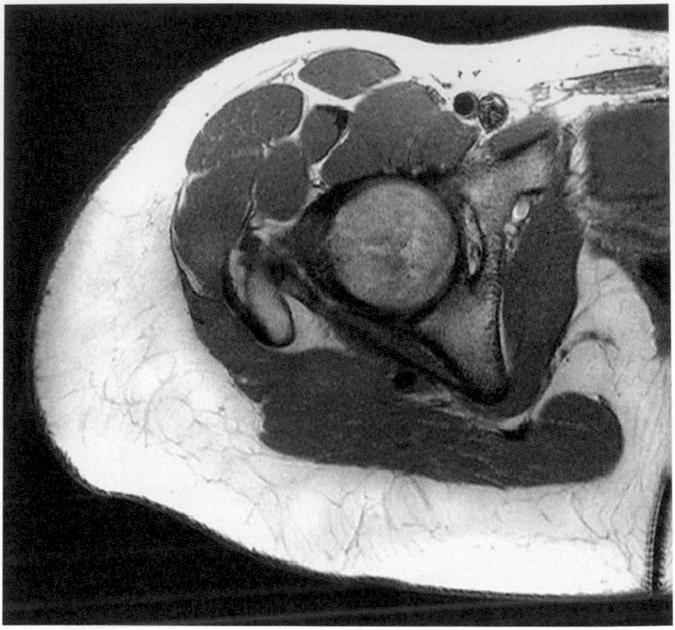

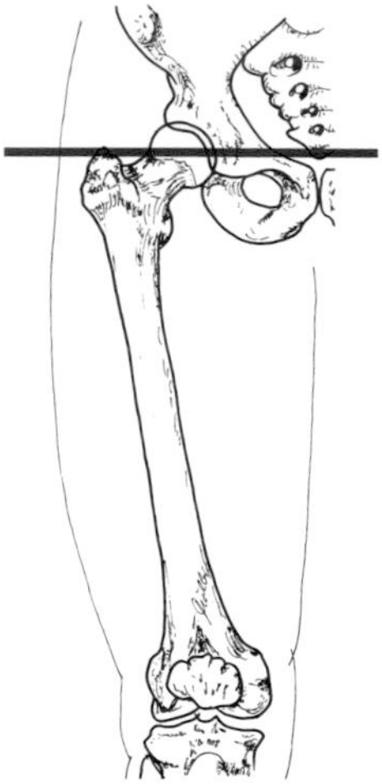

Ventral

Lateral Medial

Dorsal

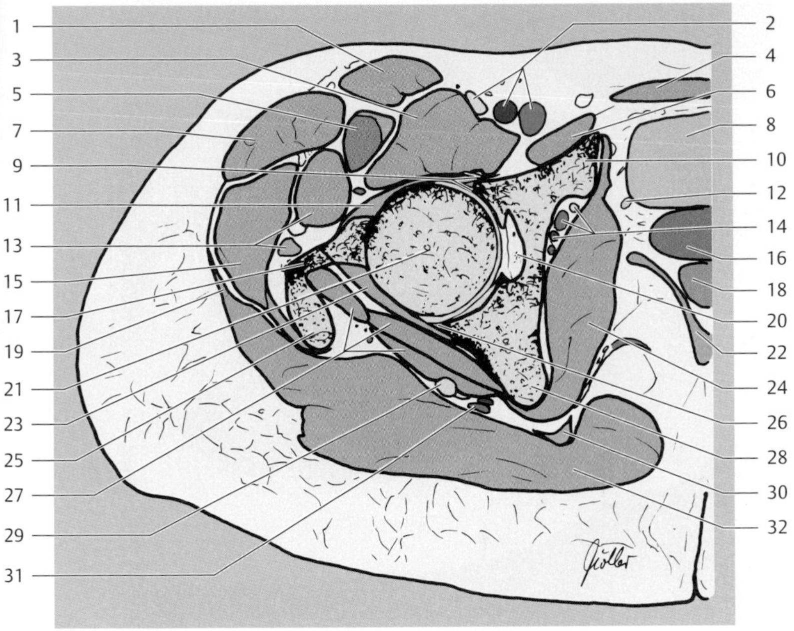

1 Sartorius muscle
2 Femoral artery, vein, and nerve
3 Iliopsoas muscle
4 Rectus abdominis muscle
5 Rectus femoris muscle (+ tendon)
6 Pectineus muscle
7 Tensor fasciae latae muscle
8 Urinary bladder
9 Anterior glenoid labrum
10 Pubis (superior ramus)
11 Iliofemoral ligament
12 Ureter
13 Gluteus minimus muscle (+ tendon)
14 Obturator artery, vein, and nerve
15 Gluteus medius muscle (+ tendon)
16 Vagina
17 Neck of femur
18 Rectum
19 Iliotibial tract
20 Acetabular fossa
21 Head of femur
22 Levator ani muscle
23 Ischiofemoral ligament and ligamentous capsule
24 Obturator internus muscle
25 Great trochanter
26 Posterior glenoid labrum
27 Gemellus inferior muscle
28 Ischium
29 Sciatic nerve
30 Sacrotuberal ligament
31 Superior gluteal artery and nerve
32 Gluteus maximus muscle

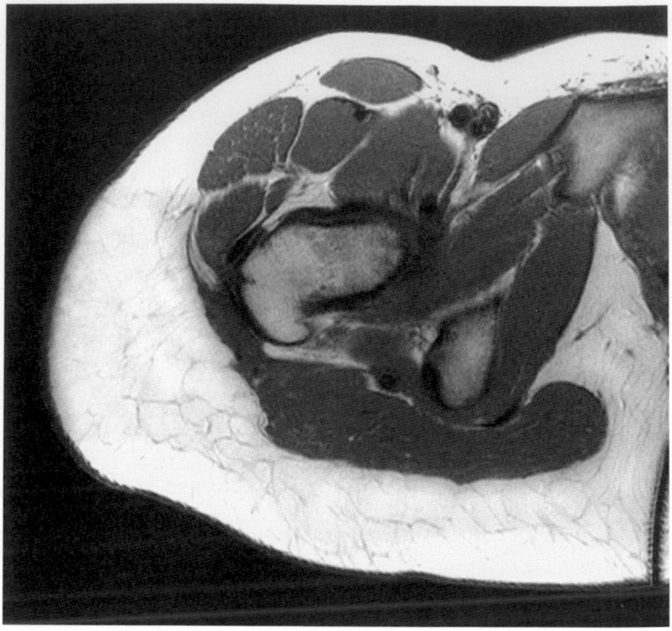

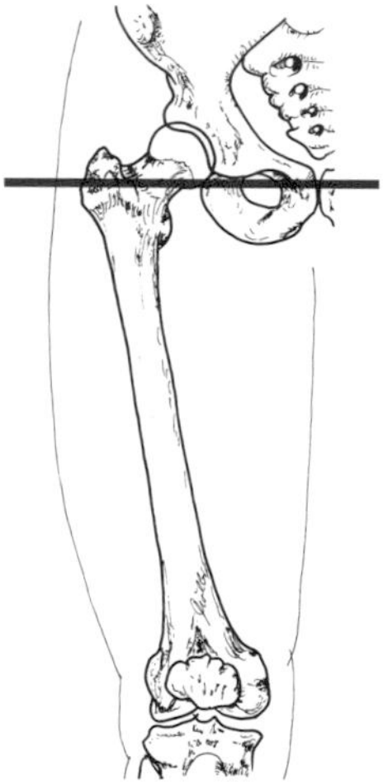

Ventral

Lateral ☐ Medial

Dorsal

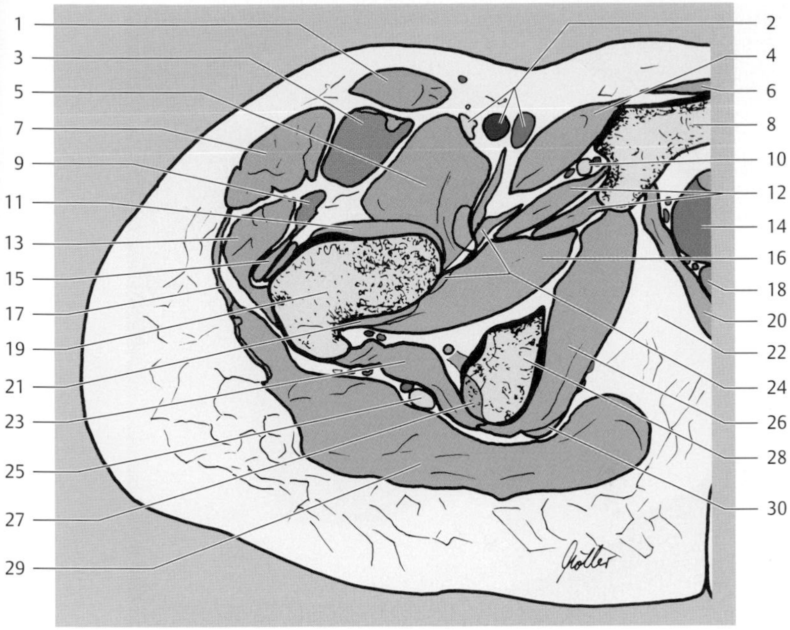

1 Sartorius muscle
2 Femoral artery, vein, and nerve
3 Rectus femoris muscle (+ tendon)
4 Pectineus muscle
5 Iliopsoas muscle
6 Rectus abdominis muscle
7 Tensor fasciae latae muscle
8 Pubis (inferior ramus)
9 Vastus lateralis muscle
10 Obturator nerve (anterior branch)
11 Iliofemoral ligament
12 Adductor brevis muscle
13 Gluteus medius muscle (+ tendon)
14 Vagina and urethra
15 Gluteus minimus muscle (tendon)
16 Obturator externus muscle
17 Iliotibial tract
18 Rectum
19 Femur
20 Levator ani muscle
21 Ischiofemoral ligament
22 Ischiorectal fossa
23 Quadratus femoris muscle
24 Pubofemoral ligament
25 Sciatic nerve
26 Obturator internus muscle
27 Tendon attachment of dorsal thigh muscles
28 Ischial tuberosity
29 Gluteus maximus muscle
30 Sacrotuberal ligament

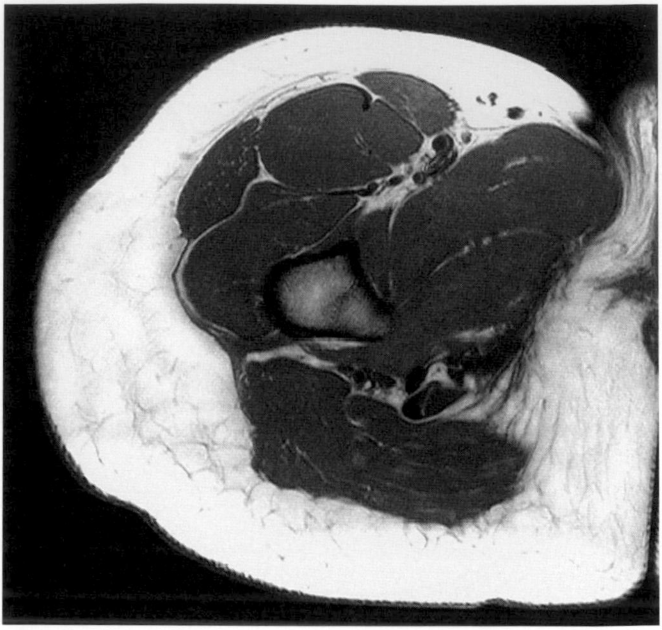

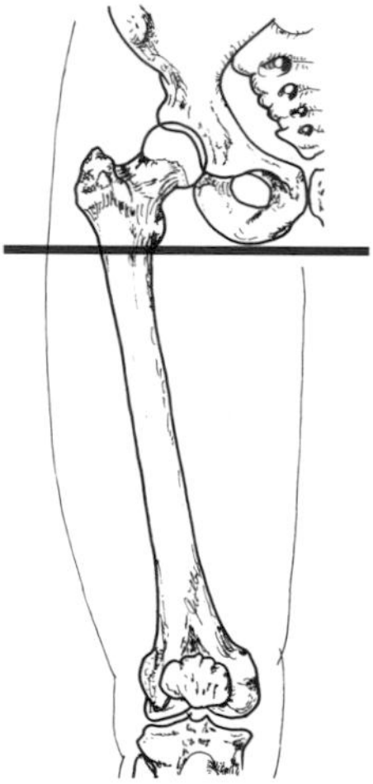

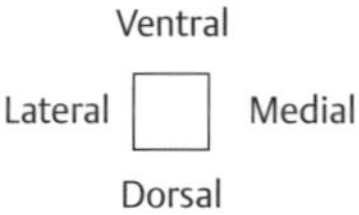
Ventral
Lateral
Medial
Dorsal

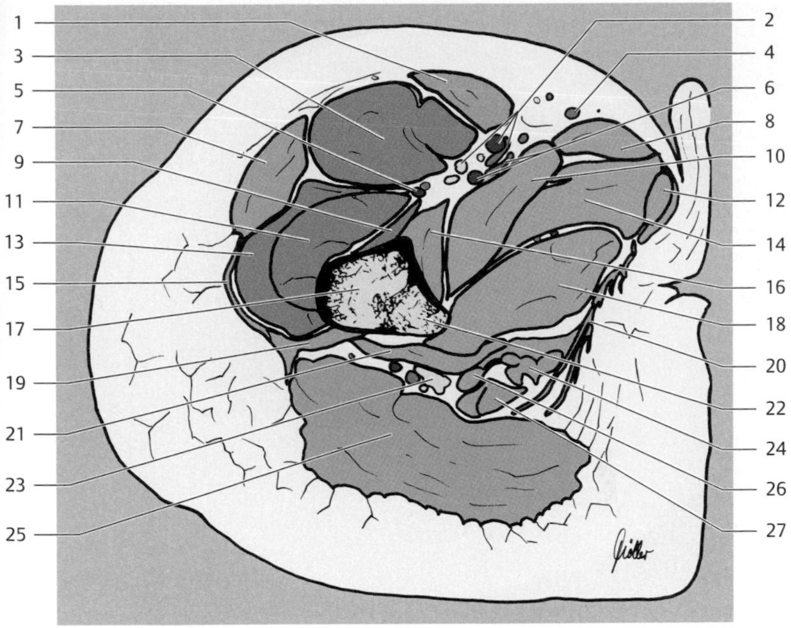

1 Sartorius muscle
2 Femoral artery, vein, and nerve
3 Rectus femoris muscle
4 Great saphenous vein
5 Circumflex femoral artery and vein
6 Deep femoral artery and vein
7 Tensor fasciae latae muscle
8 Adductor longus muscle
9 Vastus medialis muscle
10 Pectineus muscle
11 Vastus intermedius muscle
12 Gracilis muscle
13 Vastus lateralis muscle
14 Adductor brevis muscle
15 Iliotibial tract
16 Iliopsoas muscle
17 Femur
18 Adductor magnus muscle
19 Lateral femoral intermuscular septum
20 Obturator internus muscle
21 Quadratus femoris muscle
22 Lesser trochanter
23 Sciatic nerve
24 Semimembranosus muscle (tendon)
25 Gluteus maximus muscle
26 Biceps femoris muscle (tendon)
27 Semitendinosus muscle (tendon)

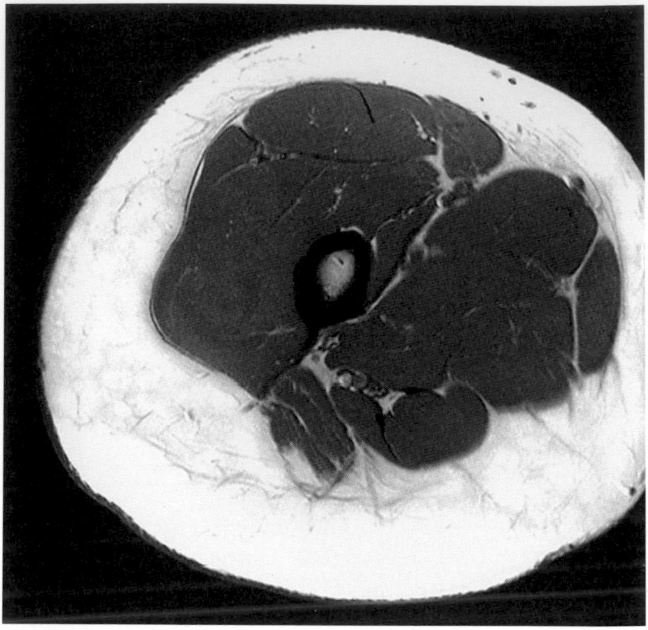

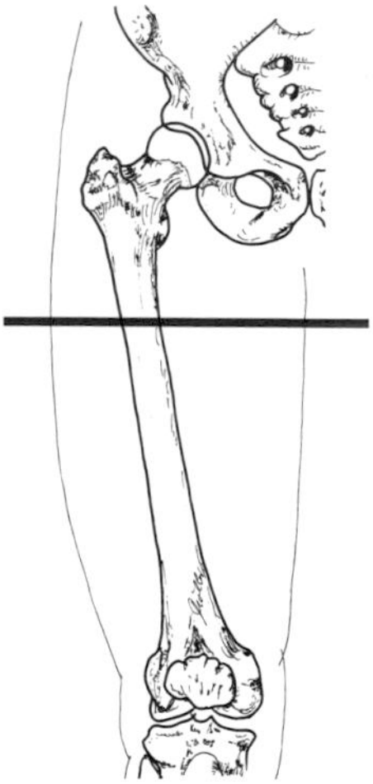

Ventral

Lateral ☐ Medial

Dorsal

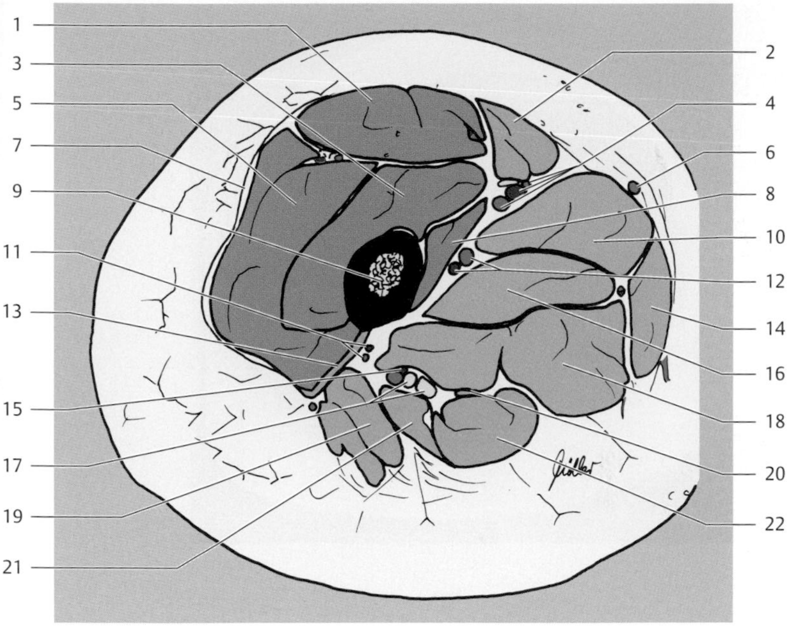

1 Rectus femoris muscle
2 Sartorius muscle
3 Vastus intermedius muscle
4 Femoral artery, vein, and nerve
5 Vastus lateralis muscle
6 Great saphenous vein
7 Iliotibial tract
8 Vastus medialis muscle
9 Femur
10 Adductor longus muscle
11 Perforating artery of deep artery of thigh (+ vein)
12 Deep artery and vein of thigh
13 Lateral femoral intermuscular septum
14 Gracilis muscle
15 Artery and vein to sciatic nerve
16 Adductor brevis muscle
17 Sciatic nerve
18 Adductor magnus muscle
19 Gluteus maximus muscle
20 Semimembranosus muscle (tendon)
21 Biceps femoris muscle
22 Semitendinosus muscle

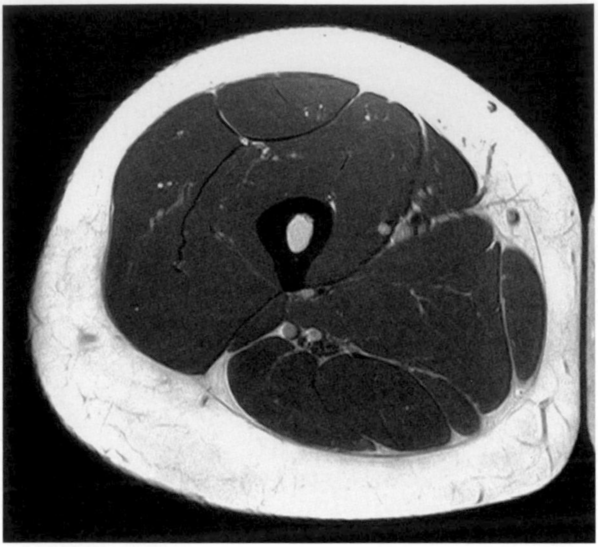

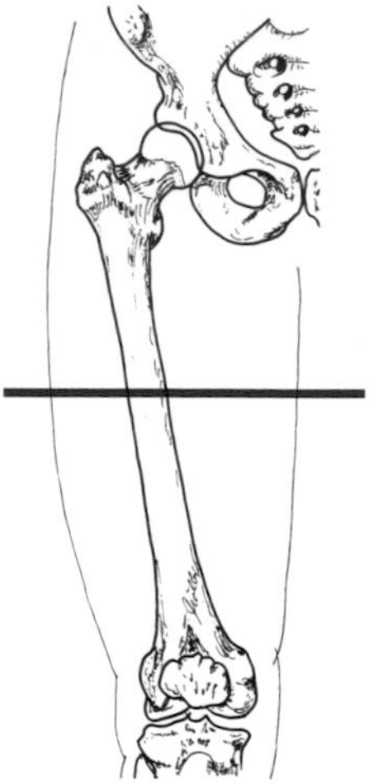

Ventral

Lateral ☐ Medial

Dorsal

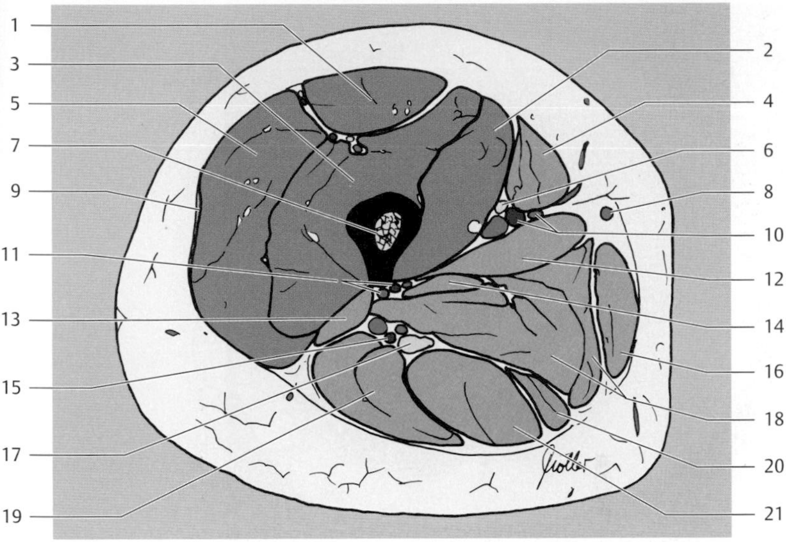

1 Rectus femoris muscle
2 Vastus medialis muscle
3 Vastus intermedius muscle
4 Sartorius muscle
5 Vastus lateralis muscle
6 Saphenous nerve
7 Femur
8 Great saphenous vein
9 Iliotibial tract
10 Femoral artery and vein
11 Deep artery and vein of thigh
12 Adductor longus muscle
13 Biceps femoris muscle (short head)
14 Adductor brevis muscle
15 Artery to sciatic nerve
16 Gracilis muscle
17 Sciatic nerve
18 Adductor magnus muscle
19 Biceps femoris muscle (long head)
20 Semimembranosus muscle
21 Semitendinosus muscle

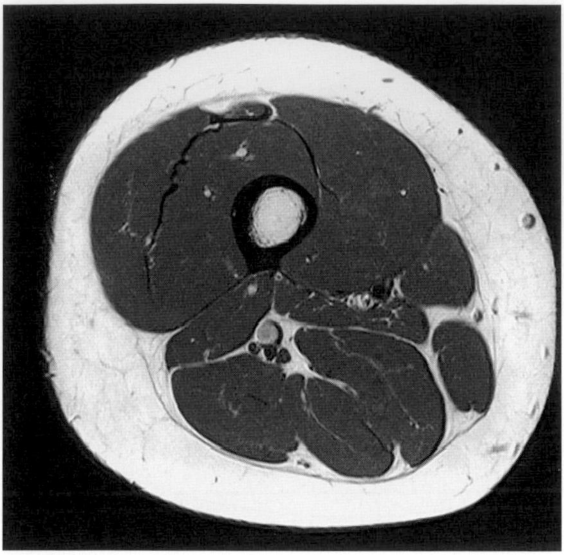

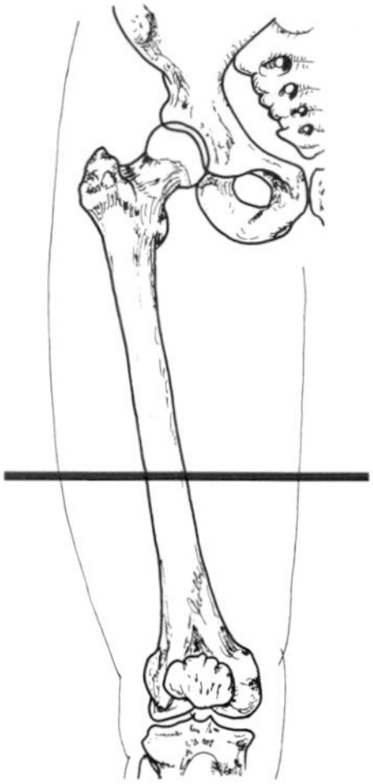

Ventral
Lateral
Medial
Dorsal

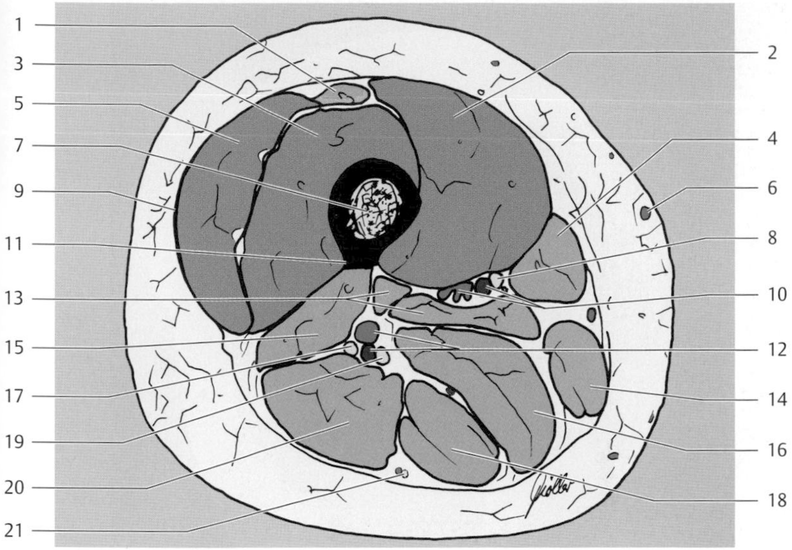

1 Rectus femoris muscle (+ tendon)
2 Vastus medialis muscle
3 Vastus intermedius muscle
4 Sartorius muscle
5 Vastus lateralis muscle
6 Great saphenous vein
7 Femur
8 Saphenous nerve
9 Iliotibial tract
10 Femoral artery and vein
11 Linea aspera
12 Perforating artery and vein of deep artery and vein of thigh
13 Adductor magnus muscle
14 Gracilis muscle
15 Biceps femoris muscle (short head)
16 Semimembranosus muscle
17 Common fibular (peroneal) nerve
18 Semitendinosus muscle
19 Tibial nerve
20 Biceps femoris muscle (long head)
21 Posterior femoral cutaneous nerve

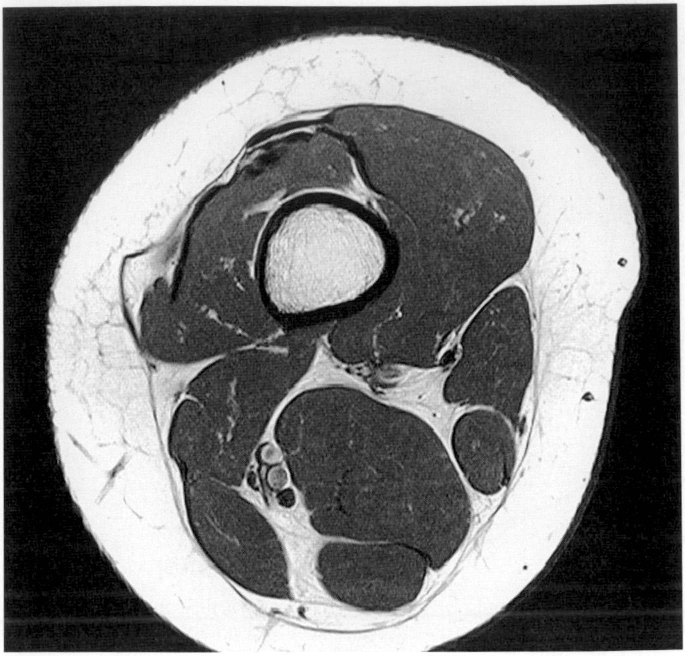

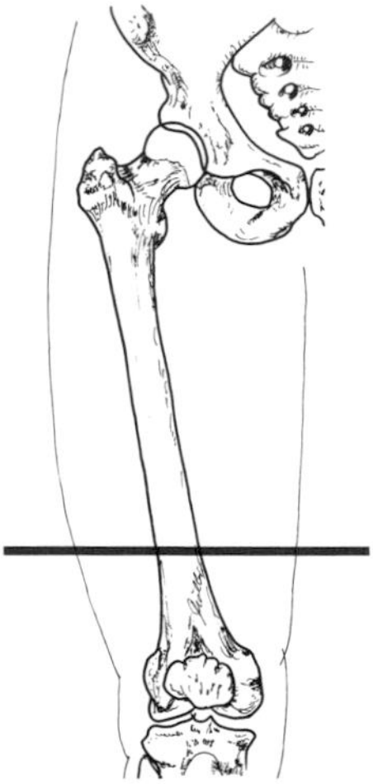

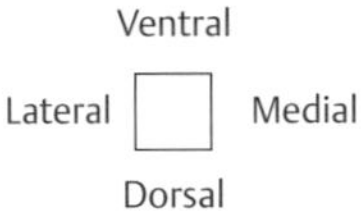
Ventral
Lateral
Medial
Dorsal

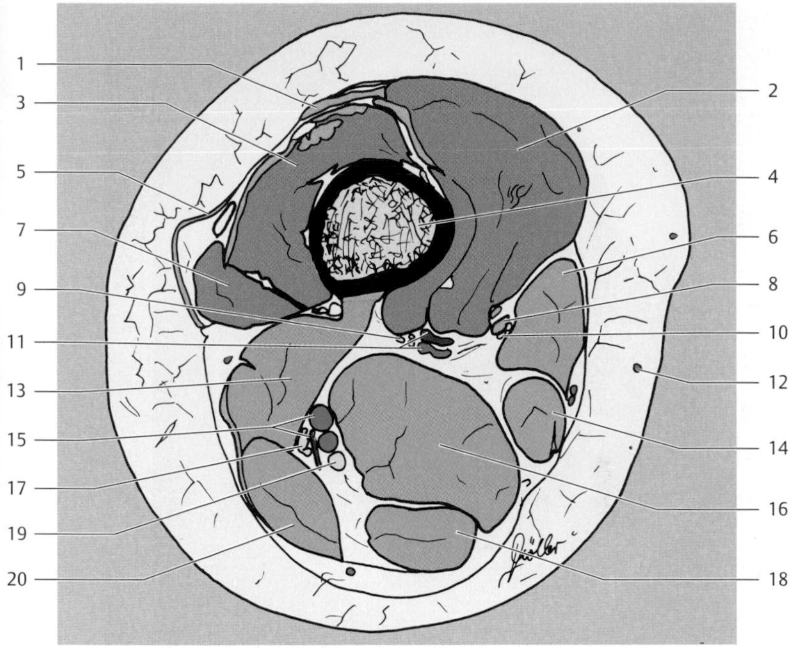

1 Rectus femoris muscle (tendon)
2 Vastus medialis muscle
3 Vastus intermedius muscle
4 Femur
5 Iliotibial tract
6 Sartorius muscle
7 Vastus lateralis muscle
8 Adductor magnus muscle (tendon)
9 Muscular branch of femoral nerve
10 Saphenous nerve
11 Femoral artery and vein
12 Great saphenous vein
13 Biceps femoris muscle (short head)
14 Gracilis muscle
15 Perforating artery and vein of deep artery and vein of thigh
16 Semimembranosus muscle
17 Common fibular (peroneal) nerve
18 Semitendinosus muscle
19 Tibial nerve
20 Biceps femoris muscle (long head)

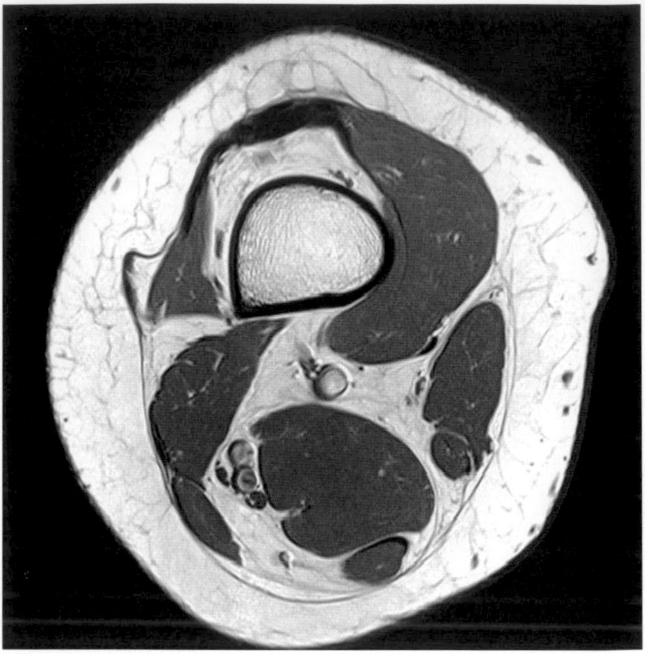

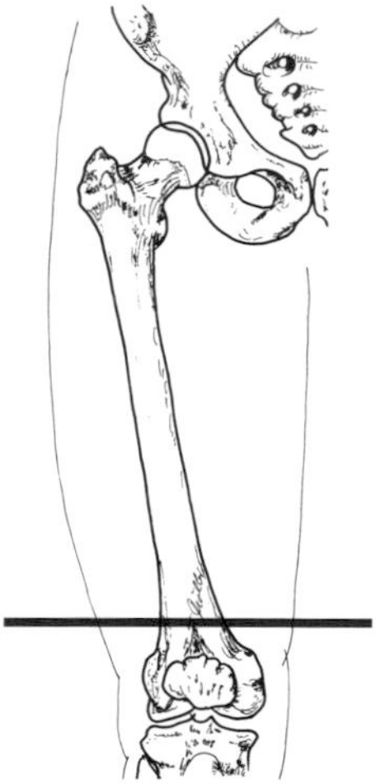

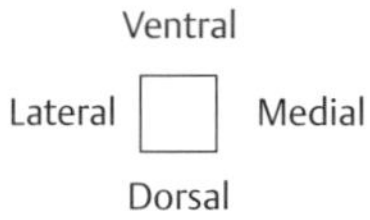
Ventral
Lateral
Medial
Dorsal

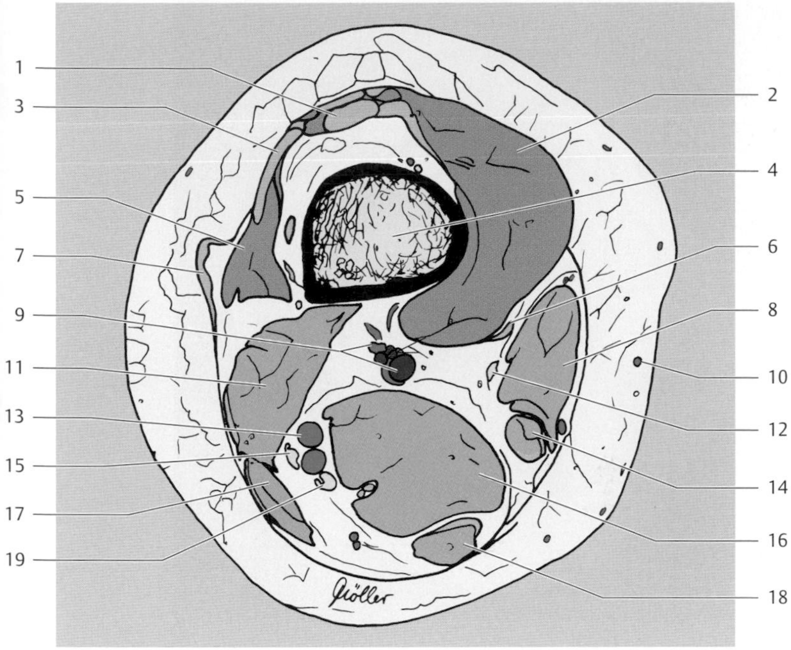

1 Rectus femoris muscle (tendon)
2 Vastus medialis muscle
3 Vastus intermedius muscle (+ tendon)
4 Femur
5 Vastus lateralis muscle
6 Adductor magnus muscle (tendon)
7 Iliotibial tract
8 Sartorius muscle
9 Femoral artery and vein
10 Great saphenous vein
11 Biceps femoris muscle (short head)
12 Saphenous nerve
13 Perforating vein of deep vein of thigh
14 Gracilis muscle
15 Common fibular (peroneal) nerve
16 Semimembranosus muscle
17 Biceps femoris muscle (long head)
18 Semitendinosus muscle
19 Tibial nerve

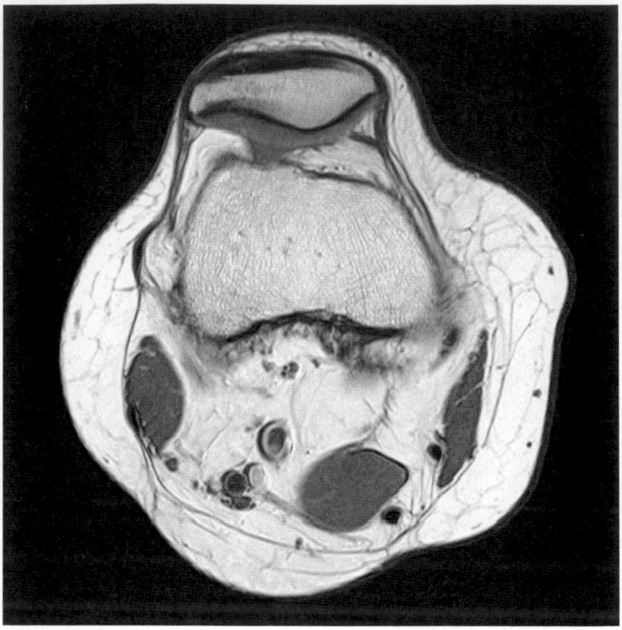

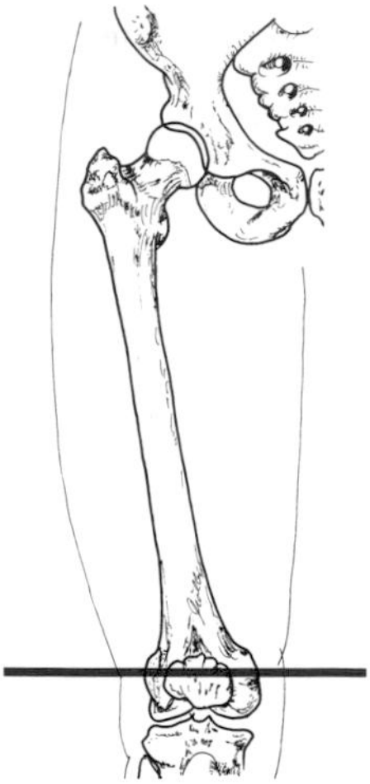

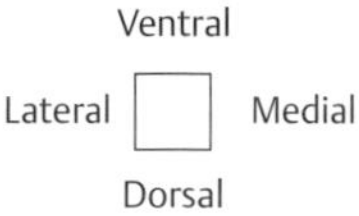
Ventral
Lateral
Medial
Dorsal

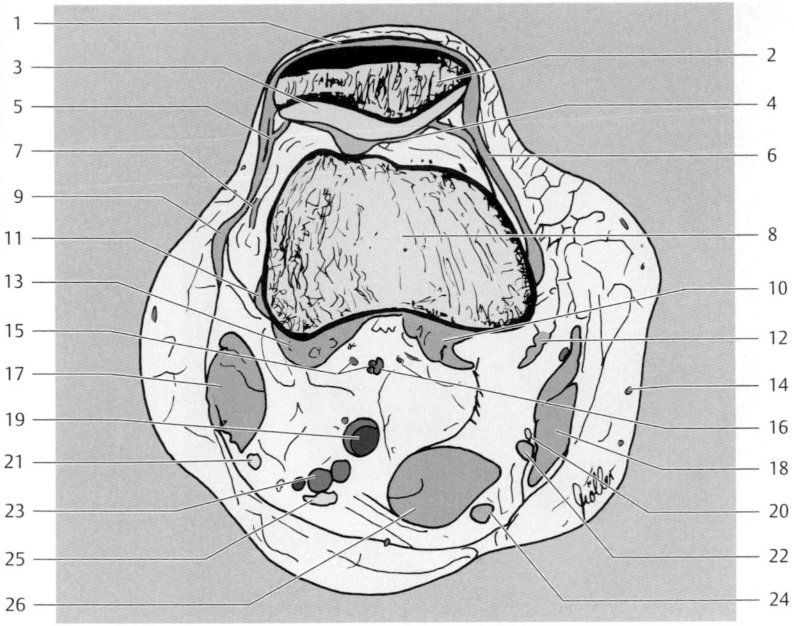

1 Patellar ligament
2 Patella
3 Retropatellar cartilage
4 Femoropatellar joint
5 Lateral patellar retinaculum
6 Medial patellar retinaculum
7 Vastus lateralis muscle (tendon)
8 Femur
9 Iliotibial tract
10 Gastrocnemius muscle (medial head, tendon)
11 Popliteus muscle (tendon)
12 Adductor magnus muscle (tendon)
13 Gastrocnemius muscle (lateral head)
14 Great saphenous vein
15 Superior lateral genicular artery and vein
16 Superior medial genicular artery and vein
17 Biceps femoris muscle (+ tendon)
18 Sartorius muscle
19 Popliteal artery and vein
20 Saphenous nerve
21 Common fibular (peroneal) nerve
22 Gracilis muscle (tendon)
23 Perforating artery of deep artery of thigh (+ vein)
24 Semimembranosus muscle (tendon)
25 Tibial nerve
26 Semitendinosus muscle

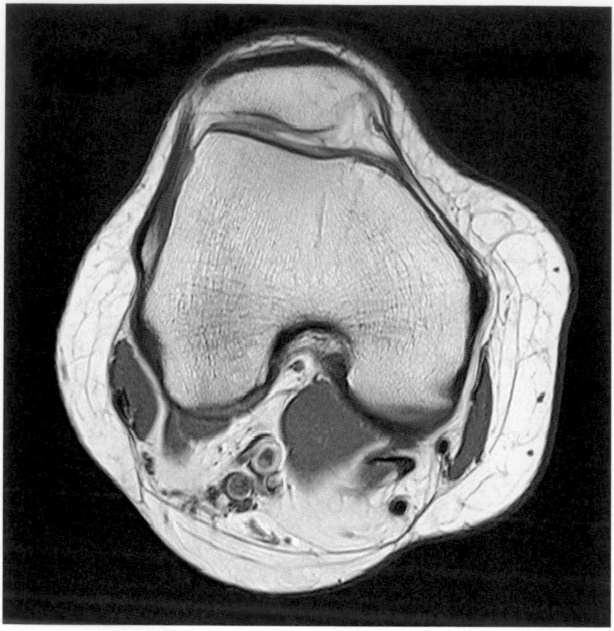

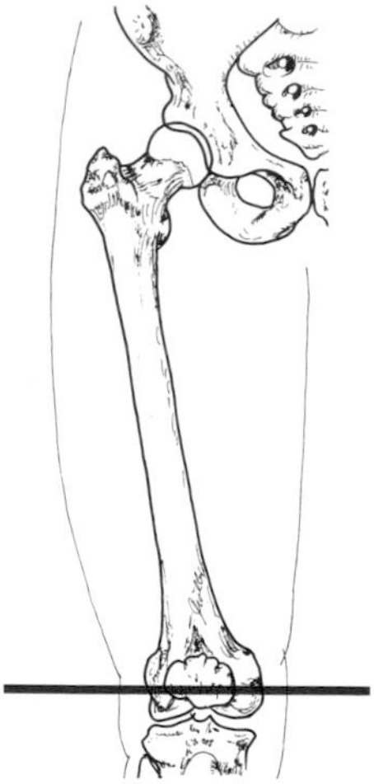

Ventral

Lateral ☐ Medial

Dorsal

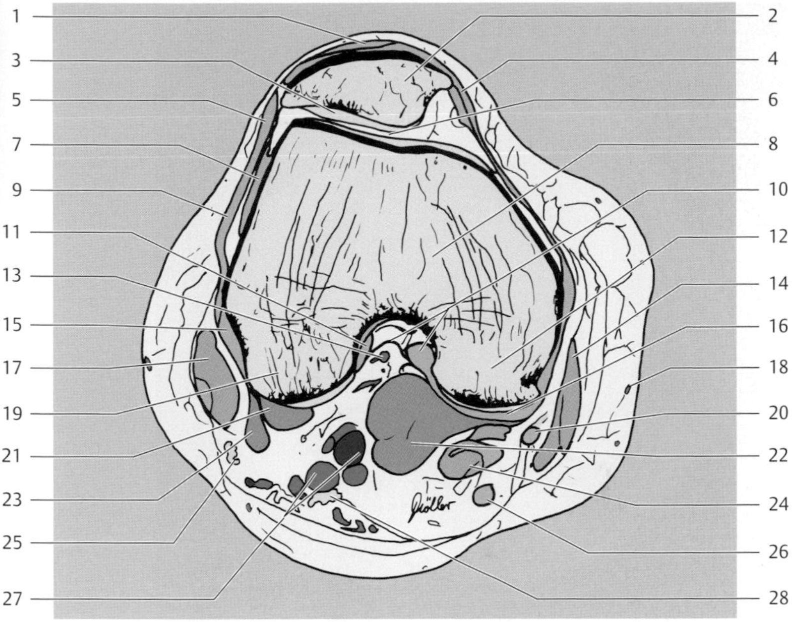

1 Patellar ligament
2 Patella
3 Retropatellar cartilage
4 Medial patellar retinaculum
5 Lateral patellar retinaculum
6 Femoropatellar joint
7 Lateral collateral ligament
8 Femur
9 Iliotibial tract
10 Joint capsule and posterior cruciate ligament (attachment)
11 Anterior cruciate ligament (attachment)
12 Medial femoral condyle
13 Middle genicular artery
14 Sartorius muscle
15 Popliteus muscle (tendon)
16 Joint capsule and oblique popliteal ligament
17 Biceps femoris muscle (+ tendon)
18 Great saphenous vein
19 Medial femoral condyle
20 Gracilis muscle (tendon)
21 Plantaris muscle
22 Gastrocnemius muscle (medial head)
23 Gastrocnemius muscle (lateral head)
24 Semimembranosus muscle (+ tendon)
25 Common fibular (peroneal) nerve
26 Semitendinosus muscle (tendon)
27 Popliteal artery and vein
28 Tibial nerve

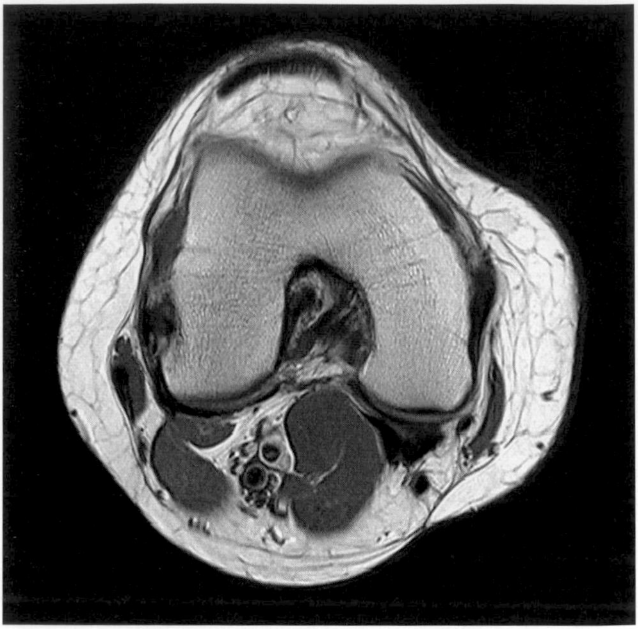

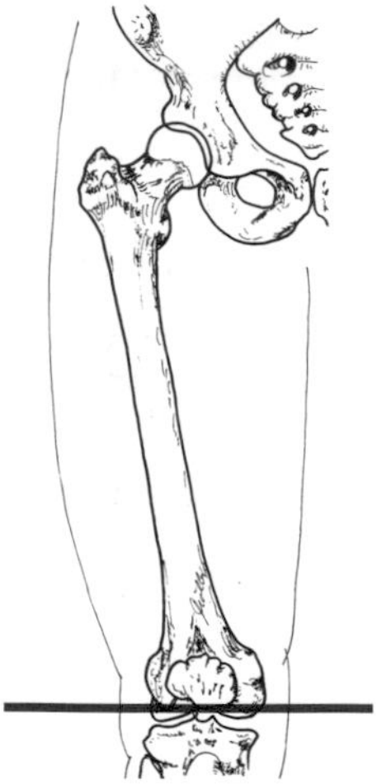

Ventral

Lateral Medial

Dorsal

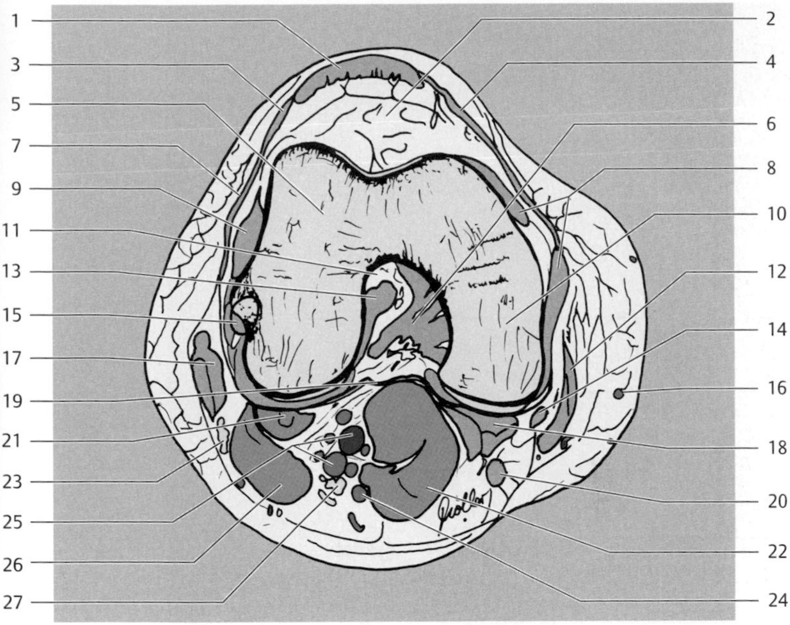

1 Patellar ligament
2 Infrapatellar fat body
3 Lateral patellar retinaculum
4 Medial patellar retinaculum
5 Lateral femoral condyle
6 Posterior cruciate ligament
7 Iliotibial tract
8 Medial collateral ligament
9 Lateral collateral ligament
10 Medial femoral condyle
11 Intercondylar fossa
12 Sartorius muscle
13 Anterior cruciate ligament
14 Gracilis muscle (tendon)
15 Popliteus muscle (tendon)
16 Great saphenous vein
17 Biceps femoris muscle (+ tendon)
18 Semimembranosus muscle (+ tendon)
19 Oblique popliteal ligament and joint capsule
20 Semitendinosus muscle (tendon)
21 Plantaris muscle
22 Gastrocnemius muscle (medial head)
23 Common fibular (peroneal) nerve
24 Popliteal vein
25 Popliteal artery and vein
26 Gastrocnemius muscle (lateral head)
27 Tibial nerve

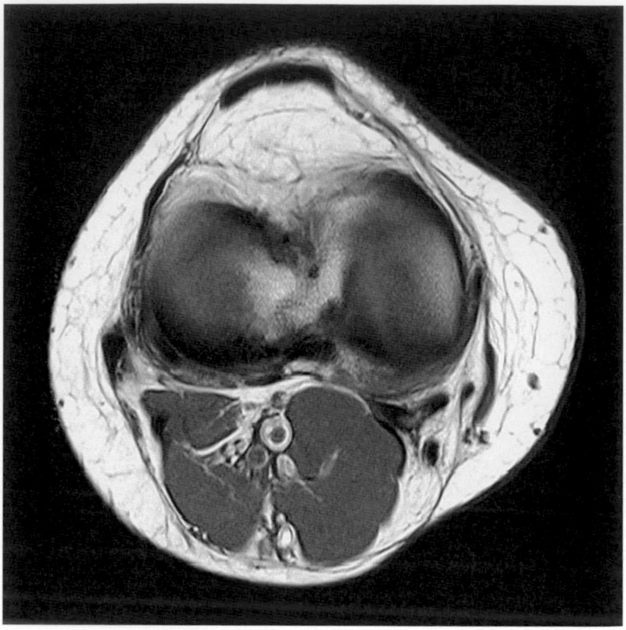

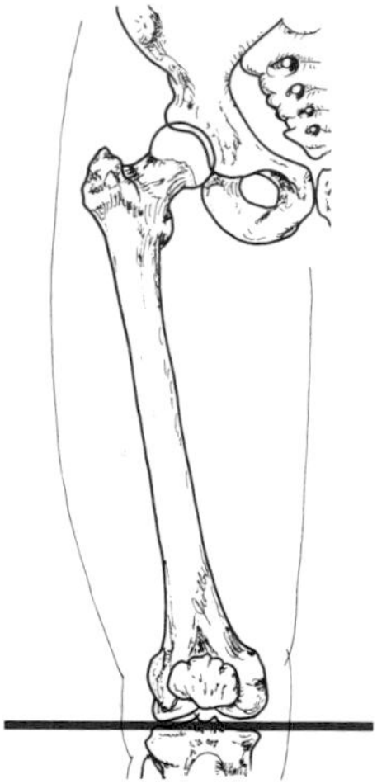

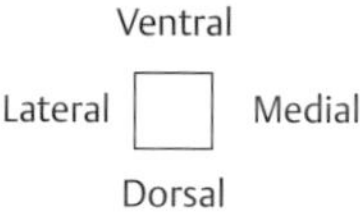
Ventral
Lateral
Medial
Dorsal

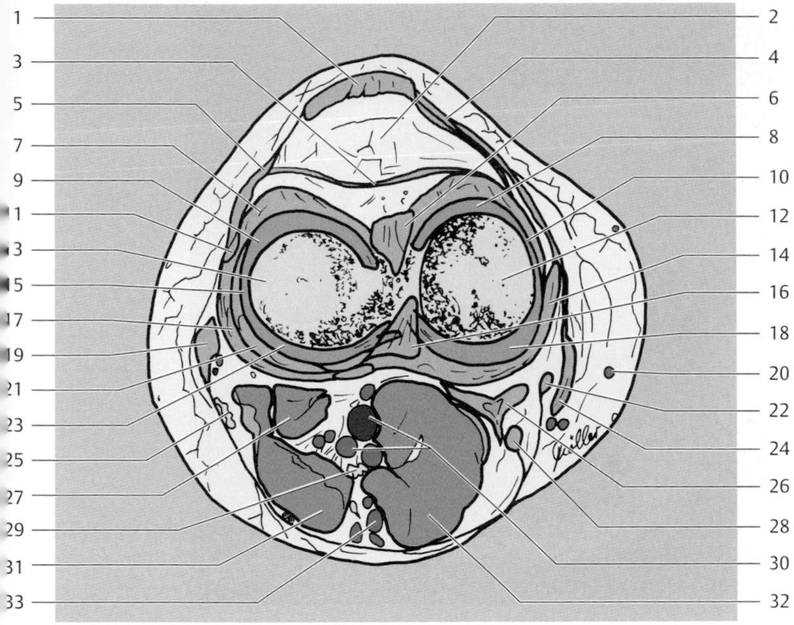

1 Patellar ligament
2 Infrapatellar fat body
3 Transverse patellar retinaculum
4 Medial patellar retinaculum
5 Lateral patellar retinaculum
6 Anterior cruciate ligament
7 Joint capsule
8 Medial meniscus (anterior horn)
9 Lateral meniscus (anterior horn)
10 Medial meniscus (intermediate part)
11 Iliotibial tract
12 Medial femoral condyle with joint cartilage
13 Lateral femoral condyle with joint cartilage
14 Medial collateral ligament
15 Lateral meniscus (intermediate portion)
16 Posterior cruciate ligament
17 Lateral collateral ligament
18 Medial meniscus (posterior horn)
19 Biceps femoris muscle (tendon)
20 Great saphenous vein
21 Popliteus muscle (tendon)
22 Gracilis muscle (tendon)
23 Lateral meniscus (posterior horn)
24 Sartorius muscle (+ tendon)
25 Common fibular (peroneal) nerve
26 Semimembranosus muscle (+ tendon)
27 Plantaris muscle
28 Semitendinosus muscle (tendon)
29 Tibial nerve
30 Popliteal artery and vein
31 Gastrocnemius muscle (lateral head, tendon)
32 Gastrocnemius muscle (medial head, tendon)
33 Popliteal vein

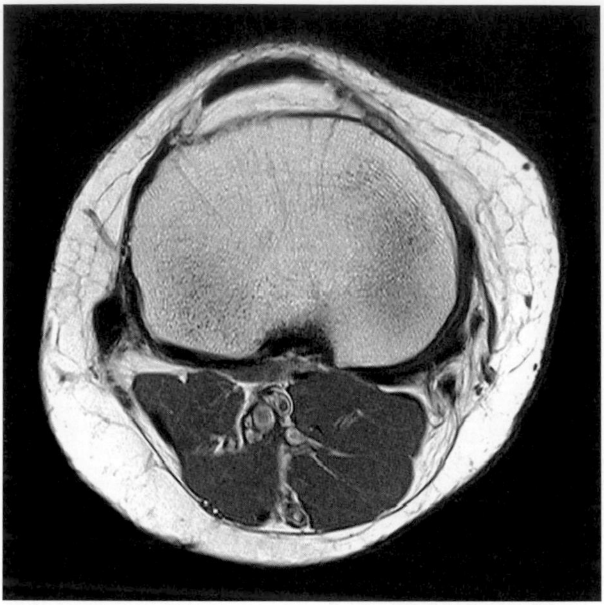

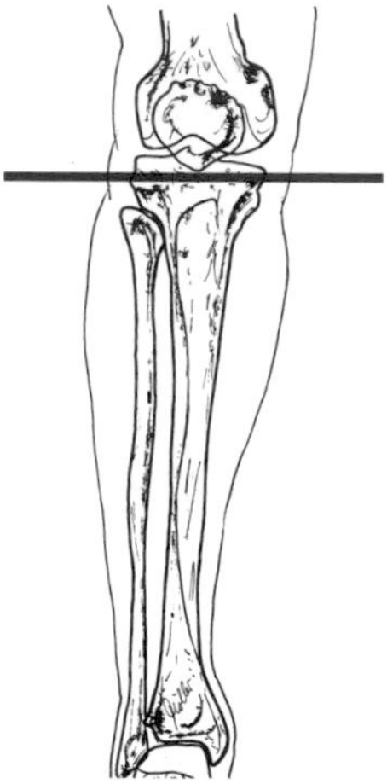

Anterior
Ventral

Lateral | Medial

Dorsal
Posterior

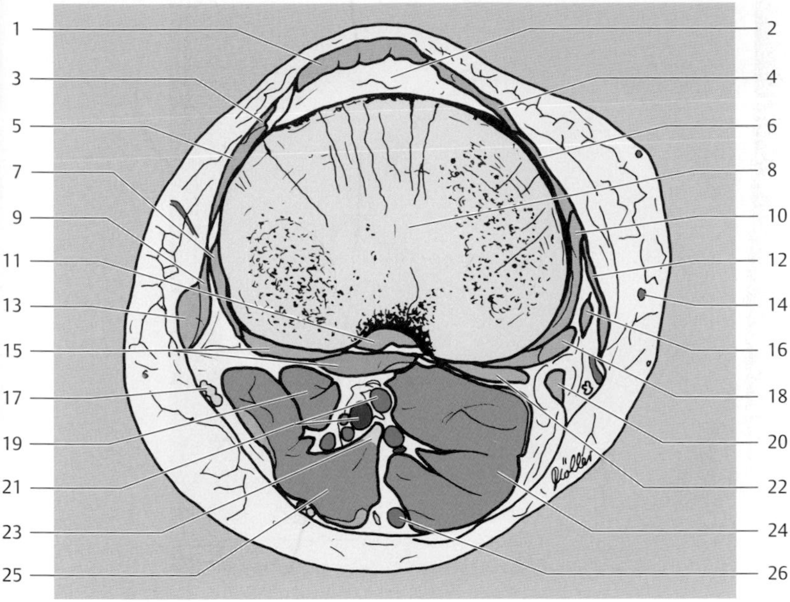

1 Patellar ligament
2 Infrapatellar fat body
3 Lateral patellar retinaculum
4 Medial patellar retinaculum
5 Iliotibial tract
6 Joint capsule
7 Lateral collateral ligament
8 Head of tibia
9 Fibular collateral ligament
10 Medial ligament
11 Posterior cruciate ligament
12 Sartorius muscle (tendon)
13 Biceps femoris muscle (tendon)
14 Great saphenous vein
15 Popliteus muscle (+ tendon)
16 Gracilis muscle (tendon)
17 Common fibular (peroneal) nerve
18 Semimembranosus muscle (+ tendon)
19 Plantaris muscle
20 Semitendinosus muscle (tendon)
21 Popliteal artery and vein
22 Oblique popliteal ligament and joint capsule
23 Tibial nerve
24 Gastrocnemius muscle (medial head, tendon)
25 Gastrocnemius muscle (lateral head, tendon)
26 Popliteal vein

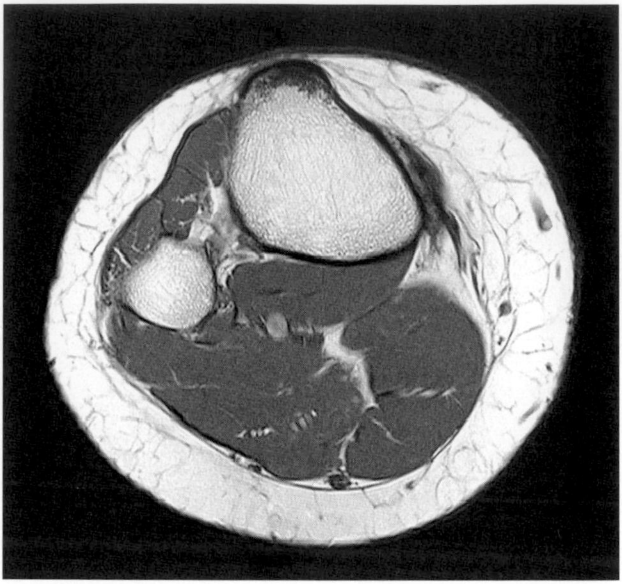

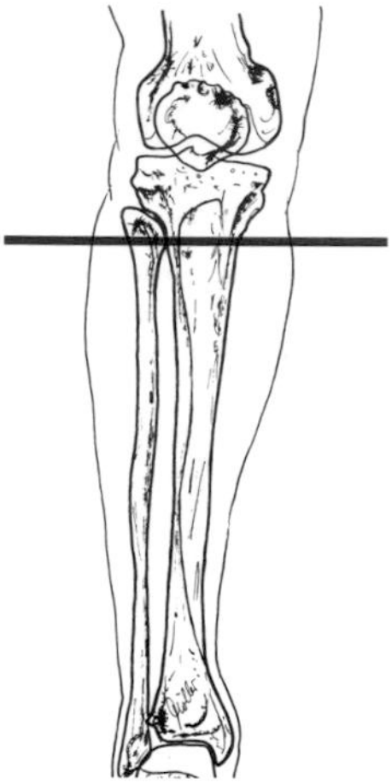

Anterior

Lateral ☐ Medial

Posterior

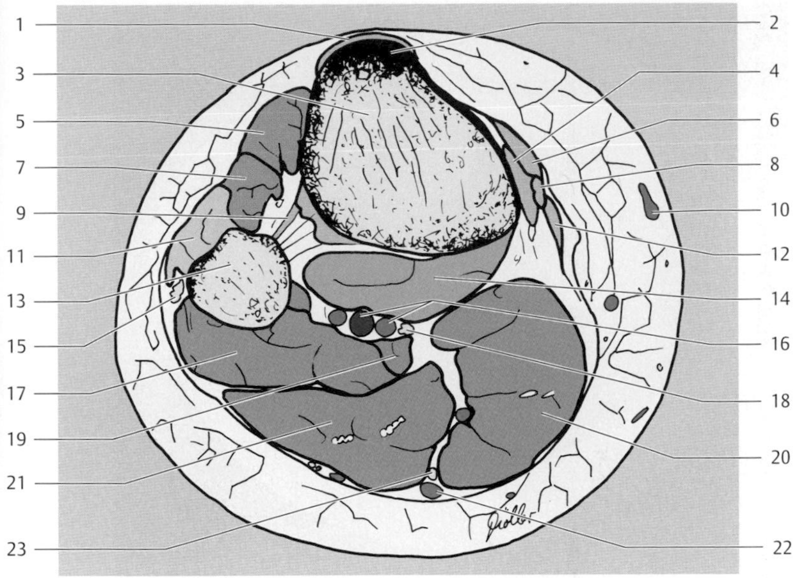

1 Patellar ligament
2 Tibial tuberosity
3 Tibia
4 Medial patellar retinaculum
5 Anterior tibial muscle
6 Sartorius muscle (tendon)
7 Extensor digitorum longus muscle
8 Gracilis muscle (tendon)
9 Interosseous membrane of leg
10 Great saphenous vein
11 Peroneus (fibularis) longus muscle
12 Semitendinosus muscle (tendon)
13 Head of fibula
14 Popliteus muscle
15 Common fibular (peroneal) nerve
16 Popliteal artery and vein
17 Plantaris muscle
18 Tibial nerve
19 Soleus muscle
20 Gastrocnemius muscle (medial head)
21 Gastrocnemius muscle (lateral head)
22 Popliteal vein
23 Medial sural cutaneous nerve

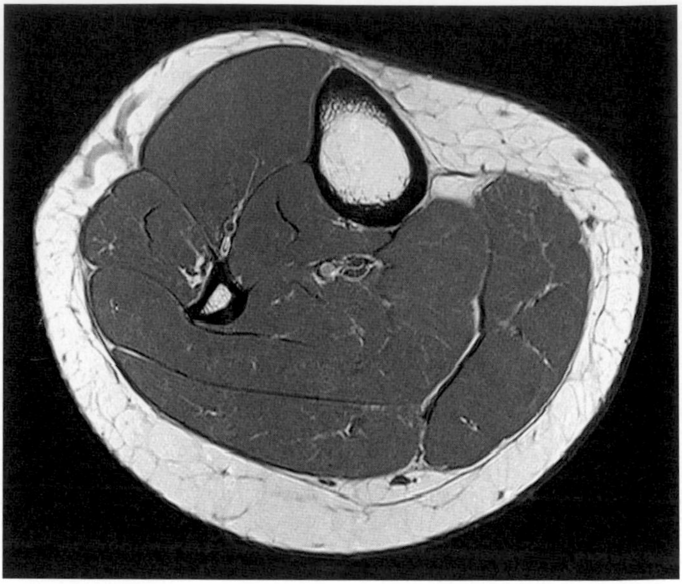

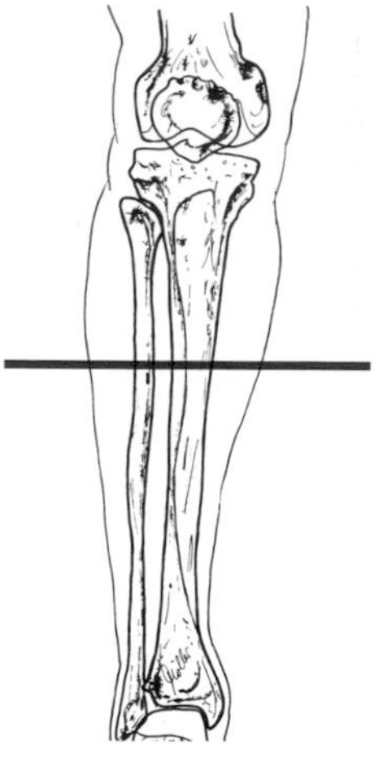

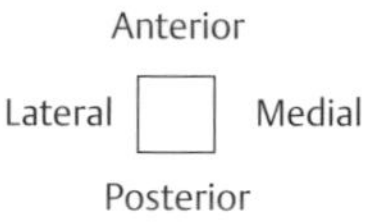
Anterior
Lateral
Medial
Posterior

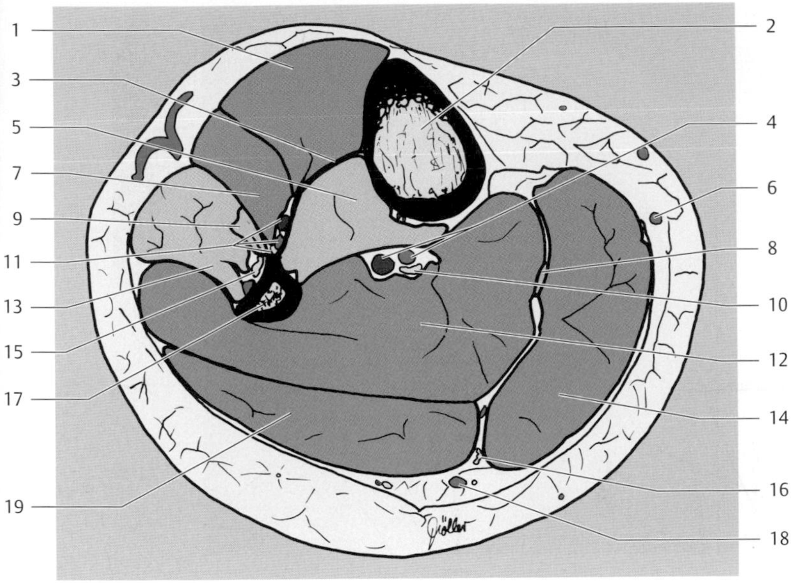

1 Tibialis anterior muscle
2 Tibia
3 Interosseous membrane of leg
4 Tibiofibular trunk (of posterior tibial and of fibular artery and vein)
5 Tibialis posterior muscle
6 Great saphenous vein
7 Extensor digitorum longus muscle
8 Plantaris muscle (tendon)
9 Peroneus (fibularis) brevis muscle
10 Tibial nerve
11 Anterior tibial artery and vein and deep fibular (peroneal) nerve
12 Soleus muscle
13 Peroneus (fibularis) longus muscle
14 Gastrocnemius muscle (medial head)
15 Superficial fibular (peroneal) nerve
16 Medial sural cutaneous nerve
17 Fibula
18 Small saphenous vein
19 Gastrocnemius muscle (lateral head)

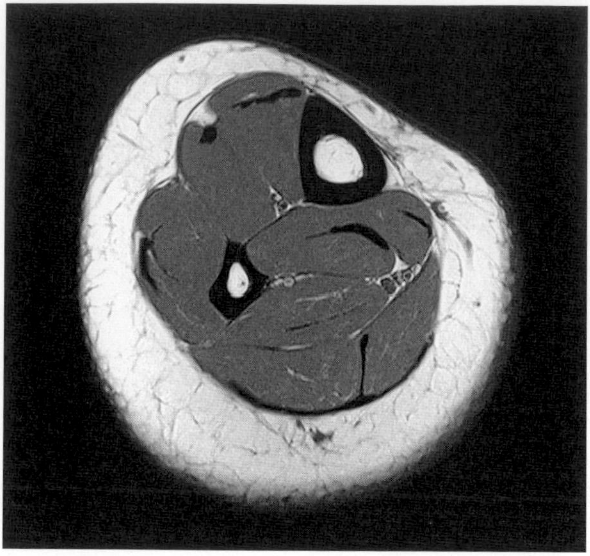

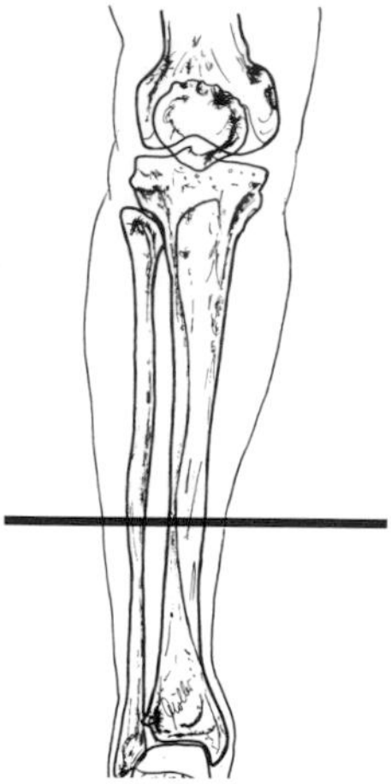

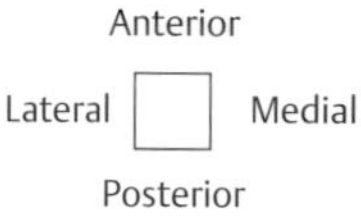
Anterior
Lateral
Medial
Posterior

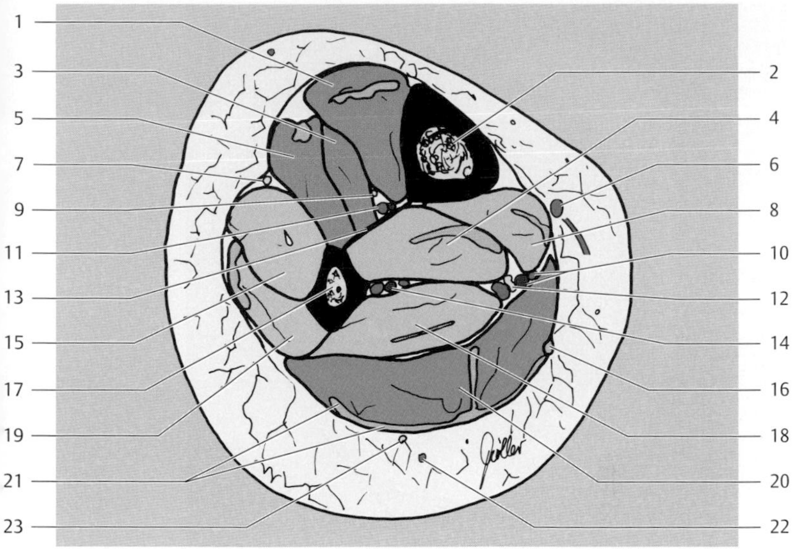

1 Tibialis anterior muscle (+ tendon)
2 Tibia
3 Extensor hallucis longus muscle
4 Tibialis posterior muscle
5 Extensor digitorum longus muscle (+ tendon)
6 Great saphenous vein
7 Superficial fibular (peroneal) nerve
8 Flexor digitorum longus muscle (+ tendon)
9 Deep fibular (peroneal) nerve
10 Posterior tibial artery and vein
11 Anterior tibial artery and vein
12 Tibial nerve
13 Interosseous membrane of leg
14 Fibular (peroneal) artery and vein
15 Peroneus (fibularis) brevis muscle
16 Plantaris muscle (tendon)
17 Fibula
18 Flexor hallucis longus muscle
19 Peroneus (fibularis) longus muscle (+ tendon)
20 Soleus muscle
21 Gastrocnemius muscle (tendon)
22 Small saphenous vein
23 Medial sural cutaneous nerve

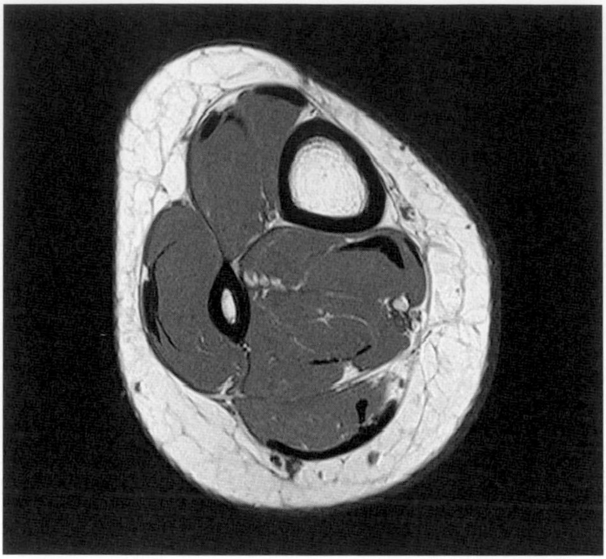

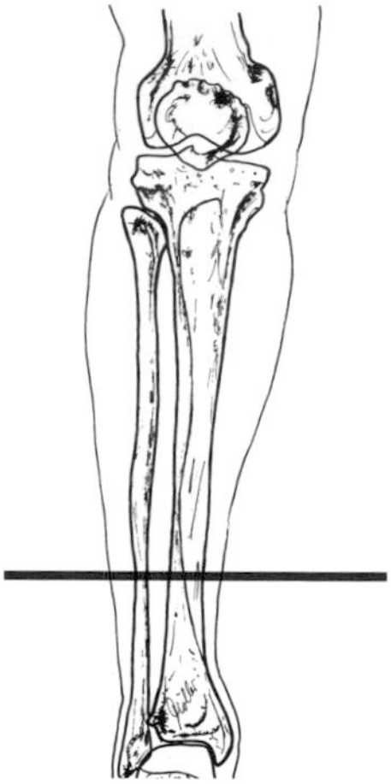

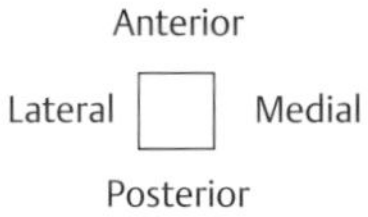
Anterior
Lateral
Medial
Posterior

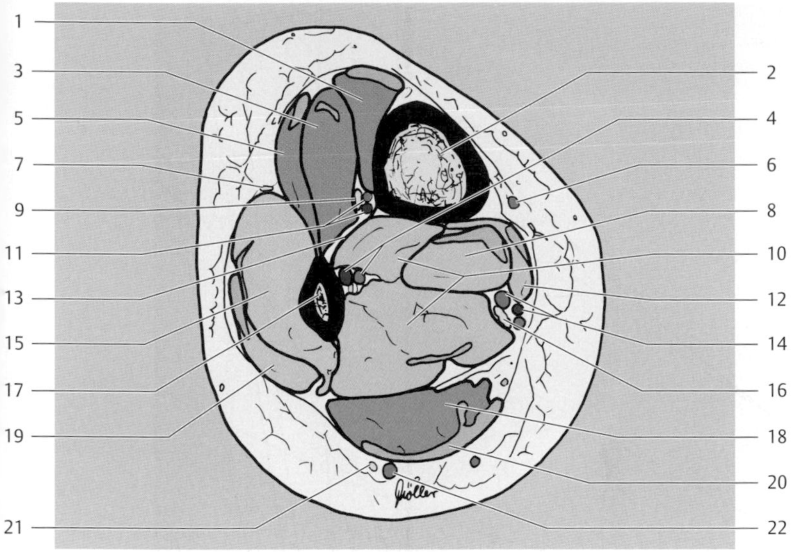

1 Tibialis anterior muscle (+ tendon)
2 Tibia
3 Extensor hallucis longus muscle
4 Fibular (peroneal) artery and vein
5 Extensor digitorum longus muscle (+ tendon)
6 Great saphenous vein
7 Superficial fibular (peroneal) nerve
8 Tibialis posterior muscle (+ tendon)
9 Deep fibular (peroneal) nerve
10 Flexor hallucis longus muscle
11 Anterior tibial artery and vein
12 Flexor digitorum longus muscle (+ tendon)
13 Interosseous membrane of leg
14 Posterior tibial artery and vein
15 Peroneus (fibularis) brevis muscle
16 Tibial nerve
17 Fibula
18 Soleus muscle
19 Peroneus (fibularis) longus muscle (+ tendon)
20 Gastrocnemius muscle (tendon, + tendon of plantaris muscle)
21 Sural nerve
22 Small saphenous vein

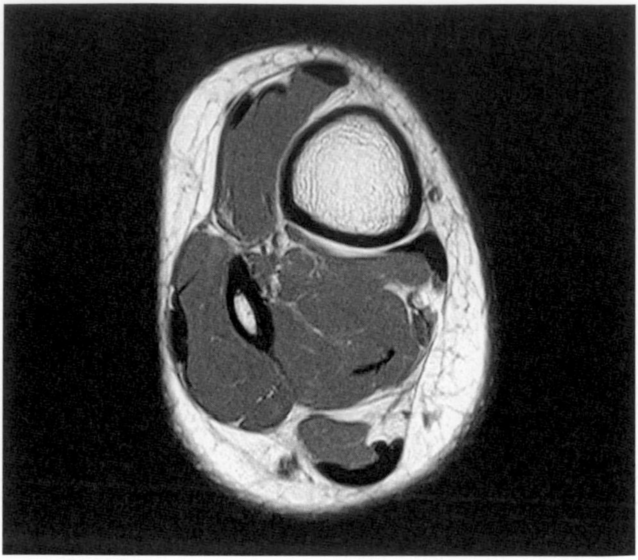

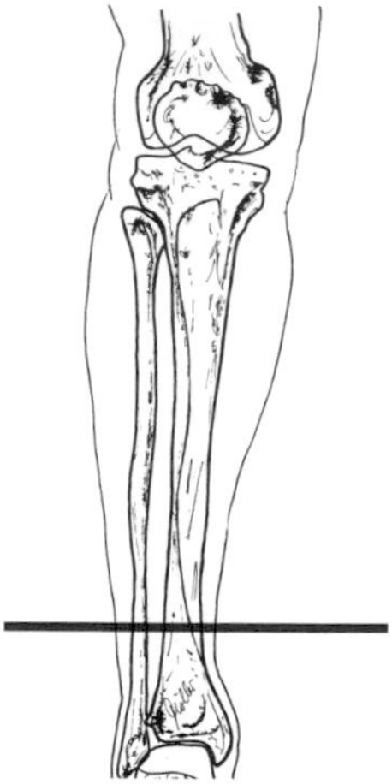

Anterior
Lateral
Medial
Posterior

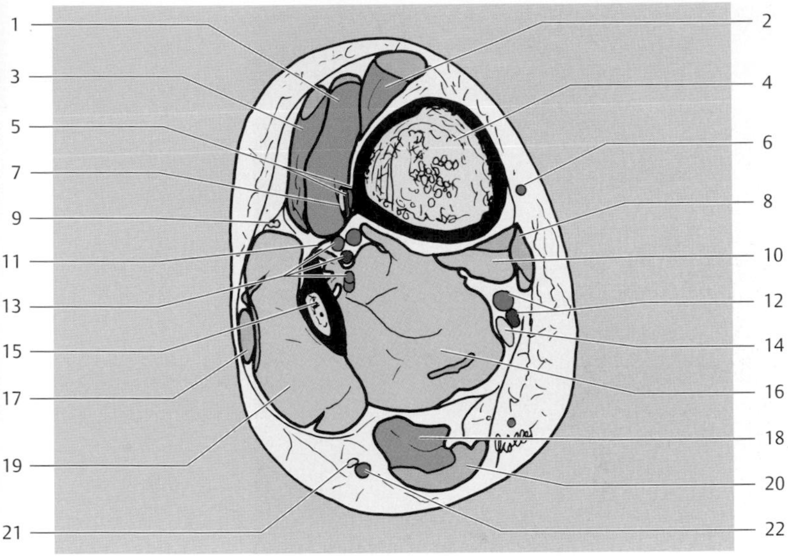

1 Extensor hallucis longus muscle (+ tendon)
2 Tibialis anterior muscle (+ tendon)
3 Extensor digitorum longus muscle (+ tendon)
4 Tibia
5 Anterior tibial artery and vein
6 Great saphenous vein
7 Deep fibular (peroneal) nerve
8 Flexor digitorum longus muscle (+ tendon)
9 Superficial fibular (peroneal) nerve
10 Tibialis posterior muscle (+ tendon)
11 Interosseous membrane of leg
12 Posterior tibial artery and vein
13 Fibular (peroneal) artery and veins
14 Tibial nerve
15 Fibula
16 Flexor hallucis longus muscle
17 Peroneus (fibularis) longus muscle (tendon)
18 Soleus muscle
19 Peroneus (fibularis) brevis muscle
20 Gastrocnemius muscle (tendon, + tendon of plantaris muscle)
21 Sural nerve
22 Small saphenous vein

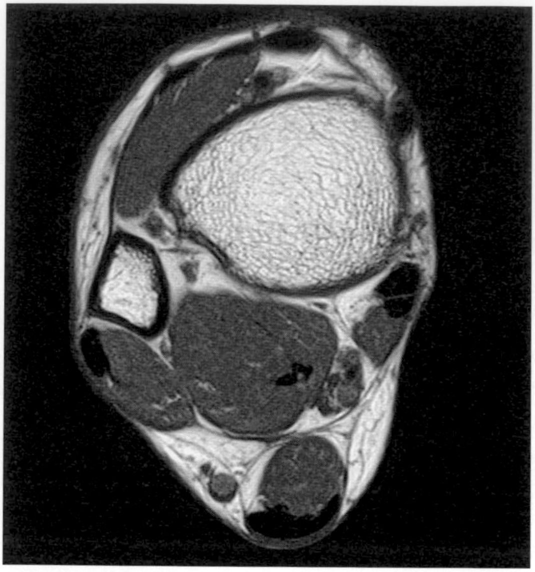

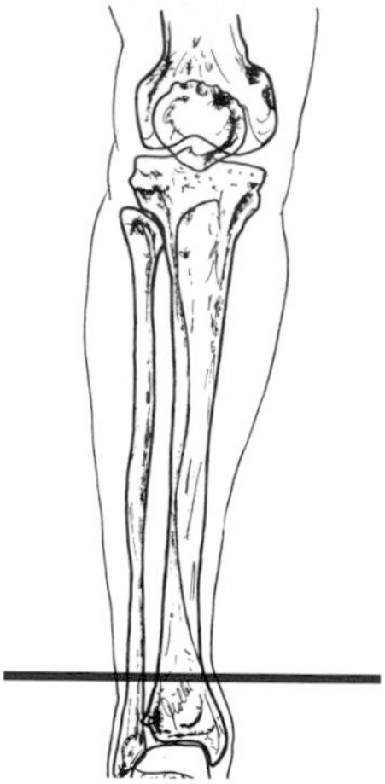

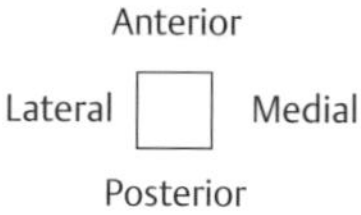
Anterior
Lateral
Medial
Posterior

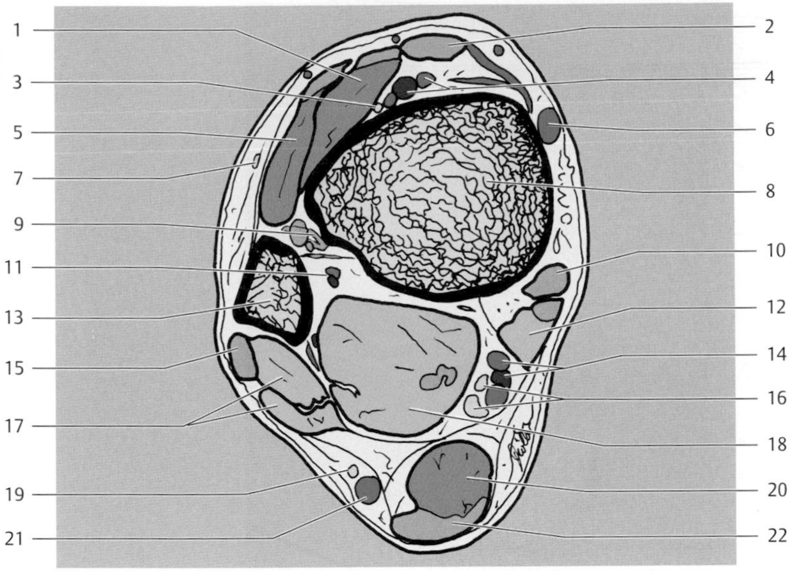

1 Extensor hallucis longus muscle (+ tendon)
2 Tibialis anterior muscle (tendon)
3 Deep fibular (peroneal) nerve
4 Anterior tibial artery and vein
5 Extensor digitorum longus muscle (+ tendon)
6 Great saphenous vein
7 Superficial fibular (peroneal) nerve
8 Tibia
9 Interosseous membrane of leg
10 Tibialis posterior muscle (tendon)
11 Fibular (peroneal) artery and vein
12 Flexor digitorum longus muscle (+ tendon)
13 Fibula
14 Posterior tibial artery and vein
15 Peroneus (fibularis) longus muscle (tendon)
16 Tibial nerve
17 Peroneus (fibularis) brevis muscle
18 Flexor hallucis longus muscle
19 Sural nerve
20 Soleus muscle
21 Small saphenous vein
22 Tendons of triceps surae and plantaris muscles

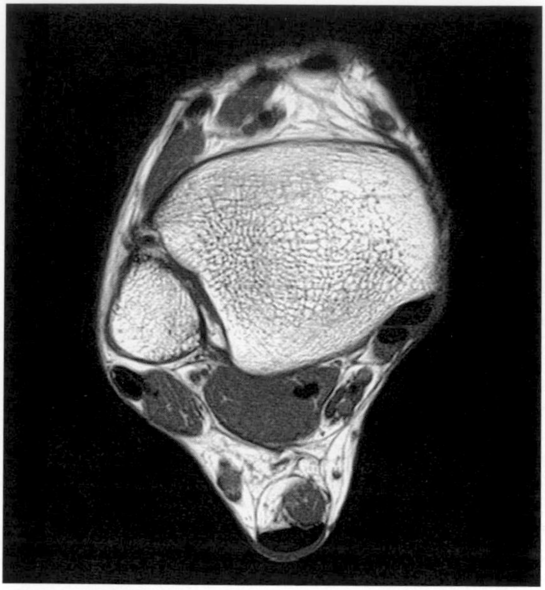

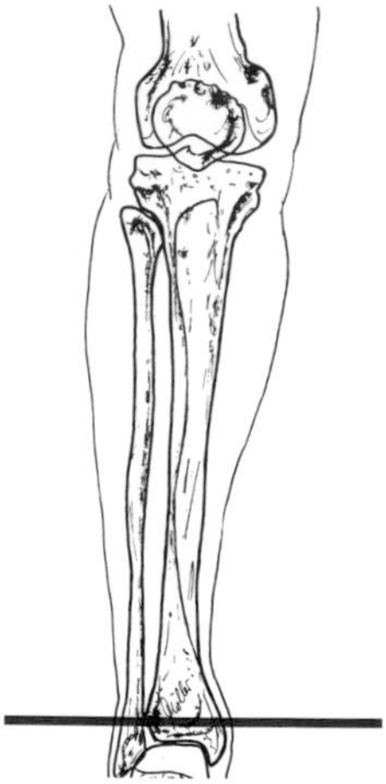

Anterior

Lateral Medial

Posterior

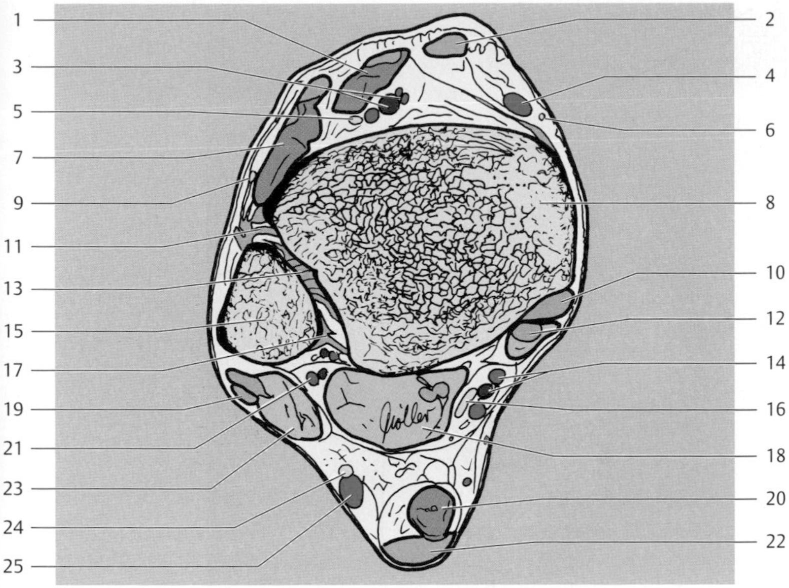

1 Extensor hallucis longus muscle (+ tendon)
2 Tibialis anterior muscle (tendon)
3 Anterior tibial artery and vein
4 Great saphenous vein
5 Deep fibular (peroneal) nerve
6 Saphenous nerve
7 Extensor digitorum longus muscle (+ tendon)
8 Tibia
9 Superficial fibular (peroneal) nerve
10 Tibialis posterior muscle (tendon)
11 Anterior tibiofibular ligament
12 Flexor digitorum longus muscle (+ tendon)
13 Inferior tibiofibular joint
14 Posterior tibial artery and vein
15 Fibula
16 Tibial nerve
17 Posterior tibiofibular ligament
18 Flexor hallucis longus muscle (+ tendon)
19 Peroneus (fibularis) longus muscle (tendon)
20 Soleus muscle
21 Fibular (peroneal) artery and vein
22 Tendons of triceps surae and plantaris muscles
23 Peroneus (fibularis) brevis muscle (+ tendon)
24 Sural nerve
25 Small saphenous vein

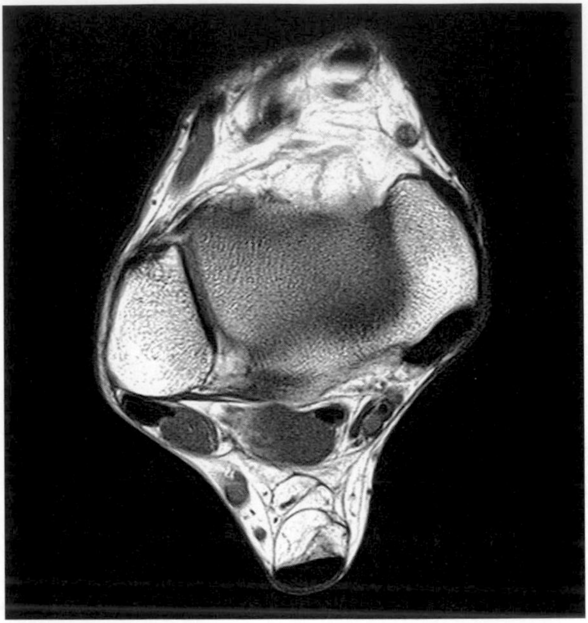

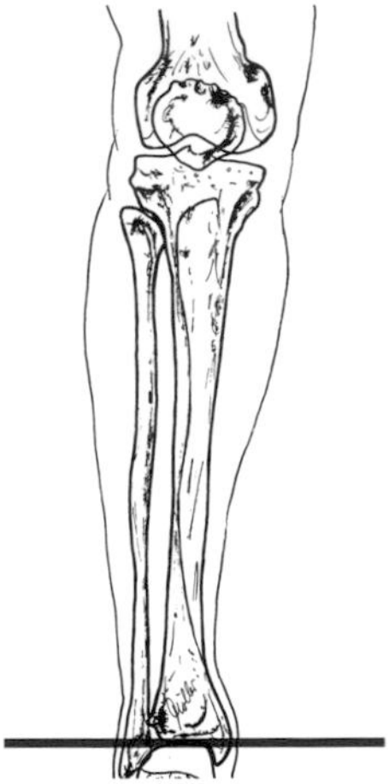

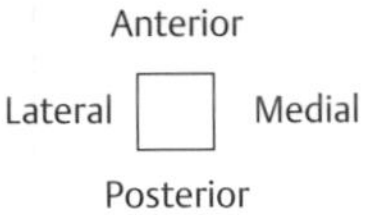
Anterior
Lateral
Medial
Posterior

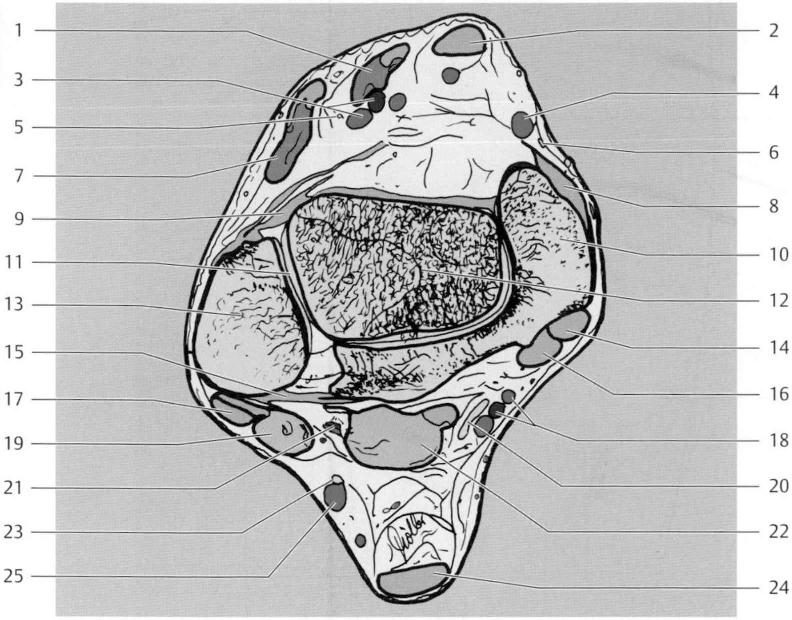

1 Extensor hallucis longus muscle (+ tendon)
2 Tibialis anterior muscle (tendon)
3 Anterior tibial artery and vein
4 Great saphenous vein
5 Deep fibular (peroneal) nerve
6 Saphenous nerve
7 Extensor digitorum longus muscle (+ tendon)
8 Deltoid ligament (tibionavicular and anterior tibiotalar parts)
9 Anterior tibiofibular ligament
10 Medial malleolus (tibia)
11 Tibiofibular syndesmosis
12 Ankle joint
13 Lateral malleolus (fibula)
14 Tibialis posterior muscle (tendon)
15 Posterior tibiofibular ligament
16 Flexor digitorum longus muscle (tendon)
17 Peroneus (fibularis) longus muscle (tendon)
18 Posterior tibial artery and vein
19 Peroneus (fibularis) brevis muscle (+ tendon)
20 Tibial nerve
21 Fibular (peroneal) artery and vein
22 Flexor hallucis longus muscle (+ tendon)
23 Sural nerve
24 Tendons of triceps surae muscle and plantaris muscle
25 Small saphenous vein

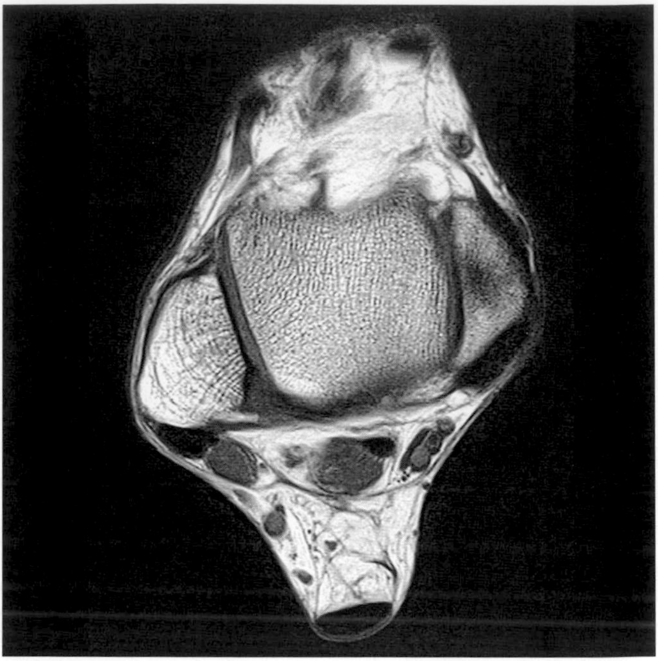

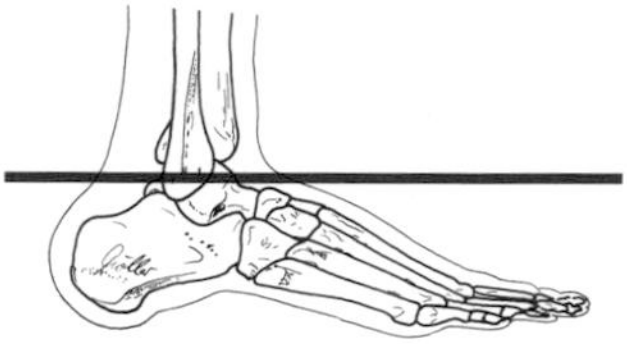

Anterior

Lateral Medial

Posterior

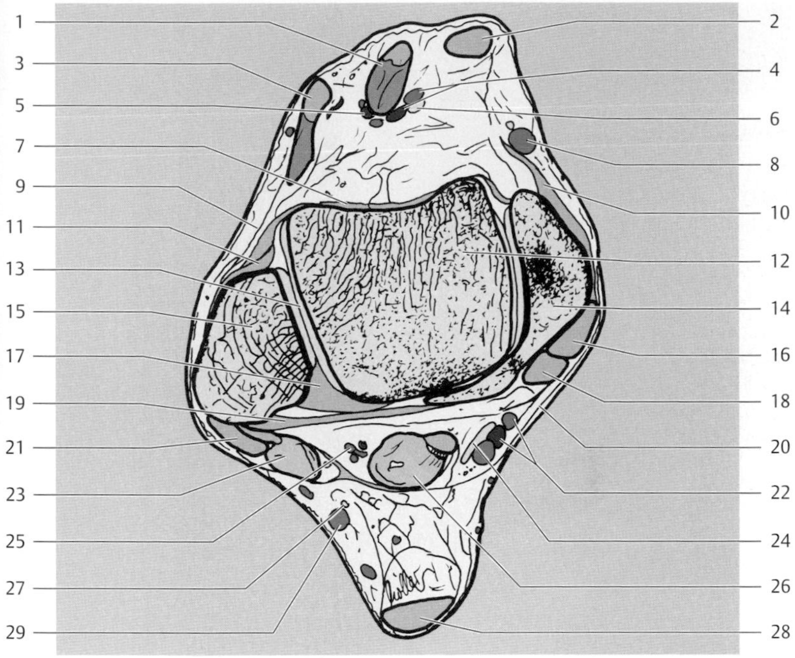

1 Extensor hallucis longus muscle (tendon)
2 Tibialis anterior muscle (tendon)
3 Extensor digitorum longus muscle (tendon)
4 Dorsalis pedis artery (+ vein)
5 Lateral tarsal artery
6 Deep fibular nerve
7 Dorsal talonavicular ligament and joint capsule
8 Great saphenous vein
9 Extensor retinaculum
10 Deltoid ligament (tibionavicular and anterior tibiotalar parts)
11 Anterior talofibular ligament
12 Talus
13 Ankle joint
14 Medial malleolus (tibia)
15 Lateral malleolus (fibula)
16 Tibialis posterior muscle (tendon)
17 Posterior talofibular ligament
18 Flexor digitorum longus muscle (tendon)
19 Posterior tibiofibular ligament
20 Flexor retinaculum
21 Peroneus (fibularis) longus muscle (tendon)
22 Posterior tibial artery and vein
23 Peroneus (fibular) brevis muscle (+ tendon)
24 Tibial nerve
25 Fibular (peroneal) artery and vein
26 Flexor hallucis longus muscle (+ tendon)
27 Sural nerve
28 Achilles tendon (calcaneal tendon)
29 Small saphenous vein

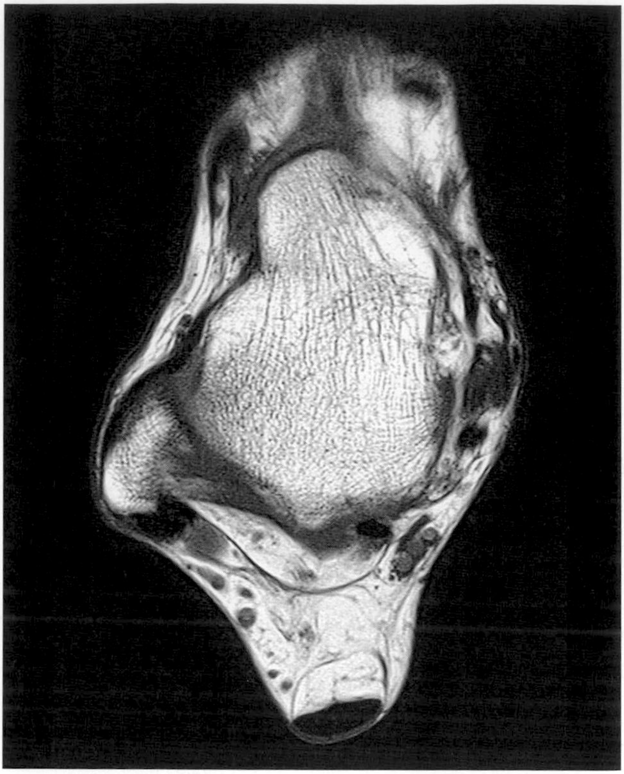

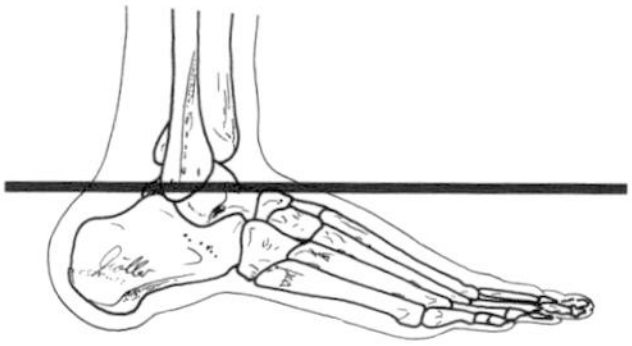

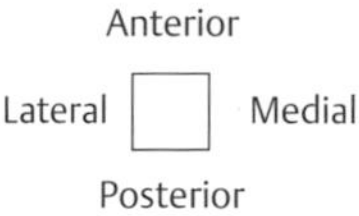

1 Extensor hallucis longus muscle (tendon)
2 Tibialis anterior muscle (tendon)
3 Dorsalis pedis artery
4 Dorsal talonavicular ligament
5 Extensor digitorum longus muscle (+ tendon)

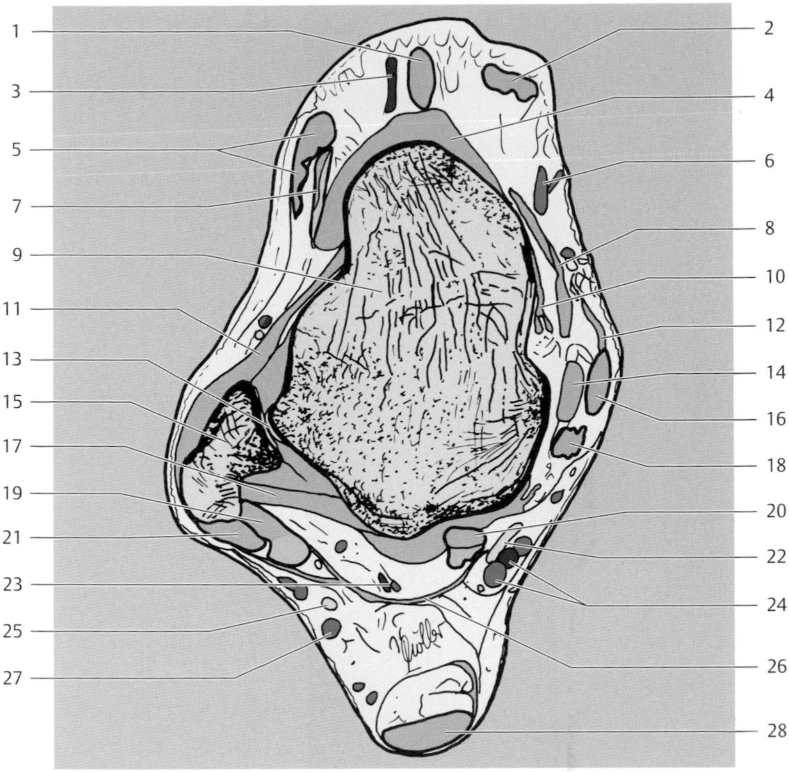

6 Great saphenous vein
7 Extensor digitorum brevis muscle (+ tendon)
8 Deltoid ligament (tibionavicular part)
9 Talus
10 Deltoid ligament (anterior tibiotalar part)
11 Anterior talofibular ligament
12 Flexor retinaculum
13 Ankle joint
14 Deltoid ligament (posterior tibiotalar part)
15 Lateral malleolus (fibula)
16 Tibialis posterior muscle (tendon)
17 Posterior talofibular ligament
18 Flexor digitorum longus muscle (tendon)
19 Peroneus (fibularis) brevis muscle (+ tendon)
20 Flexor hallucis longus muscle (+ tendon)
21 Peroneus (fibularis) longus muscle (tendon)
22 Tibial nerve
23 Fibular (peroneal) artery and vein
24 Posterior tibial artery and vein
25 Sural nerve
26 Superior peroneal retinaculum
27 Small saphenous vein
28 Achilles tendon (calcaneal tendon)

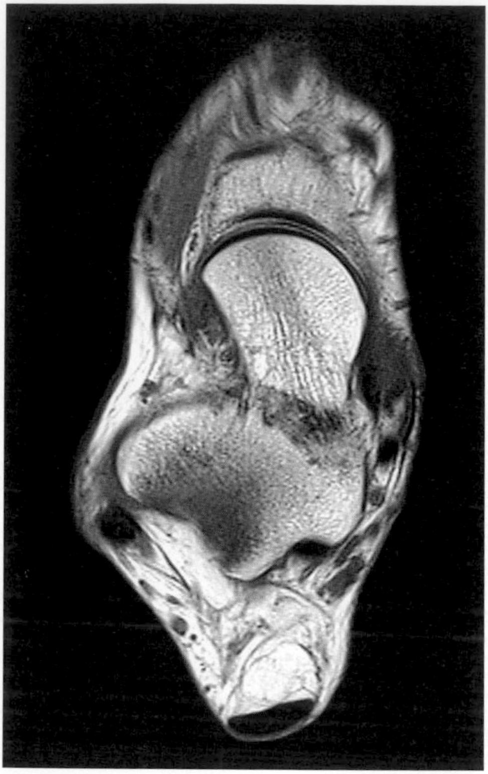

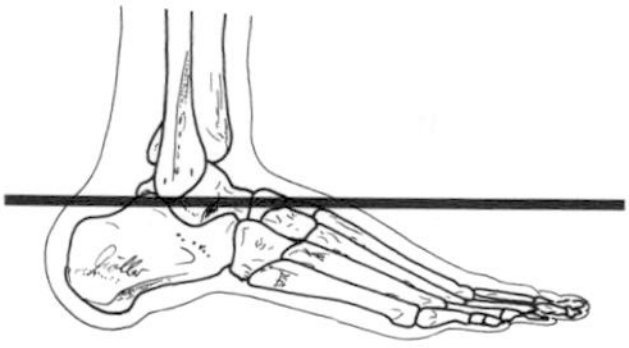

Anterior

Lateral ☐ Medial

Posterior

1 Dorsalis pedis artery
2 Extensor hallucis longus muscle (tendon)
3 Dorsal tarsal ligaments
4 Tibialis anterior muscle (tendon)
5 Extensor digitorum longus muscle (tendon)

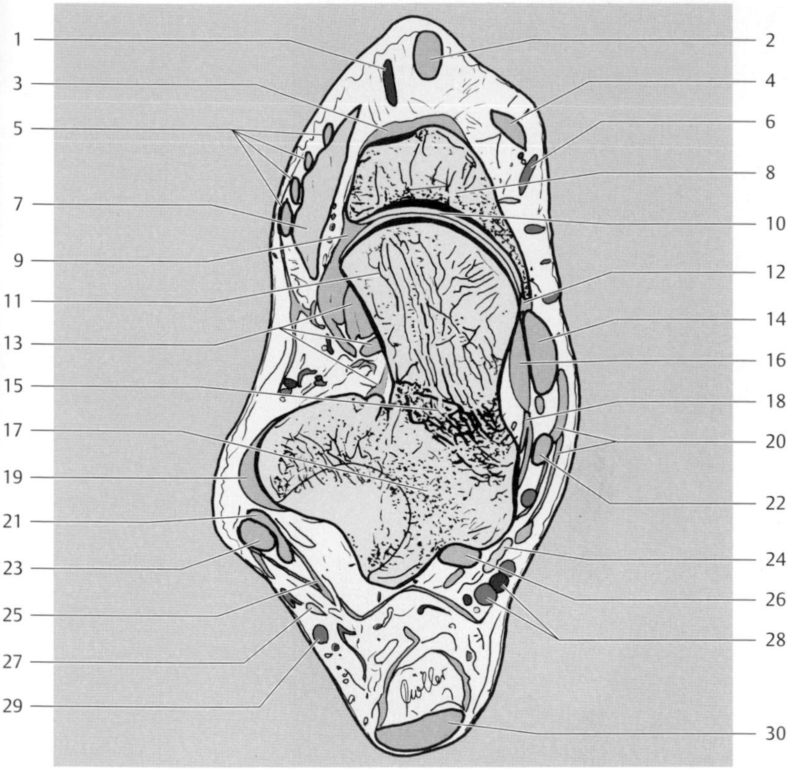

6 Great saphenous vein
7 Extensor digitorum brevis muscle
8 Navicular
9 Dorsal talonavicular ligament
10 Talonavicular joint
11 Head of talus
12 Deltoid ligament (tibionavicular part)
13 Interosseous talocalcaneal ligament
14 Tibialis posterior muscle (tendon)
15 Neck of talus
16 Deltoid ligament (tibiocalcaneal part)
17 Talus (body)
18 Deltoid ligament (posterior tibiotalar part)
19 Calcaneofibular ligament
20 Flexor retinaculum
21 Peroneus (fibularis) brevis muscle (tendon)
22 Flexor digitorum longus muscle (tendon)
23 Peroneus (fibularis) longus muscle (tendon)
24 Tibial nerve
25 Superior fibular (peroneal) retinaculum
26 Flexor hallucis longus muscle (tendon)
27 Sural nerve
28 Posterior tibial artery and vein
29 Small saphenous vein
30 Achilles tendon (calcaneal tendon)

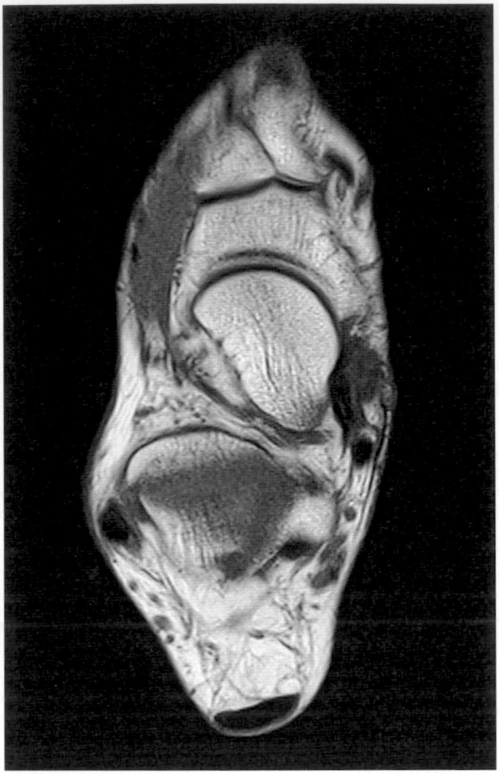

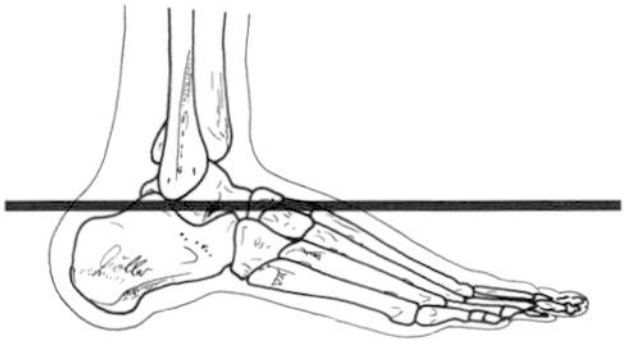

Anterior

Lateral Medial

Posterior

1 Dorsalis pedis artery
2 Extensor hallucis longus muscle (tendon)
3 Intermediate cuneiform
4 Medial cuneiform
5 Extensor digitorum longus muscle (tendons)

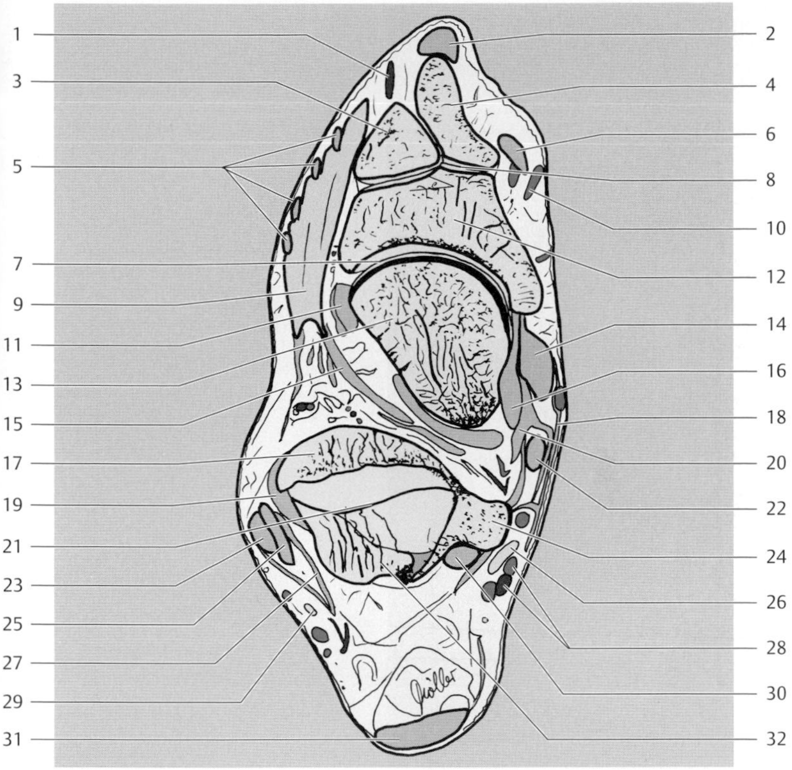

6 Tibialis anterior muscle (tendon)
7 Talonavicular joint
8 Cuneonavicular joint
9 Extensor digitorum brevis muscle
10 Great saphenous vein
11 Bifurcate ligament
12 Navicular
13 Talus (head)
14 Tibialis posterior muscle (tendon)
15 Interosseous talocalcaneal ligament
16 Deltoid ligament (tibiocalcaneal and tibionavicular part)
17 Talus (body)
18 Flexor retinaculum
19 Calcaneofibular ligament
20 Talocalcaneal ligament (medial)
21 Subtalar (talocalcaneal) joint
22 Flexor digitorum longus muscle (tendon)
23 Peroneus (fibularis) longus muscle (tendon)
24 Talus (posterior process)
25 Peroneus (fibularis) brevis muscle (tendon)
26 Tibial nerve
27 Peroneal retinaculum
28 Posterior tibial artery and vein
29 Dorsal lateral cutaneous nerve
30 Flexor hallucis longus muscle (tendon)
31 Achilles tendon (calcaneal tendon)
32 Calcaneus

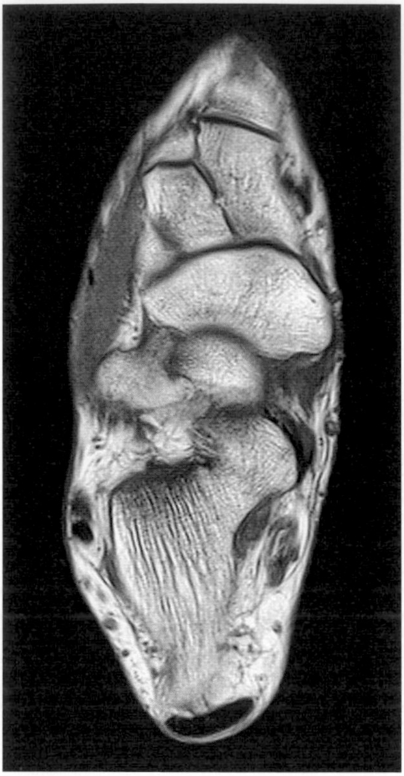

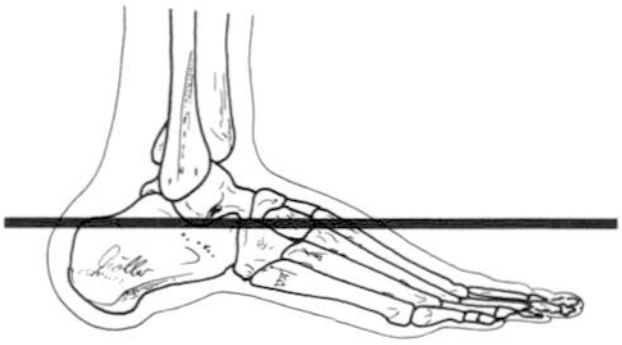

Anterior

Lateral Medial

Posterior

1 Extensor hallucis longus muscle (tendon)
2 Metatarsal I (base)
3 Dorsalis pedis artery
4 First tarsometatarsal joint
5 Metatarsal II (base)

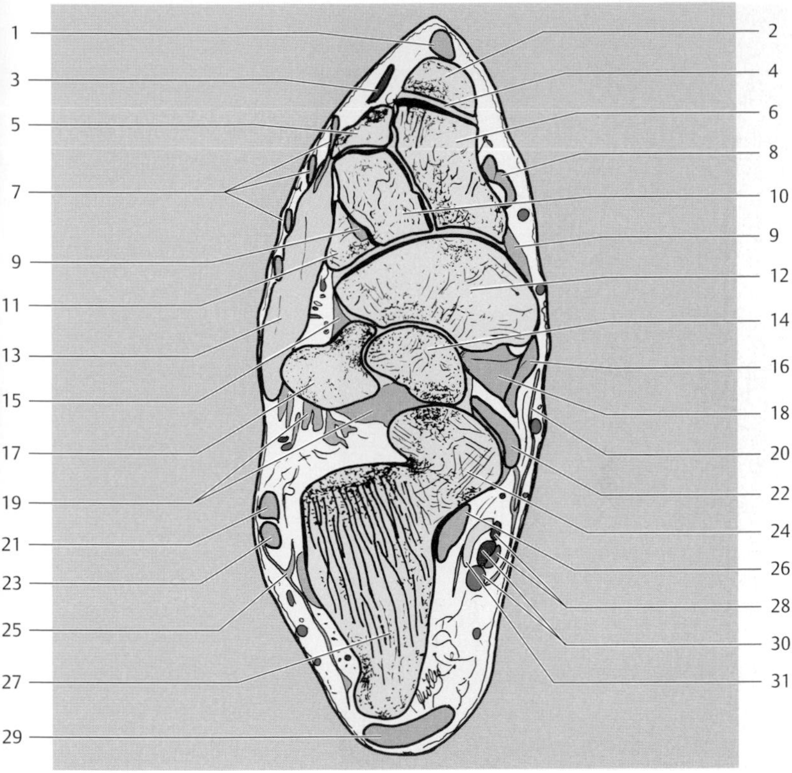

6 Medial cuneiform
7 Extensor digitorum longus muscle (tendons)
8 Tibialis anterior muscle (tendon)
9 Dorsal tarsal ligaments
10 Intermediate cuneiform
11 Lateral cuneiform
12 Navicular
13 Extensor digitorum brevis muscle
14 Talus (head)
15 Bifurcate ligament
16 Deltoid ligament (tibionavicular part)
17 Calcaneus
18 Tibialis posterior muscle (tendon)
19 Interosseous talocalcaneal ligament
20 Flexor retinaculum
21 Peroneus (fibularis) brevis muscle (tendon)
22 Flexor digitorum longus muscle (tendon)
23 Peroneus (fibularis) longus muscle (tendon)
24 Calcaneus (talar shelf)
25 Peroneal retinaculum
26 Flexor hallucis longus muscle (tendon)
27 Calcaneal tuberosity
28 Medial plantar artery and vein
29 Achilles tendon (calcaneal tendon)
30 Lateral plantar artery and vein
31 Tibial nerve

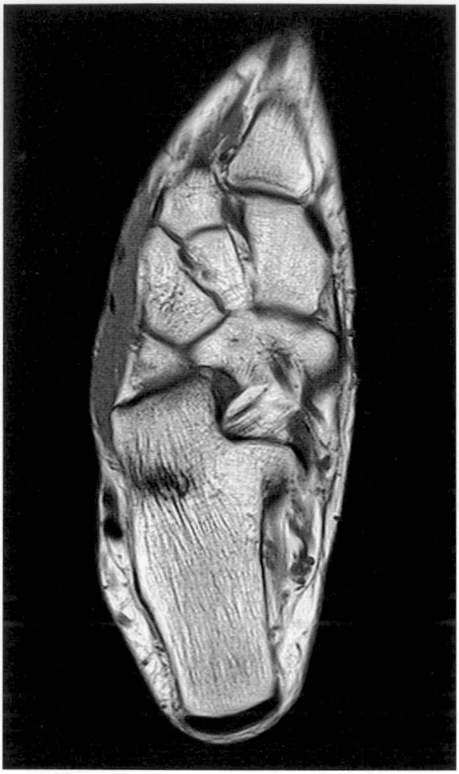

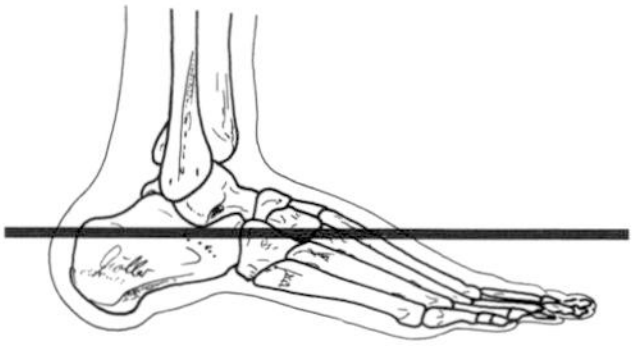

Anterior

Lateral Medial

Posterior

1 Extensor hallucis longus muscle (tendon)
2 Metatarsal I (base)
3 Dorsalis pedis artery
4 Metatarsal II (base)
5 Dorsal interosseous muscles
6 Interosseous cuneometatarsal ligaments

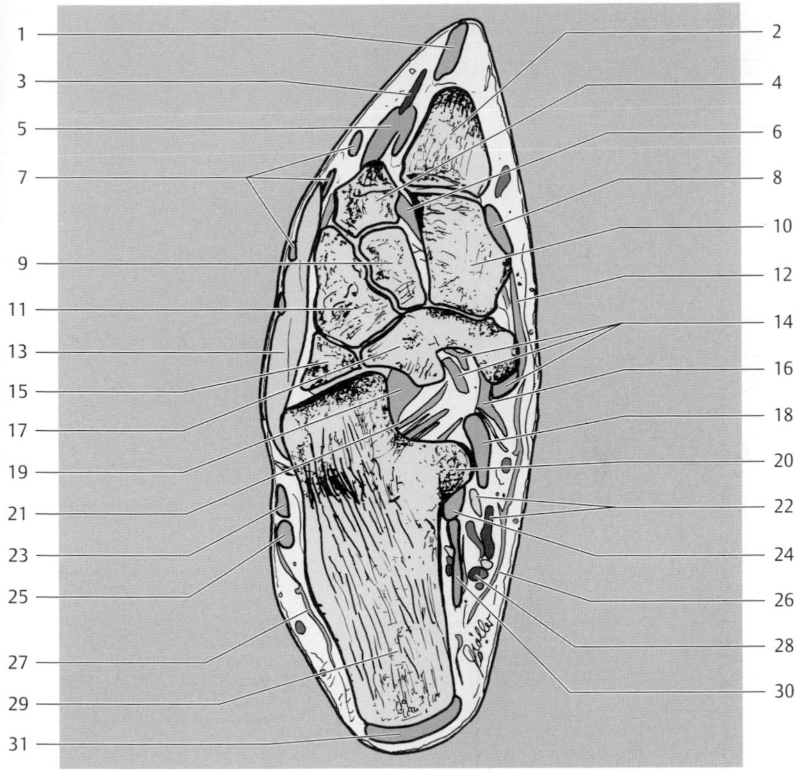

7 Extensor digitorum longus muscle (tendons)
8 Tibialis anterior muscle (tendon)
9 Intermediate cuneiform
10 Medial cuneiform
11 Lateral cuneiform
12 Dorsal tarsal ligaments
13 Extensor digitorum brevis muscle
14 Tibialis posterior muscle (tendon)
15 Cuboid
16 Spring ligament (plantar calcaneonavicular ligament)
17 Navicular
18 Flexor digitorum longus muscle (tendon)
19 Spring ligament (plantar calcaneonavicular ligament)
20 Calcaneus (talar shelf)
21 Long plantar ligament
22 Medial plantar artery, vein and nerve
23 Peroneus (fibularis) brevis muscle (tendon)
24 Flexor hallucis longus muscle (tendon)
25 Peroneus (fibularis) longus muscle (tendon)
26 Flexor retinaculum
27 Peroneal retinaculum
28 Lateral plantar artery and vein
29 Calcaneus (calcaneal tuberosity)
30 Quadratus plantae muscle
31 Achilles tendon (calcaneal tendon)

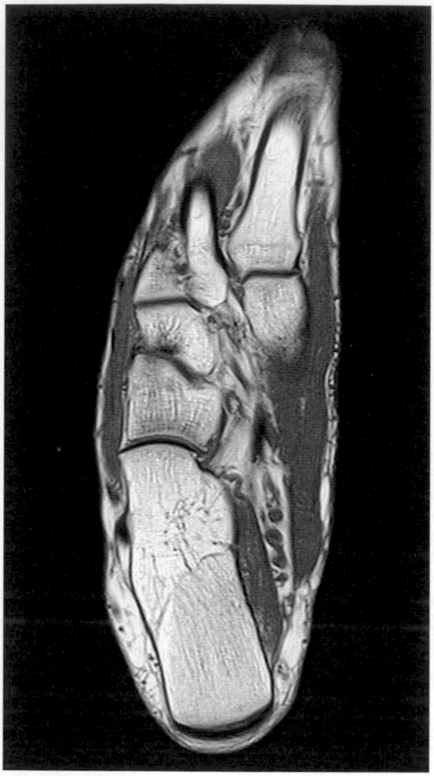

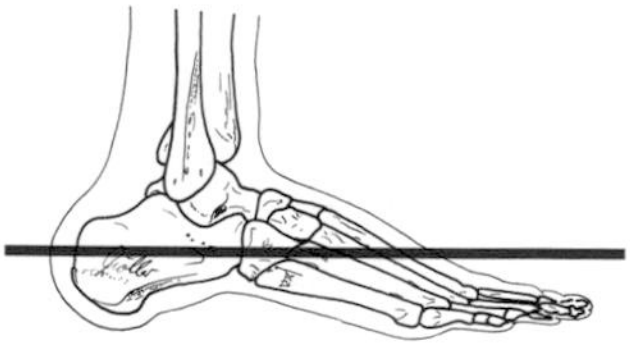

Anterior
Lateral
Medial
Posterior

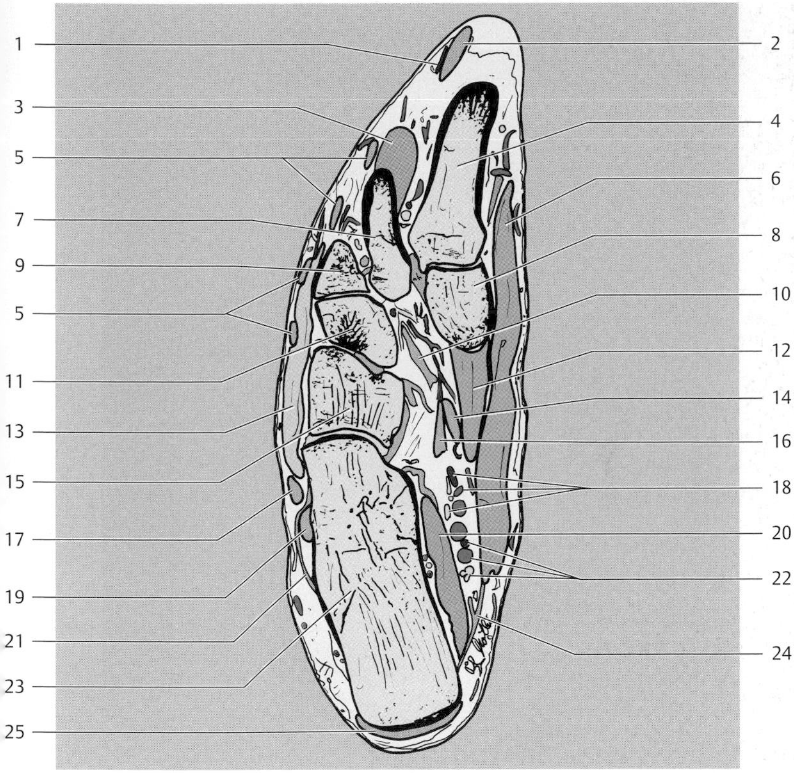

1 Dorsalis pedis artery
2 Extensor hallucis longus muscle (tendon)
3 Dorsal interosseous muscles
4 Metatarsal I (base)
5 Extensor digitorum longus muscle (tendons)
6 Abductor hallucis muscle
7 Metatarsal II (base)
8 Medial cuneiform
9 Metatarsal III (base)
10 Tibialis posterior muscle (tendon)
11 Lateral cuneiform
12 Flexor hallucis brevis muscle
13 Extensor digitorum brevis muscle
14 Flexor hallucis longus muscle (tendon)
15 Cuboid
16 Flexor digitorum longus muscle (tendon)
17 Peroneus (fibularis) brevis muscle (tendon)
18 Medial plantar artery, vein, and nerve
19 Peroneus (fibularis) brevis muscle (tendon)
20 Quadratus plantae muscle
21 Inferior fibular (peroneal) retinaculum
22 Lateral plantar artery, vein, and nerve
23 Calcaneus
24 Flexor retinaculum
25 Achilles tendon (calcaneal tendon) (attachment)

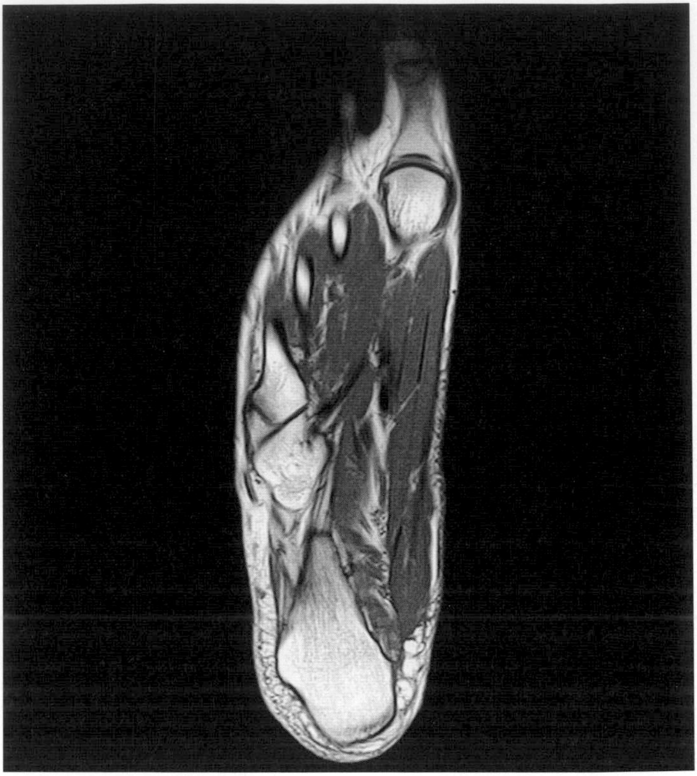

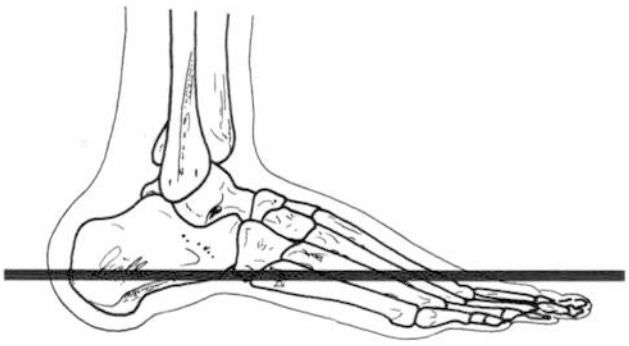

Anterior

Lateral ☐ Medial

Posterior

1 Extensor digitorum longus muscle (tendons)
2 Proximal phalanx I
3 Dorsal and plantar interosseous muscles
4 Metacarpophalangeal joint

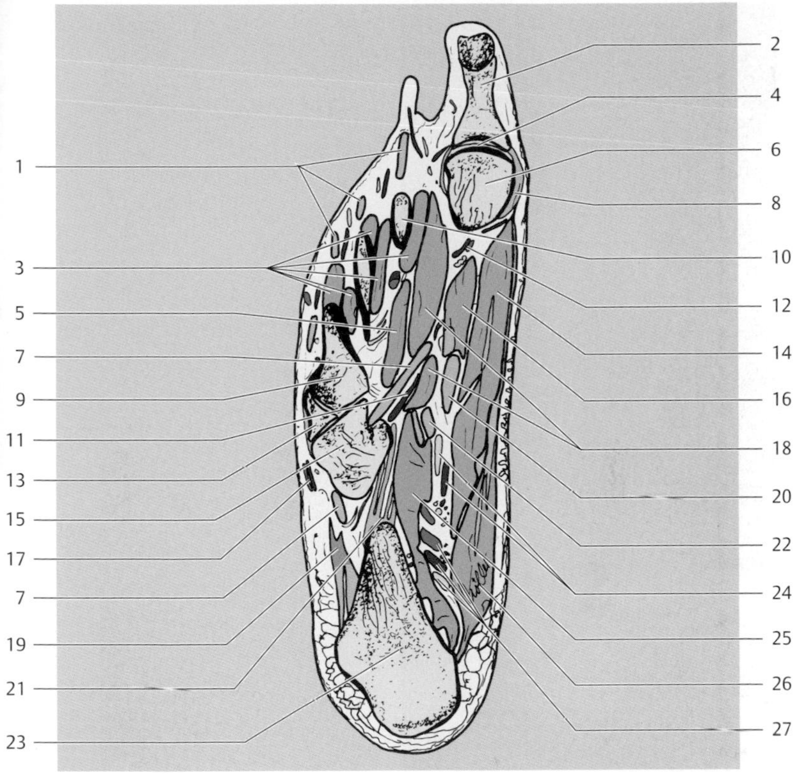

5 Adductor hallucis brevis muscle (oblique head)
6 Metatarsal I (head)
7 Peroneus (fibularis) longus muscle (tendon)
8 Joint capsule
9 Metatarsal IV (base)
10 Metatarsal II
11 Plantar arch
12 Plantar metatarsal artery, vein, and nerve
13 Lateral cuneiform
14 Flexor hallucis brevis muscle (medial head)
15 Cuboid
16 Flexor hallucis brevis muscle (lateral head)
17 Fifth plantar digital artery, vein, and nerve
18 Adductor hallucis brevis muscle
19 Abductor digiti minimi muscle
20 Flexor hallucis longus muscle (tendon)
21 Long plantar ligament
22 Flexor digitorum longus muscle (tendon)
23 Calcaneus (calcaneal tuberosity)
24 Medial plantar artery and nerve
25 Quadratus plantae muscle
26 Abductor hallucis muscle
27 Lateral plantar artery, vein, and nerve

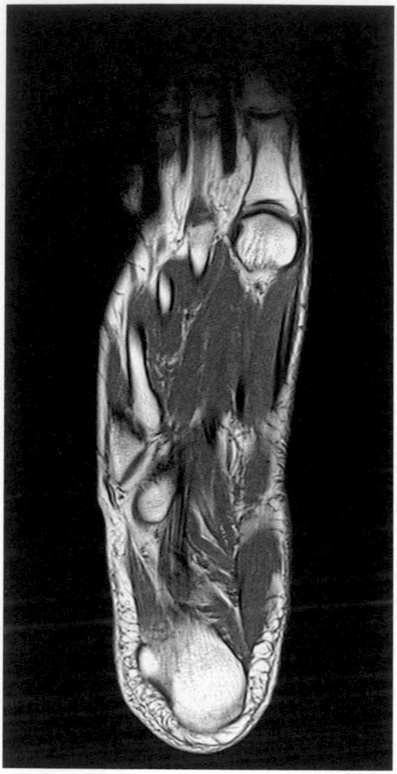

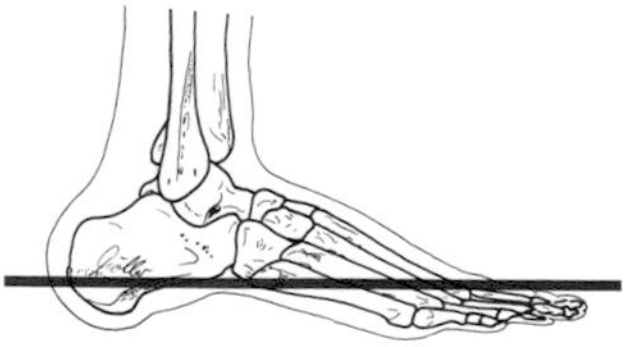

Anterior

Lateral Medial

Posterior

1 Extensor digitorum longus muscle (tendon)
2 Distal phalanx I
3 Plantar digital arteries
4 Proximal phalanx I

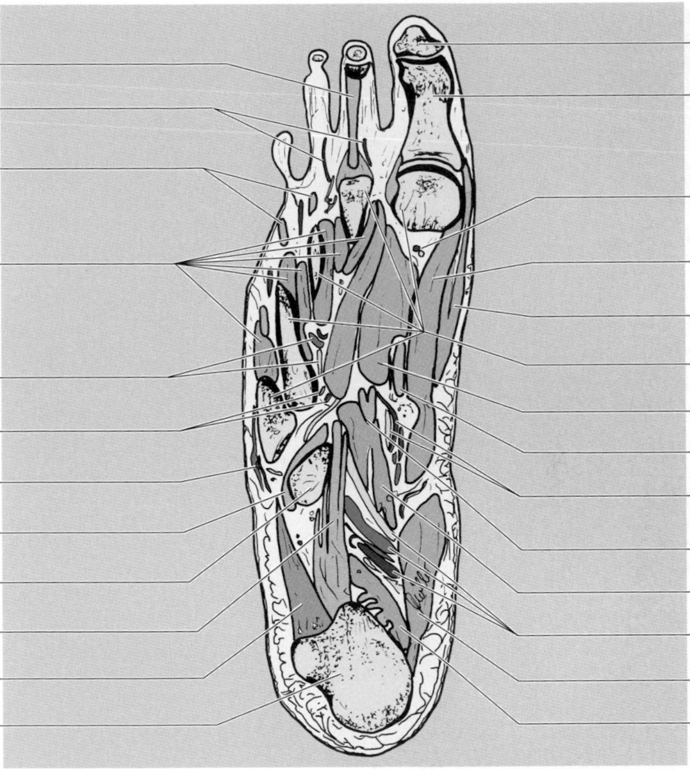

5 Dorsal and plantar interosseous muscles
6 Plantar metatarsal artery and medial plantar hallucis nerve
7 Lateral plantar artery, vein and nerve (superficial branch)
8 Flexor hallucis brevis muscle (medial head)
9 Lateral plantar artery and vein (deep branch)
10 Abductor hallucis muscle (tendon)
11 Fifth plantar digital artery, vein, and nerve
12 Metatarsals
13 Peroneus (fibularis) longus muscle (tendon)
14 Flexor hallucis brevis muscle (lateral head)
15 Cuboid
16 Flexor hallucis longus muscle (tendon)
17 Long plantar ligament
18 Medial plantar artery, vein, and nerve
19 Abductor digiti minimi muscle
20 Flexor digitorum longus muscle (tendon)
21 Calcaneus (calcaneal tuberosity)
22 Quadratus plantae muscle
23 Lateral plantar artery, vein, and nerve
24 Abductor hallucis muscle

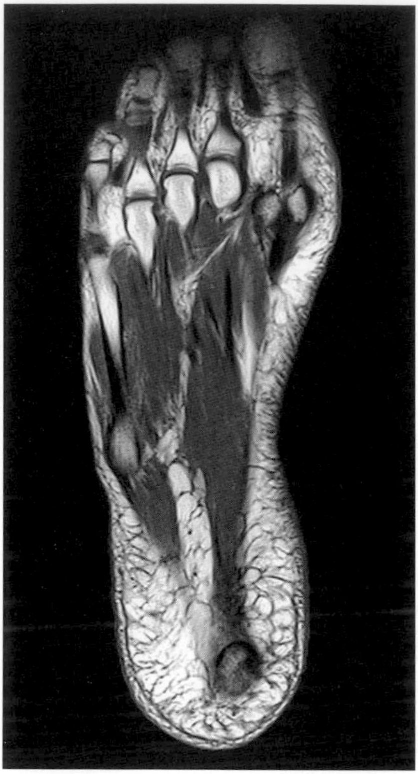

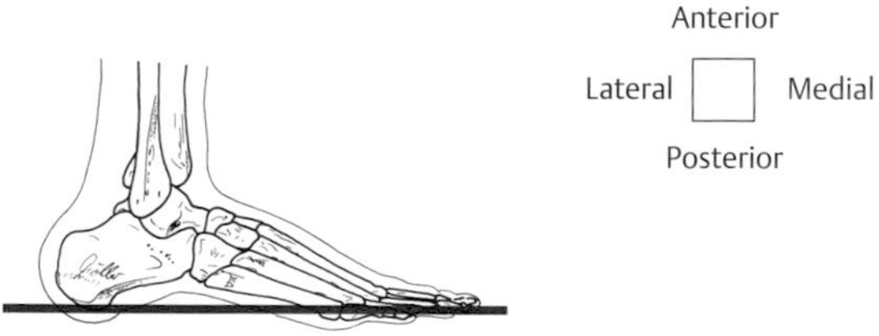
Anterior
Lateral
Medial
Posterior

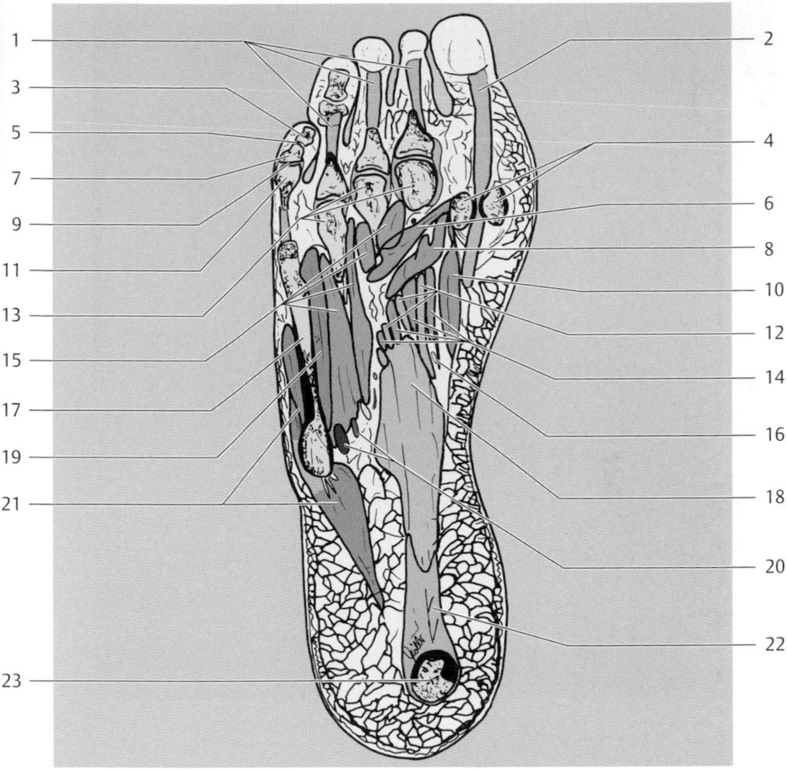

1 Flexor digitorum muscles (tendons)
2 Flexor hallucis longus muscle (tendon)
3 Distal phalanx V
4 Sesamoid bones
5 Fifth distal interphalangeal joint (DIP)
6 Adductor hallucis muscle (transverse head)
7 Medial phalanx V
8 Adductor hallucis muscle (oblique head)
9 Fifth proximal interphalangeal joint (PIP)
10 Flexor hallucis brevis muscle
11 Proximal phalanx V
12 Flexor digitorum longus muscle (tendons)
13 Metatarsal bones (heads)
14 Lumbrical muscles
15 Dorsal and plantar interosseous muscles
16 Medial plantar artery, vein, and nerve (deep branch)
17 Metatarsal V
18 Flexor digitorum brevis muscle
19 Flexor digiti minimi brevis muscle
20 Lateral plantar artery and vein
21 Abductor digiti minimi muscle
22 Plantar aponeurosis
23 Calcaneus (calcaneal tuberosity)

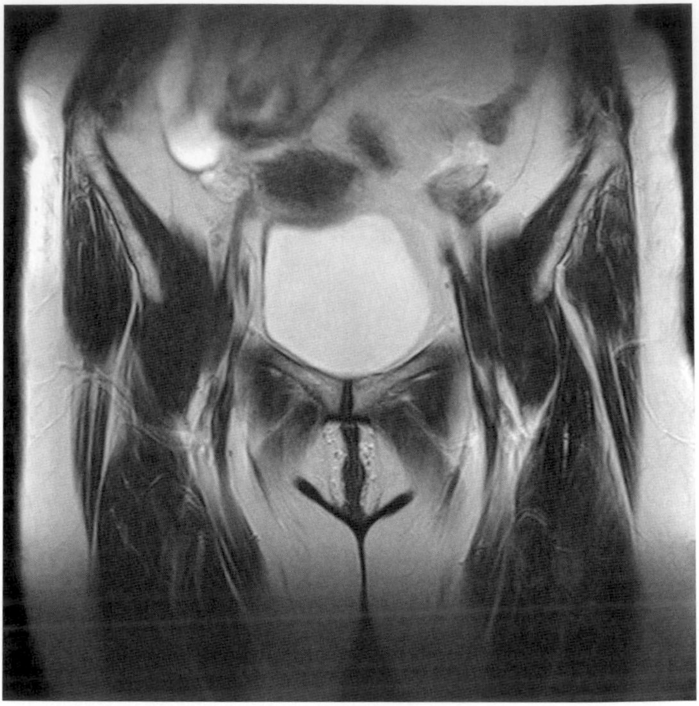

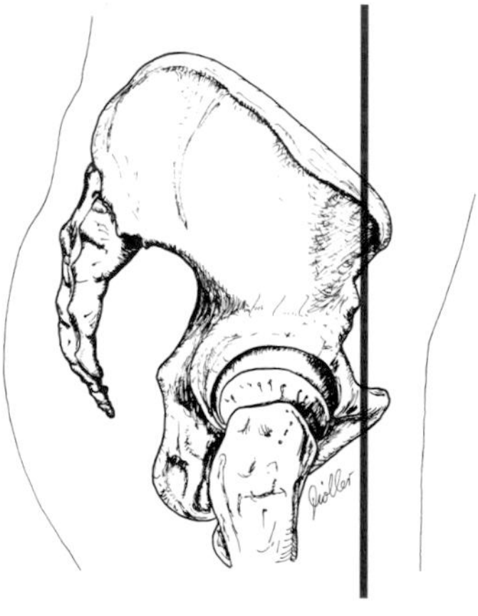

Cranial
(Proximal)

Right ☐ Left

Caudal
(Distal)

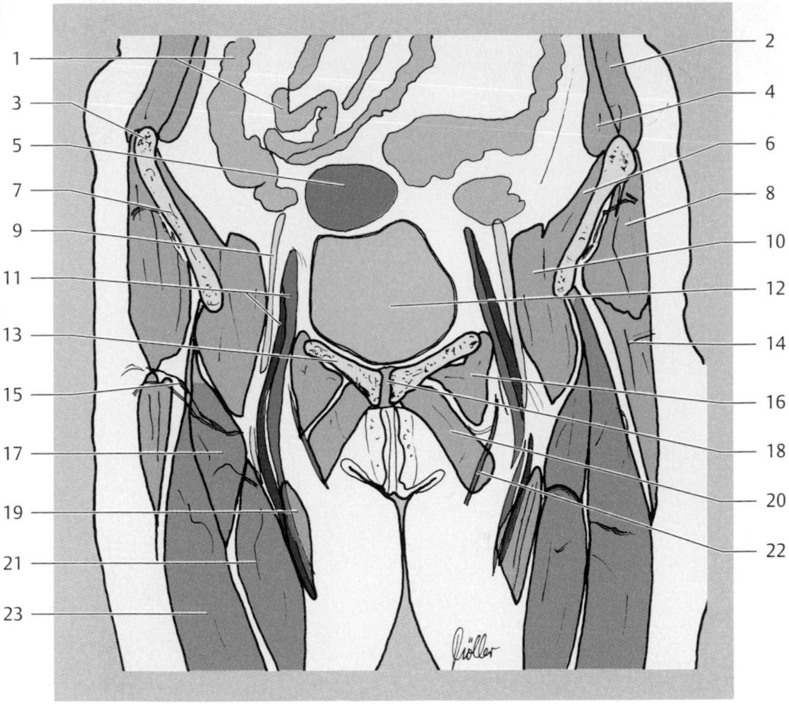

1 Small intestine
2 External oblique and internal oblique abdominal muscles
3 Anterior superior iliac spine
4 Transversus abdominis muscle
5 Uterus
6 Iliacus muscle
7 Ilium
8 Gluteus medius muscle
9 Femoral nerve
10 Iliopsoas muscle
11 Femoral artery and vein
12 Urinary bladder
13 Pubis
14 Tensor fasciae latae muscle
15 Lateral circumflex femoral artery (ascending branch)
16 Pectineus muscle
17 Rectus femoris muscle
18 Symphysis
19 Sartorius muscle
20 Adductor longus muscle
21 Vastus medialis muscle
22 Great saphenous vein
23 Vastus lateralis muscle

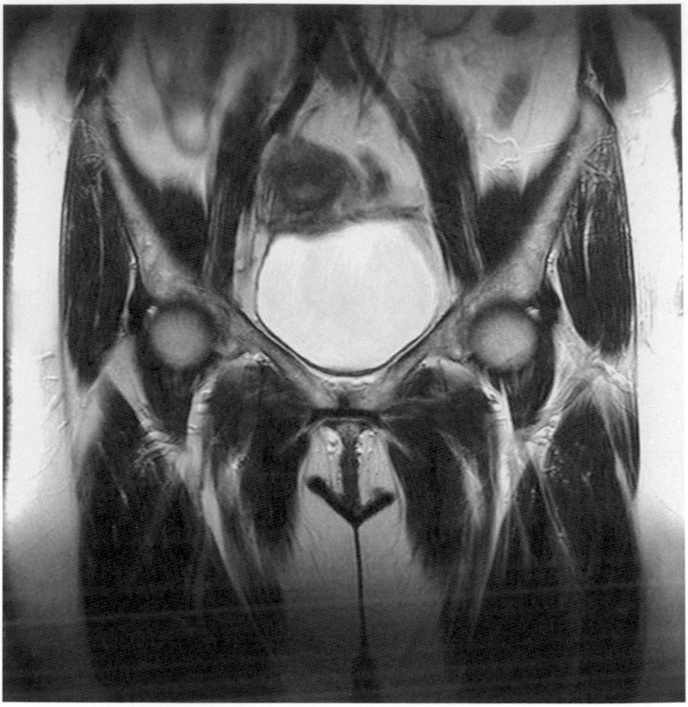

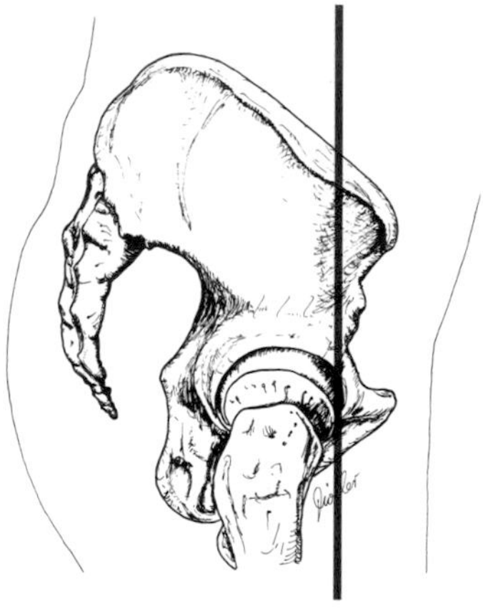

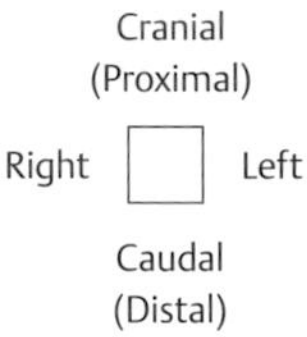

1 Inferior vena cava
2 Aorta (bifurcation)
3 Small intestine
4 Internal oblique muscle of abdomen
5 (Right) Common iliac artery
6 Transversus abdominis muscle

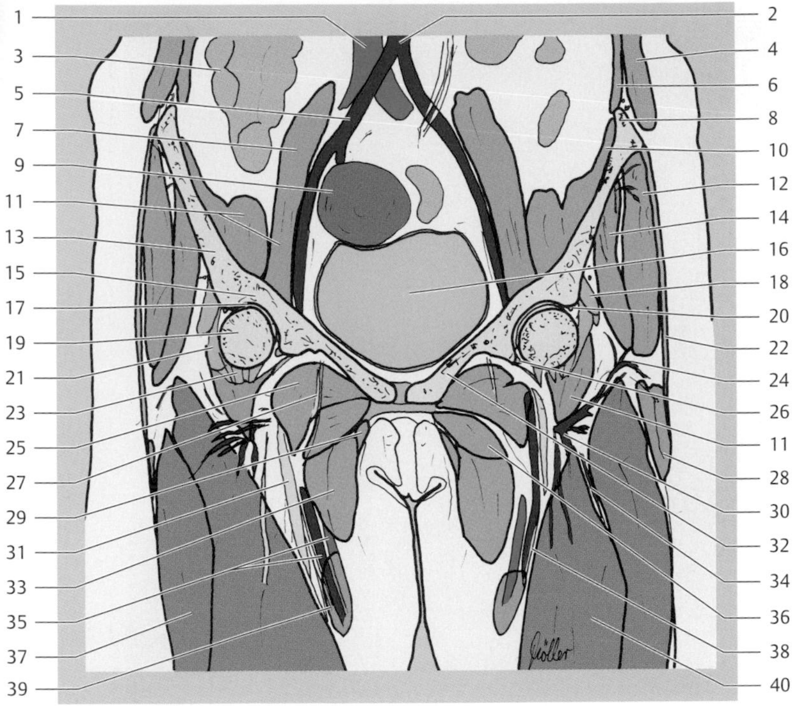

7 Psoas muscle
8 Anterior superior iliac spine
9 Uterus
10 Iliac muscle
11 Iliopsoas muscle
12 Gluteus medius muscle
13 Ilium
14 Gluteus minimus muscle
15 Roof of acetabulum
16 Urinary bladder
17 Hip joint
18 Rectus femoris muscle (tendon)
19 Head of femur
20 Superior glenoid labrum
21 Iliofemoral ligament (transverse part)
22 Iliotibial tract
23 Iliofemoral ligament (descending part)
24 Lateral circumflex femoral artery (ascending branch)
25 Pectineus muscle
26 Inferior glenoid labrum
27 Obturator nerve
28 Tensor fasciae latae muscle
29 Gracilis muscle
30 Deep artery of thigh
31 Femoral nerve
32 Pubis
33 Adductor longus muscle
34 Lateral circumflex femoral artery (descending branch)
35 (Superficial) Femoral artery and vein
36 Adductor brevis muscle
37 Vastus lateralis muscle
38 Saphenous nerve
39 Sartorius muscle
40 Vastus intermedius muscle

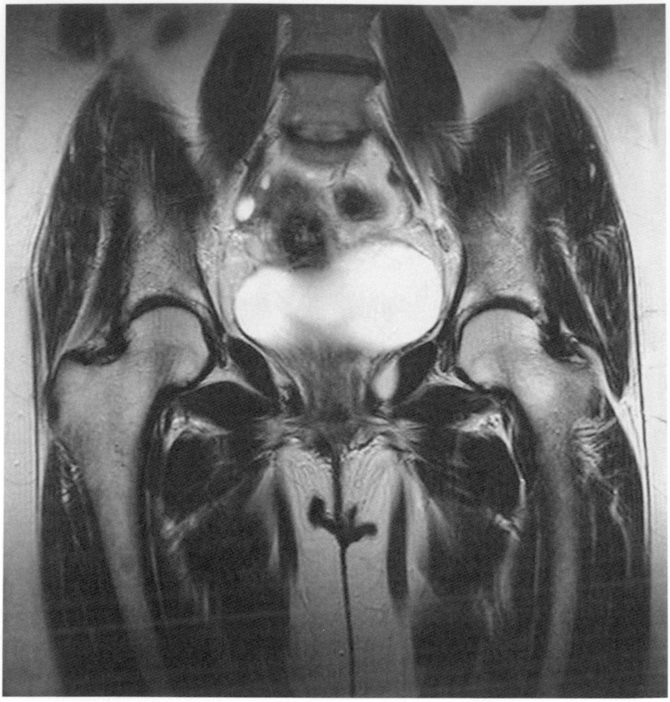

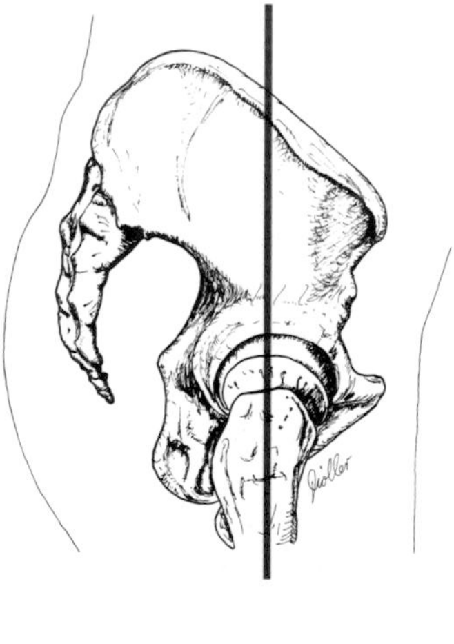

Cranial
(Proximal)

Right Left

Caudal
(Distal)

1 External oblique and internal oblique muscles of abdomen
2 Fourth lumbar vertebra
3 Psoas muscle
4 Anterior superior iliac spine
5 Iliacus muscle

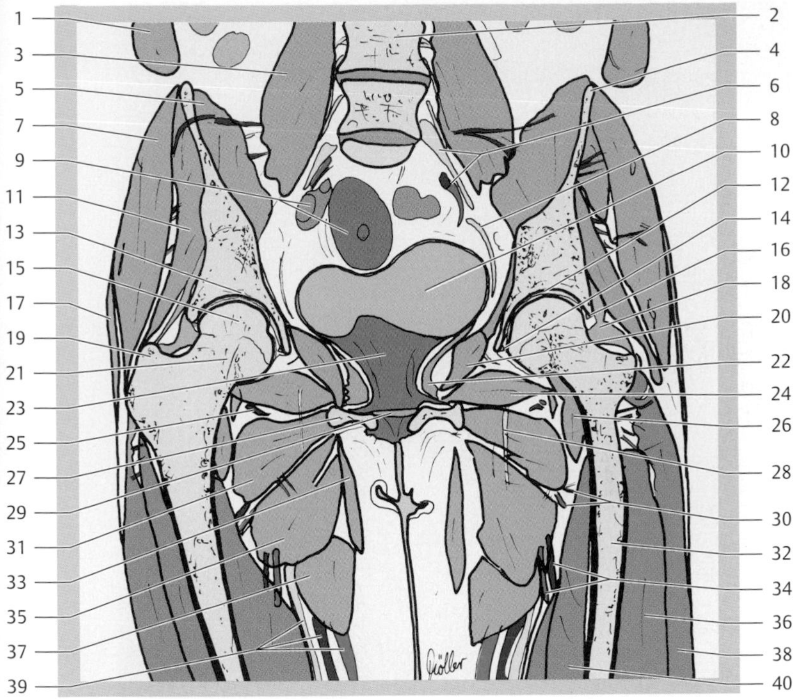

6 Sacral plexus and (left) internal iliac artery and vein
7 Gluteus medius muscle
8 Obturator nerve
9 Ovary and uterus
10 Urinary bladder
11 Gluteus minimus muscle
12 Hip joint
13 Roof of acetabulum
14 Inferior glenoid labrum
15 Head of femur
16 Superior glenoid labrum
17 Iliotibial tract
18 Iliofemoral ligament
19 Greater trochanter
20 Obturator internus muscle
21 Femur (neck)
22 Levator ani muscle
23 Vagina
24 Obturator externus muscle
25 Medial circumflex femoral artery
26 Iliopsoas muscle
27 Pubis
28 Obturator nerve
29 Deep transverse perineal muscle
30 Lateral circumflex femoral artery and vein (descending branch) and femoral nerve (anterior cutaneous branch)
31 Pectineus muscle
32 Femur (shaft)
33 Gracilis muscle
34 Deep artery and vein of thigh
35 Adductor brevis muscle
36 Vastus intermedius muscle
37 Adductor longus muscle
38 Vastus lateralis muscle
39 (Superficial) Femoral artery and vein, and saphenous nerve
40 Vastus medialis muscle

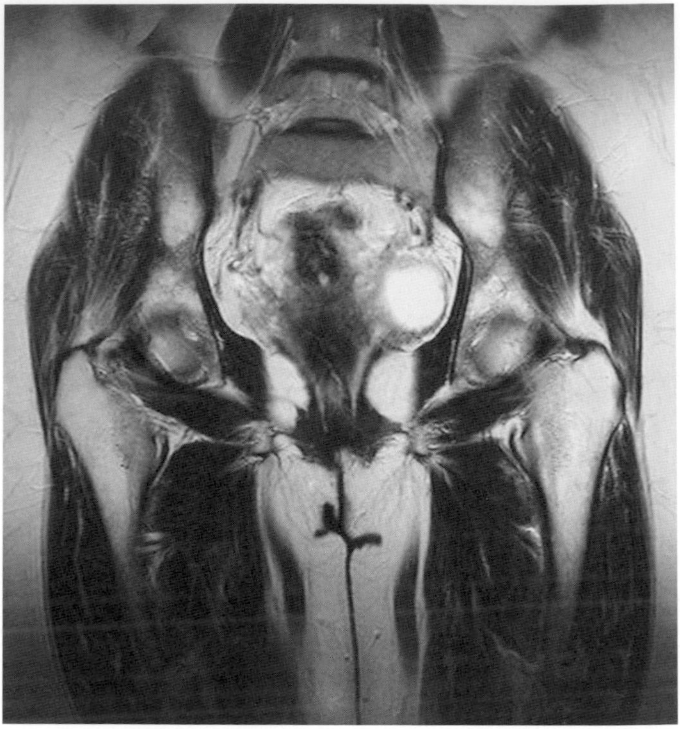

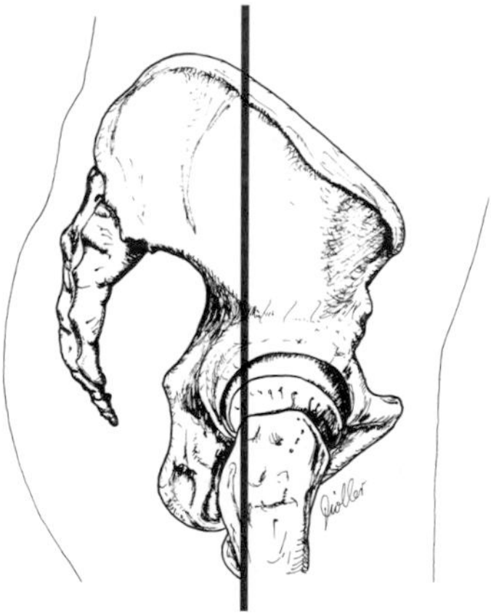

1 Lumbar plexus
2 Psoas muscle
3 Iliac crest
4 Superior gluteal artery and vein
5 Iliacus muscle
6 Sacrum

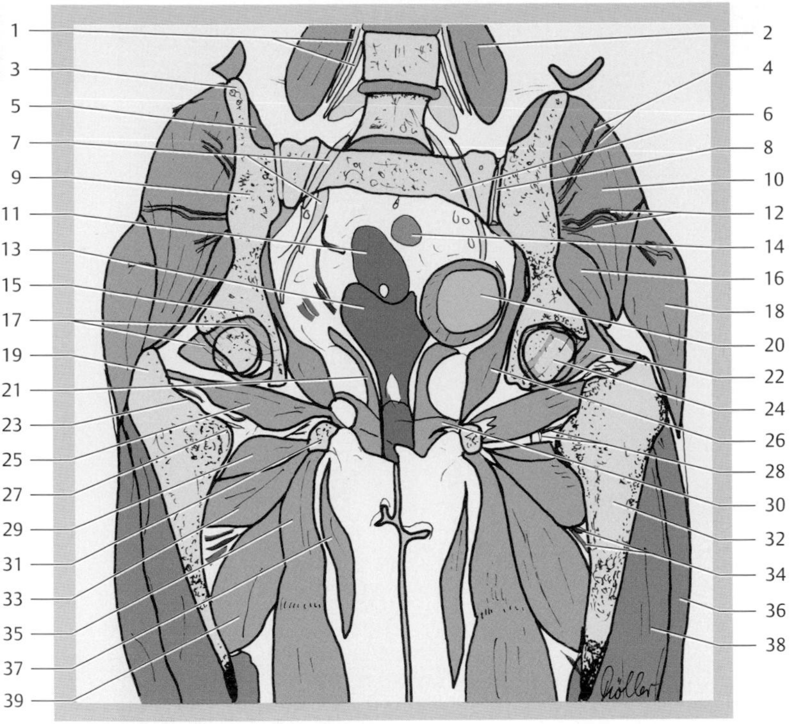

7 Sacral plexus
8 Sacro-iliac joint
9 Ilium
10 Gluteus medius muscle
11 Uterus
12 Inferior gluteal artery and vein
13 Vagina
14 Sigmoid colon
15 Roof of acetabulum
16 Gluteus minimus muscle
17 Zona orbicularis
18 Gluteus maximus muscle
19 Greater trochanter
20 Urinary bladder
21 Levator ani muscle
22 Ischiofemoral ligament
23 Intertrochanteric crest
24 Head of femur
25 Obturator externus muscle
26 Obturator internus muscle
27 Lesser trochanter
28 Medial circumflex femoral artery and vein
29 Adductor minimus muscle
30 Transversus perinei profundus muscle
31 Pubis (inferior ramus)
32 Femur (shaft)
33 Adductor brevis muscle
34 Deep femoral artery and vein
35 Adductor magnus muscle
36 Vastus lateralis muscle
37 Gracilis muscle
38 Vastus intermedius muscle
39 Adductor brevis muscle

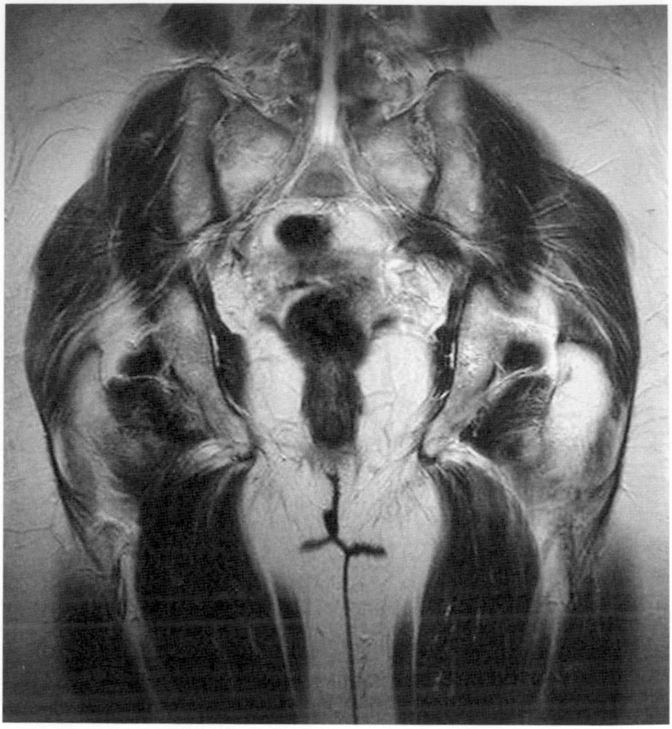

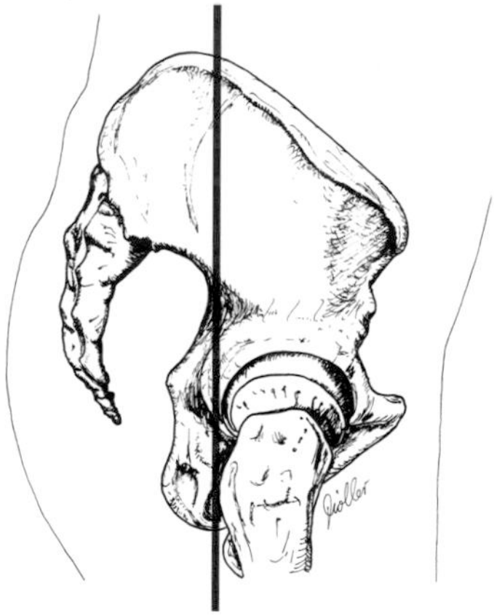

Cranial
(Proximal)

Right Left

Caudal
(Distal)

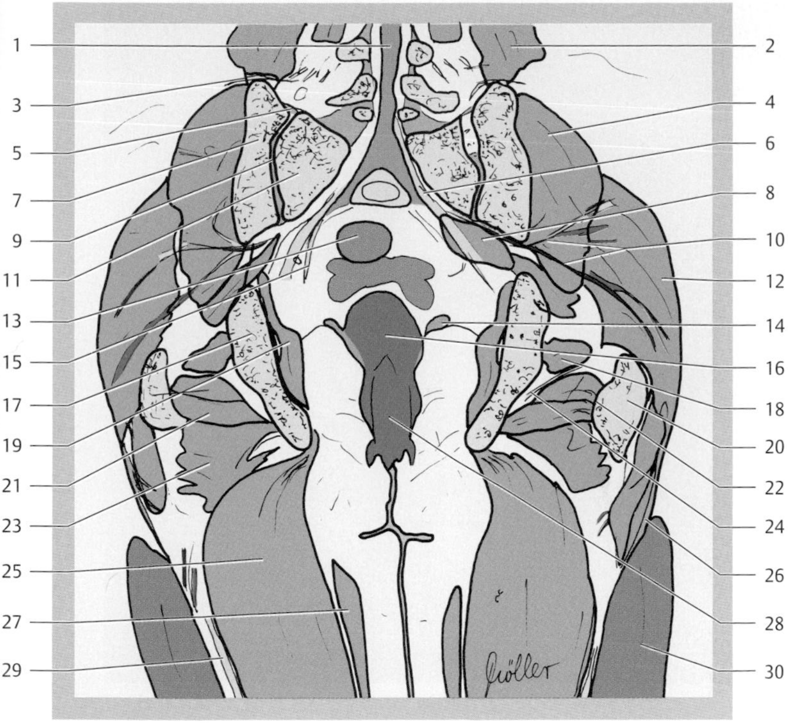

1 Spinal canal
2 External oblique and internal oblique muscles of abdomen
3 Superior clunial nerves
4 Gluteus medius muscle
5 Sacro-iliac ligament
6 Sciatic nerve
7 Ilium
8 Piriformis muscle
9 Sacro-iliac joint
10 Inferior gluteal artery, vein, and nerve
11 Sacrum (lateral mass)
12 Gluteus maximus muscle
13 Sigmoid colon
14 Levator ani muscle
15 Pudendal nerve
16 Uterus
17 Ischium
18 Gemellus superior muscle
19 Obturator internus muscle
20 Greater trochanter
21 Gemellus interior muscle
22 Intertrochanteric crest
23 Quadratus femoris muscle
24 Muscular nerve
25 Adductor magnus muscle
26 Iliotibial tract
27 Gracilis muscle
28 Vagina
29 Sciatic nerve
30 Vastus lateralis muscle

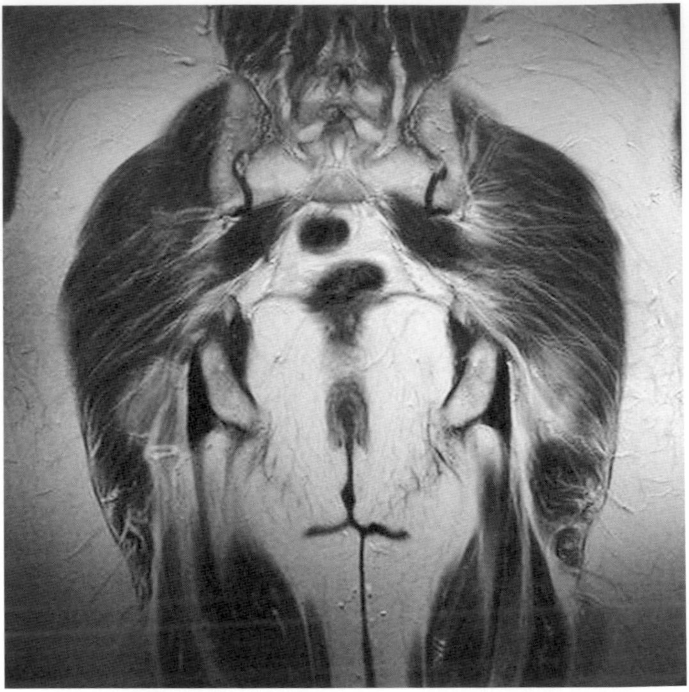

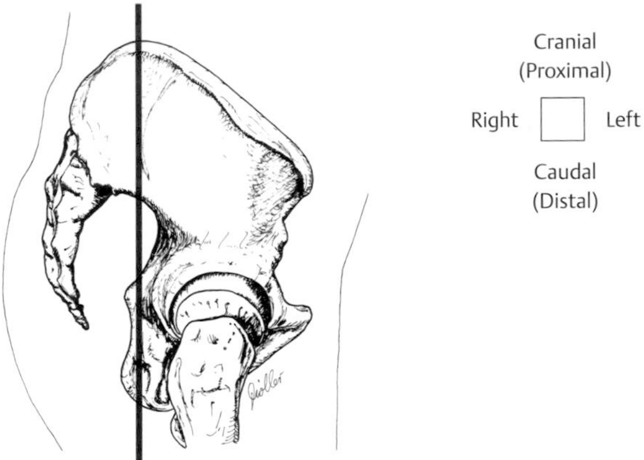
Cranial
(Proximal)
Right
Left
Caudal
(Distal)

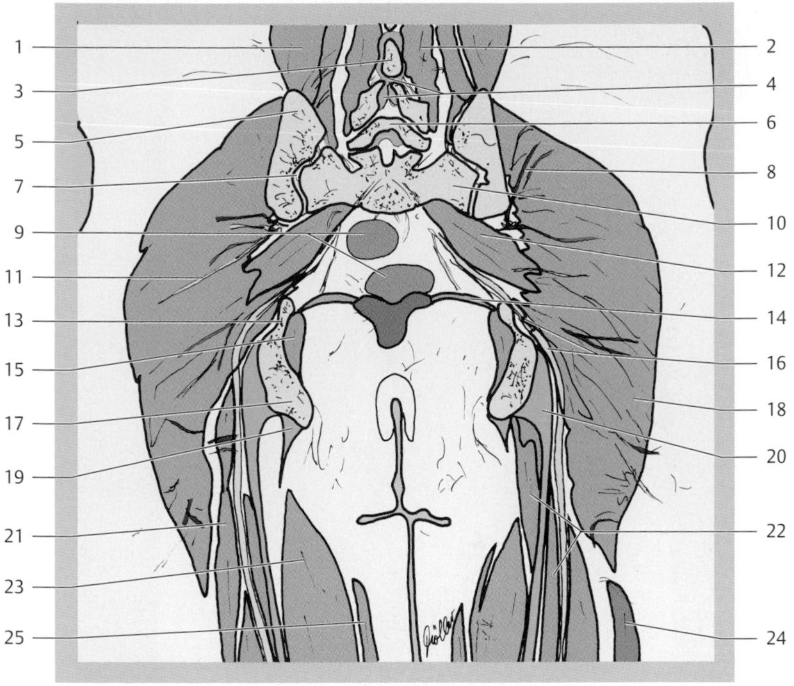

1 Iliocostalis lumborum muscle
2 Multifidus muscle
3 Spinous process
4 Interspinal ligament
5 Ilium
6 Vertebral arch
7 Sacro-iliac joint
8 Superior gluteal artery, vein, and nerve
9 Rectum
10 Sacrum (lateral mass)
11 Inferior gluteal artery, vein, and nerve
12 Piriformis muscle
13 Ischial spine
14 Levator ani muscle
15 Obturator internus muscle
16 Sciatic nerve
17 Ischial tuberosity
18 Gluteus maximus muscle
19 Adductor magnus muscle (attachment)
20 Semitendinosus and biceps femoris muscles (common tendon attachment)
21 Biceps femoris muscle (long head)
22 Semitendinosus muscle
23 Adductor magnus muscle
24 Vastus lateralis muscle
25 Gracilis muscle

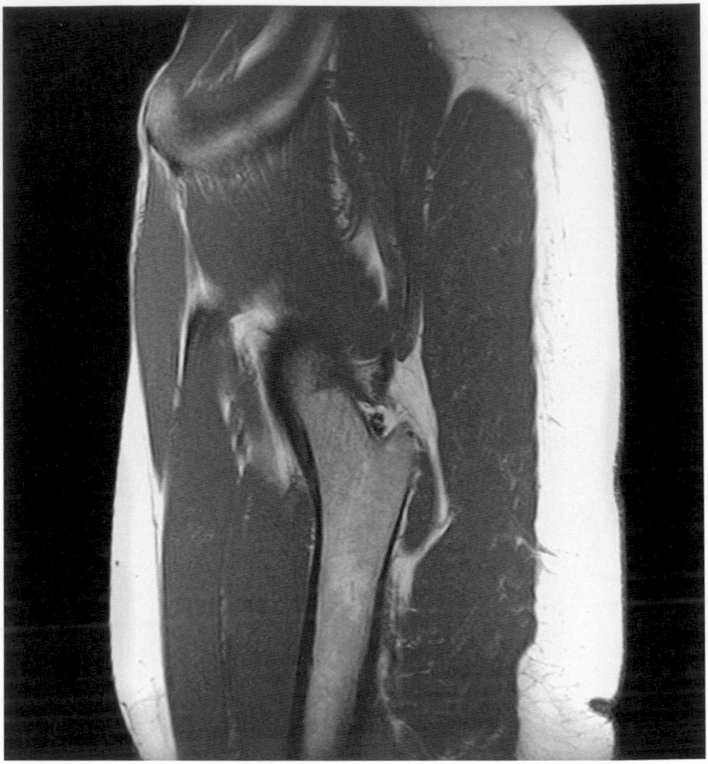

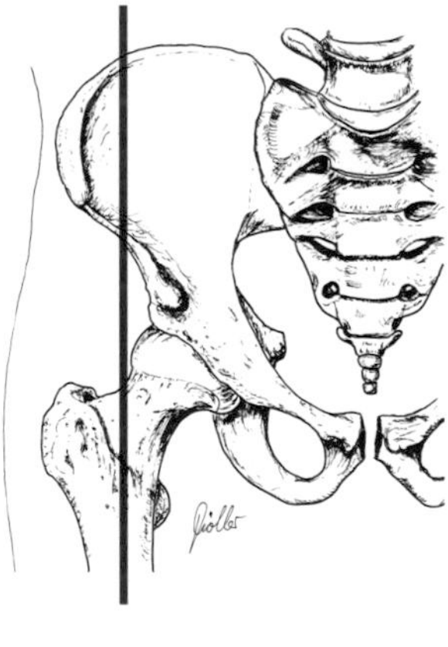

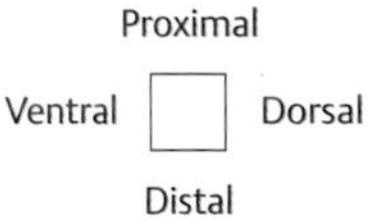
Proximal
Ventral
Dorsal
Distal

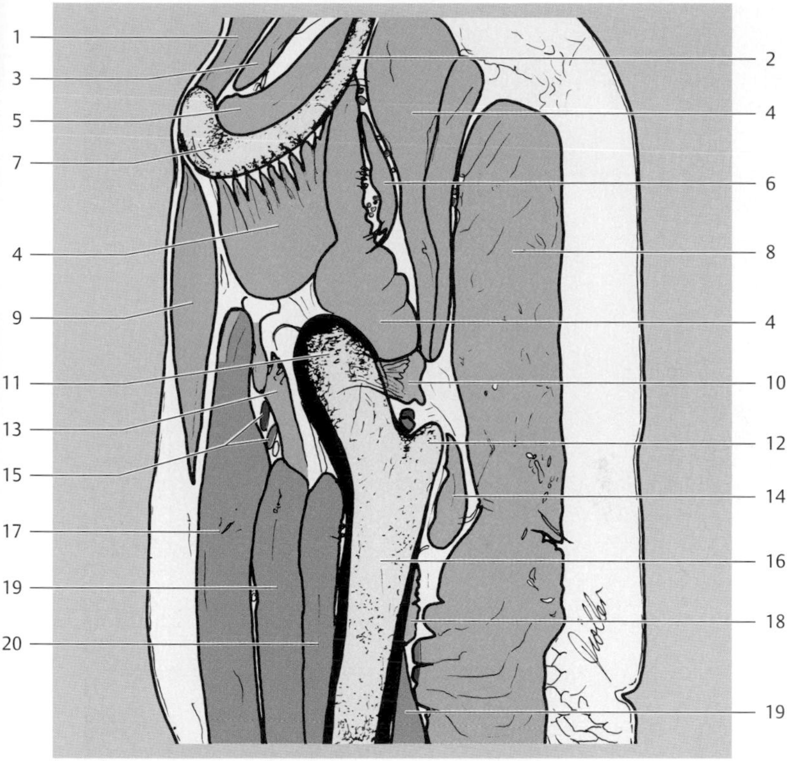

1 External oblique and internal oblique abdominal muscles
2 Ilium (wing)
3 Transversus abdominis muscle
4 Gluteus medius muscle
5 Iliopsoas muscle
6 Gluteus minimus muscle
7 Anterior superior iliac spine
8 Gluteus maximus muscle
9 Sartorius muscle
10 Obturator internus muscle and gemellus muscles
11 Femur (neck)
12 Greater trochanter
13 Iliopsoas muscle
14 Quadratus femoris muscle
15 Lateral circumflex femoral artery and vein
16 Femur (shaft)
17 Rectus femoris muscle
18 Adductor magnus muscle (tendon attachment)
19 Vastus intermedius muscle
20 Vastus medialis muscle

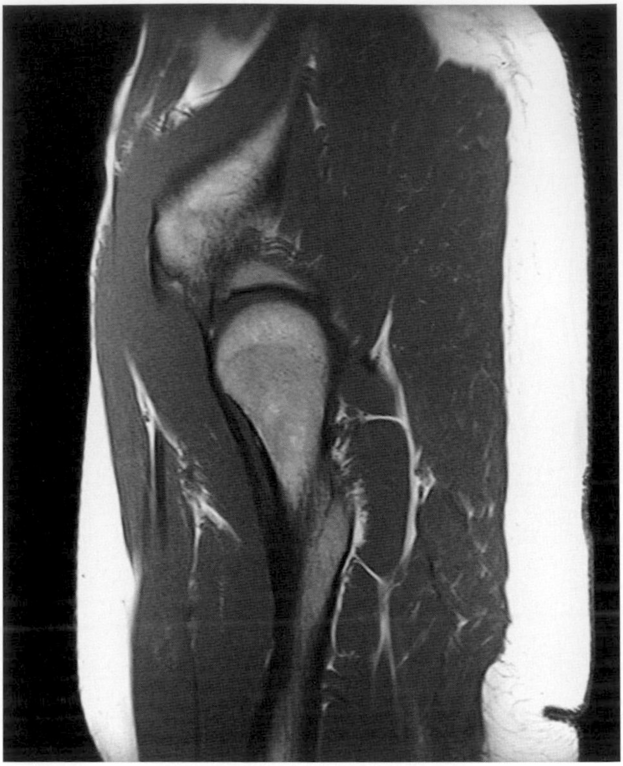

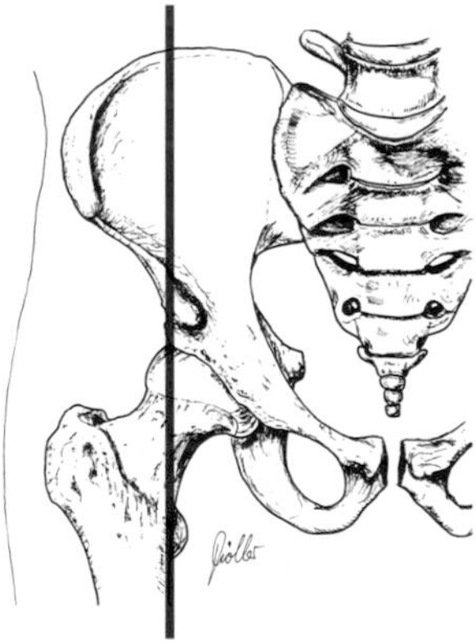

Proximal

Ventral ☐ Dorsal

Distal

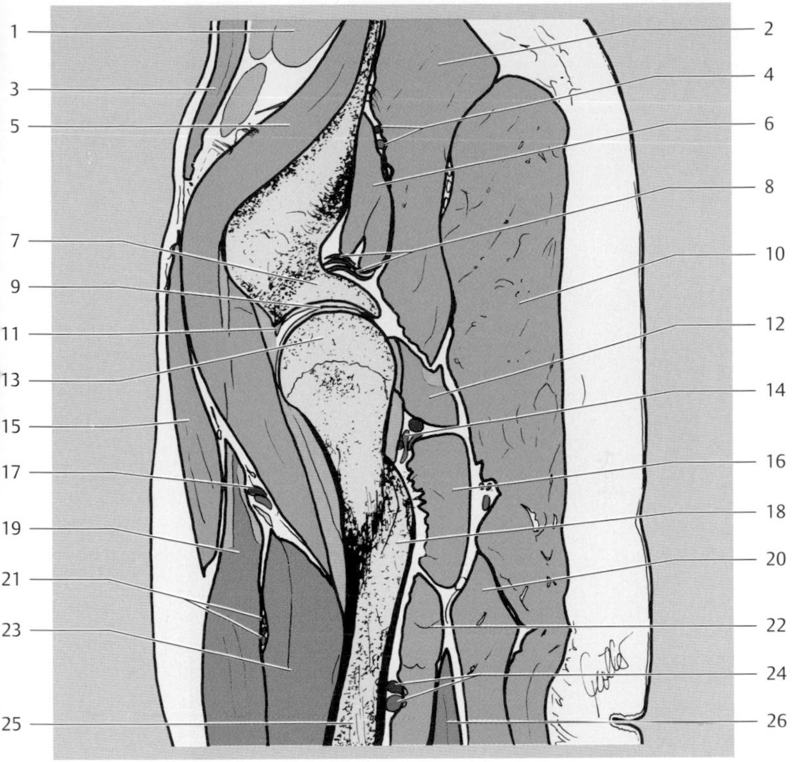

1 Small intestine
2 Gluteus medius muscle
3 Rectus abdominis muscle
4 Superior gluteal artery and vein
5 Iliopsoas muscle
6 Gluteus minimus muscle
7 Ilium (roof of acetabulum)
8 Superficial circumflex iliac artery
9 Hip joint
10 Gluteus maximus muscle
11 Superior glenoid labrum
12 Obturator internus muscle and gemellus muscles
13 Femur (head)
14 Medial circumflex femoral artery
15 Sartorius muscle
16 Quadratus femoris muscle
17 Lateral circumflex femoral artery (ascending branch)
18 Lesser trochanter
19 Rectus femoris muscle
20 Biceps femoris muscle (long head)
21 Lateral circumflex femoral artery (descending branch)
22 Adductor magnus muscle
23 Vastus intermedius muscle
24 Perforating artery and vein
25 Femur (shaft)
26 Vastus lateralis muscle

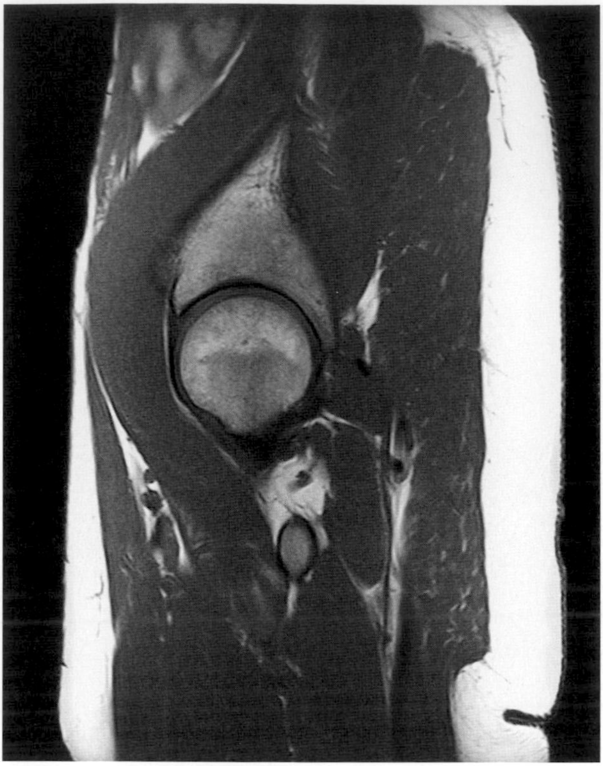

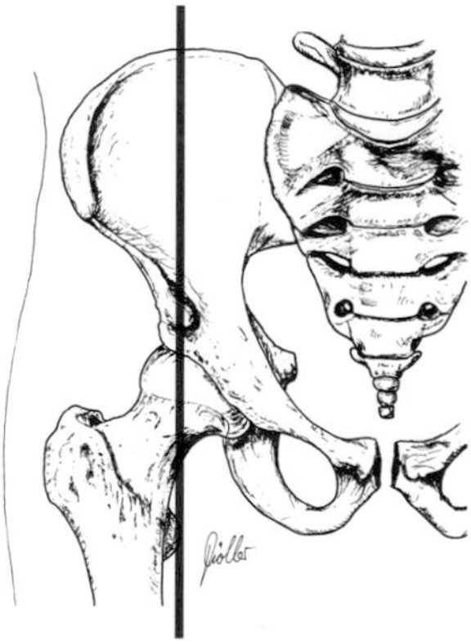

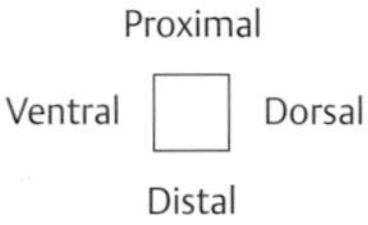
Proximal
Ventral
Dorsal
Distal

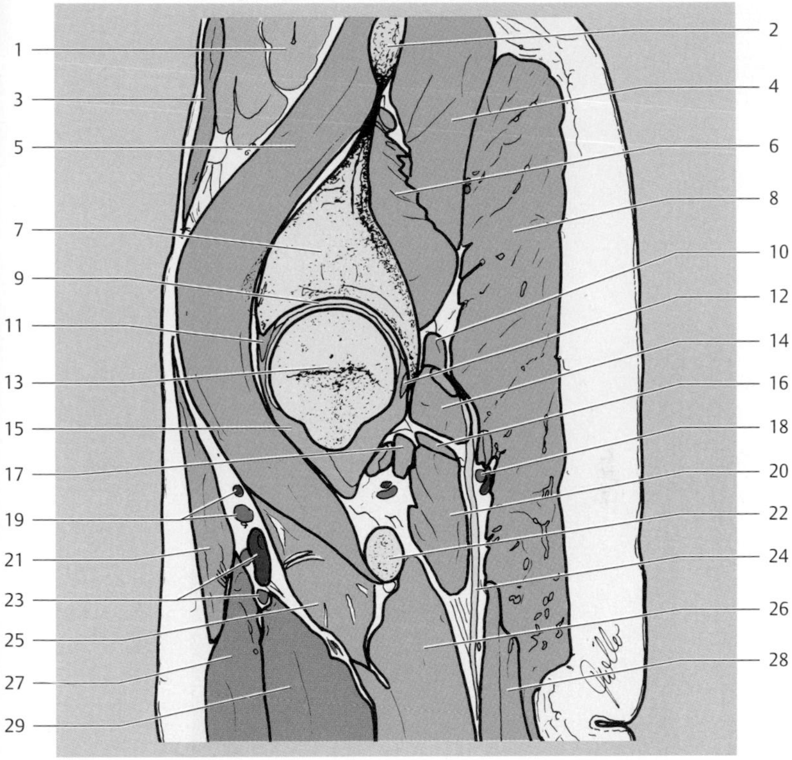

1 Small intestine
2 Ilium
3 Rectus abdominis muscle
4 Gluteus medius muscle
5 Iliopsoas muscle
6 Gluteus minimus muscle
7 Ilium (roof of acetabulum)
8 Gluteus maximus muscle
9 Hip joint
10 Piriformis muscle
11 Superior glenoid labrum
12 Inferior glenoid labrum
13 Femur (head)
14 Obturator internus muscle and gemellus muscles
15 Joint capsule
16 Adductor minimus muscle
17 Obturator externus muscle
18 Inferior gluteal artery and vein
19 Lateral circumflex femoral artery and vein (ascending branch)
20 Quadratus femoris muscle
21 Sartorius muscle
22 Lesser trochanter
23 Lateral circumflex femoral artery and vein (descending branch)
24 Sciatic nerve
25 Pectineus muscle
26 Adductor magnus muscle
27 Rectus femoris muscle
28 Biceps femoris muscle
29 Vastus medialis muscle

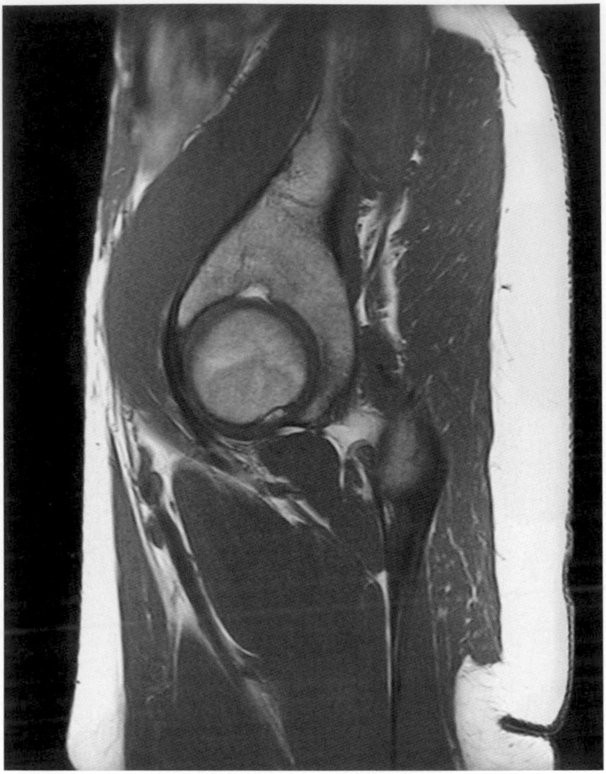

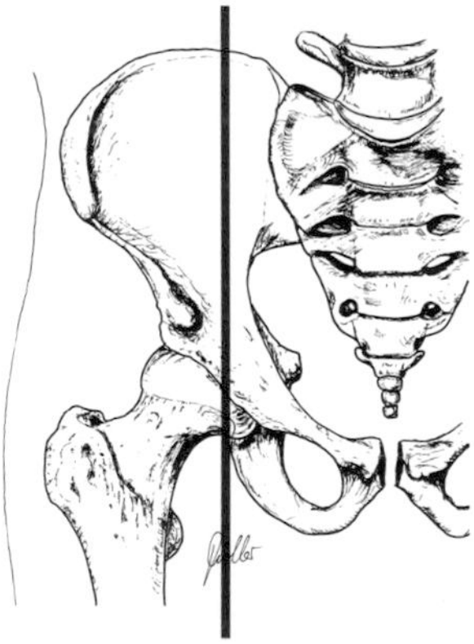

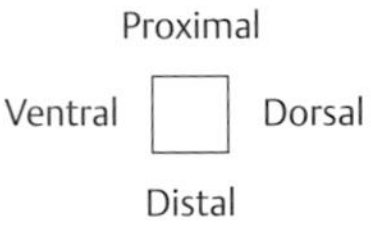

1 Small intestine
2 Gluteus medius muscle
3 Rectus abdominis muscle
4 Ilium
5 Iliopsoas muscle

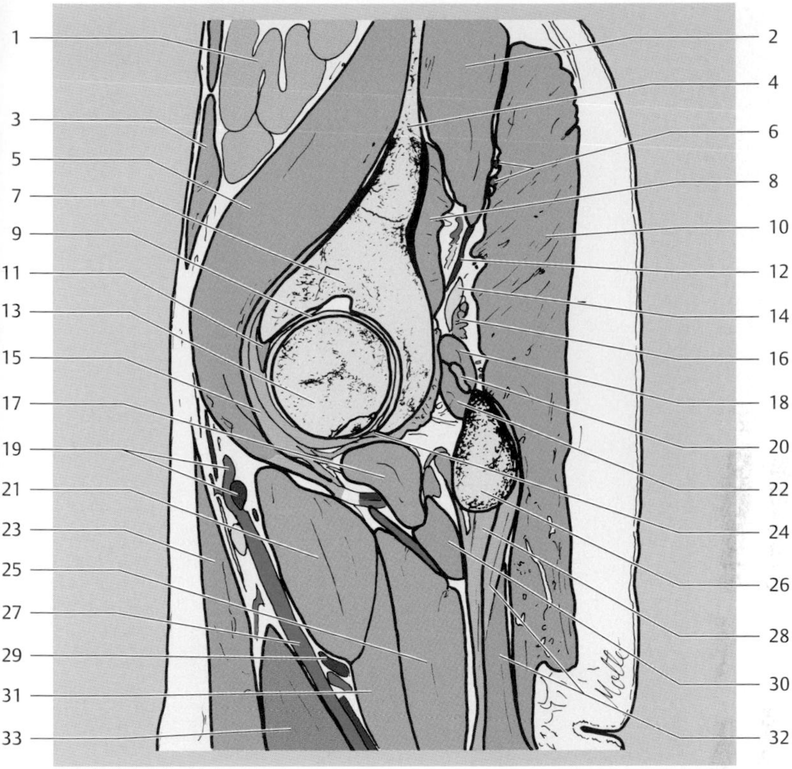

6 Superior gluteal artery, vein, and nerve
7 Ilium (roof of acetabulum)
8 Gluteus minimus muscle
9 Hip joint
10 Gluteus maximus muscle
11 Superior glenoid labrum
12 Superior gluteal artery and vein, inferior gluteal nerve
13 Femur (head)
14 Sciatic nerve
15 Joint capsule
16 Piriformis
17 Obturator externus
18 Obturator internus and gemellus muscles
19 Lateral circumflex femoris artery and vein (ascending branch)
20 Obturator internus muscle (tendon)
21 Pectineus muscle
22 Gemellus inferior muscle
23 Sartorius muscle
24 Inferior glenoid labrum
25 Adductor magnus muscle
26 Ischium
27 Deep artery and vein of thigh
28 Semimembranosus and semitendinosus muscles (tendon attachment)
29 Perforating arteries
30 Quadratus femoris muscle
31 Adductor brevis muscle
32 Biceps femoris muscle (+ tendon)
33 Vastus medialis muscle

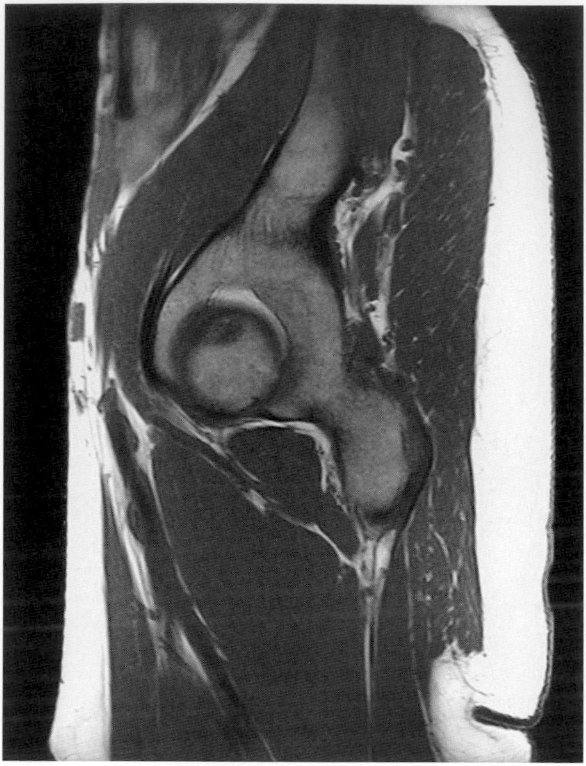

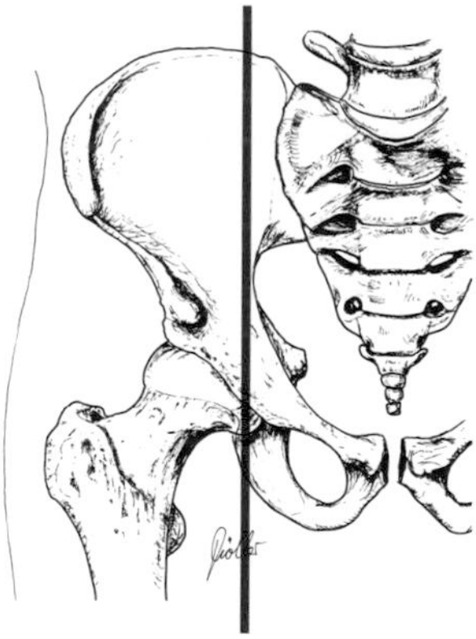

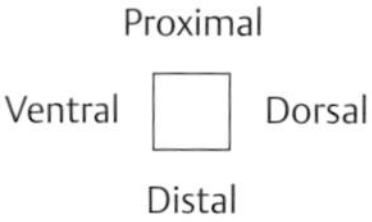
Proximal
Ventral
Dorsal
Distal

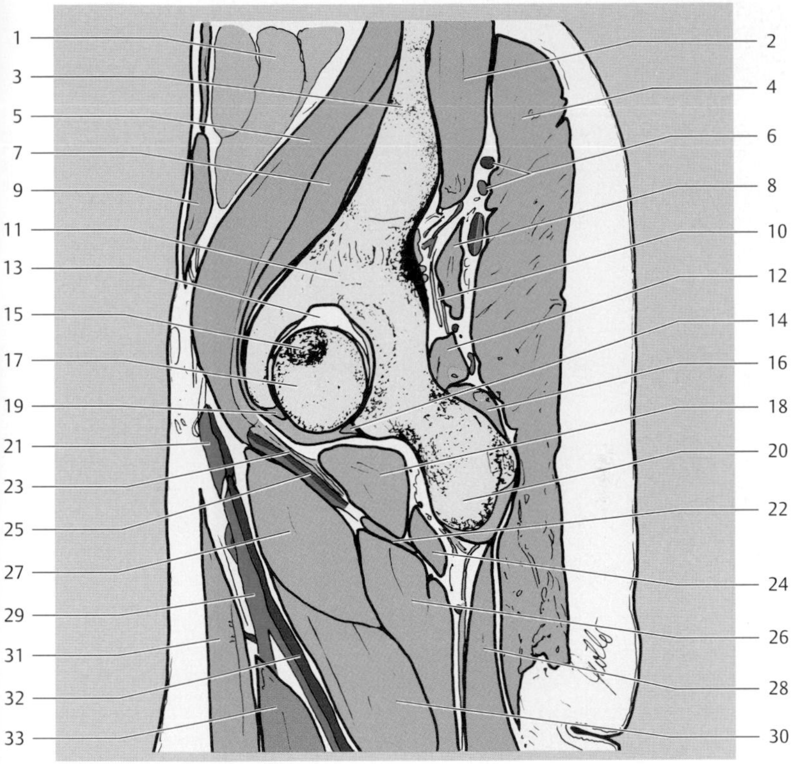

1 Small intestine
2 Gluteus medius muscle
3 Ilium
4 Gluteus maximus muscle
5 Psoas muscle
6 Superior gluteal artery, vein, and nerve
7 Iliacus muscle
8 Piriformis muscle
9 Rectus abdominis muscle
10 Sciatic nerve
11 Ilium (roof of acetabulum)
12 Gemellus superior muscle
13 Acetabular fossa
14 Inferior glenoid labrum
15 Fovea
16 Gemellus inferior muscle
17 Femur (head)
18 Obturator externus muscle
19 Superior glenoid labrum
20 Ischium
21 Lateral circumflex femoral artery and vein
22 Adductor minimus muscle
23 Ischiofemoral ligament
24 Quadratus femoris muscle
25 Lateral circumflex femoral artery
26 Adductor magnus muscle
27 Pectineus muscle
28 Biceps femoris muscle
29 (Superficial) Femoral artery and vein
30 Adductor brevis muscle
31 Sartorius muscle
32 Deep artery and vein of thigh
33 Vastus medialis muscle

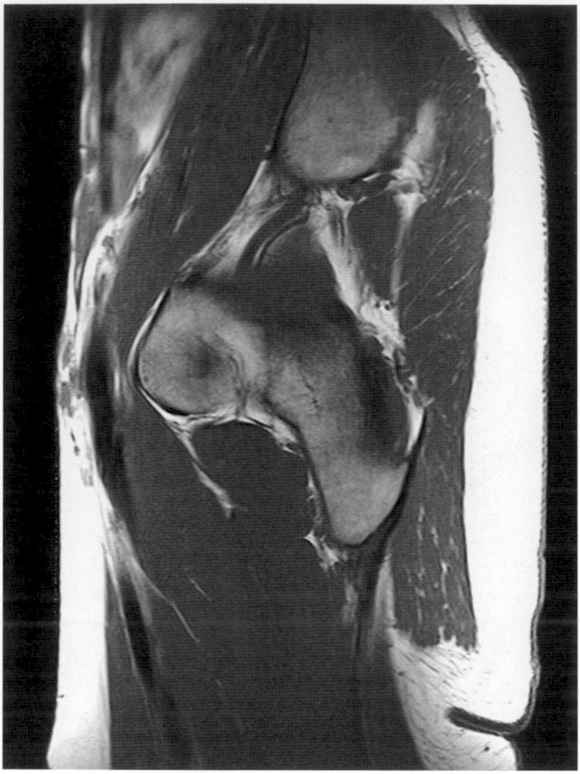

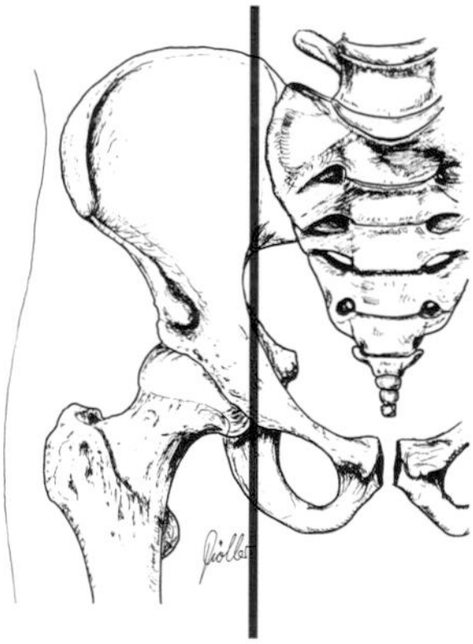

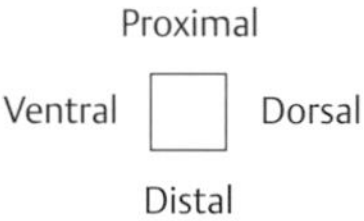
Proximal
Ventral
Dorsal
Distal

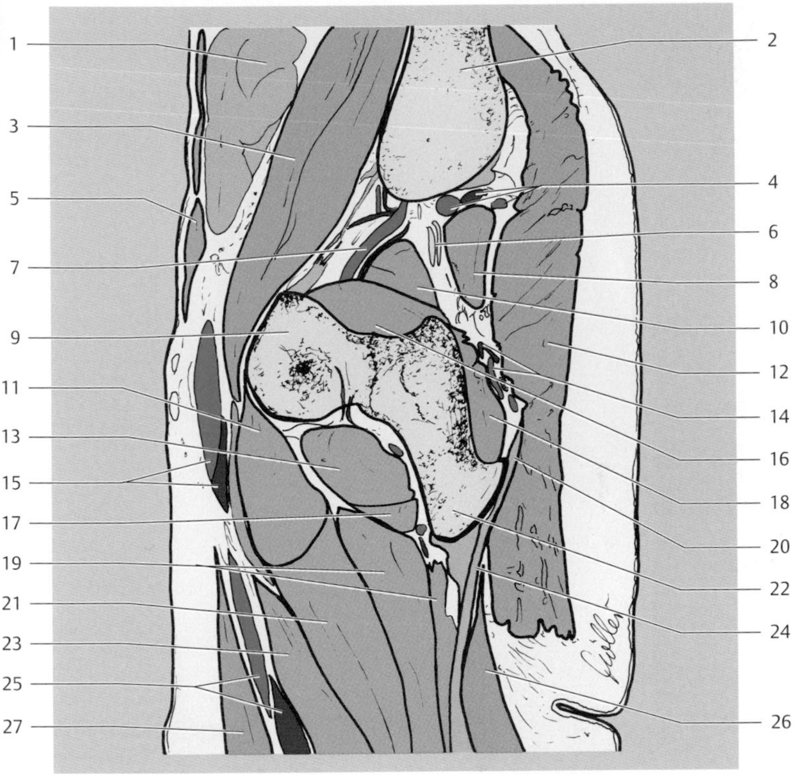

1 Small intestine
2 Ilium
3 Iliopsoas muscle
4 Superior gluteal artery, vein, and nerve
5 Rectus abdominis muscle
6 Sciatic nerve
7 Internal iliac artery and vein
8 Piriformis muscle
9 Ilium (joint socket)
10 Gemellus superior muscle
11 Pectineus muscle
12 Gluteus maximus muscle
13 Obturator externus muscle
14 Inferior gluteal artery and nerve
15 Femoral artery and vein
16 Obturator internus muscle
17 Adductor minimus muscle
18 Gemellus inferior muscle
19 Adductor magnus muscle
20 Sacrotuberous ligament
21 Adductor brevis muscle
22 Ischial tuberosity
23 Adductor longus muscle
24 Biceps femoris muscle (common tendon)
25 (Superficial) Femoral artery and vein
26 Biceps femoris muscle
27 Sartorius muscle

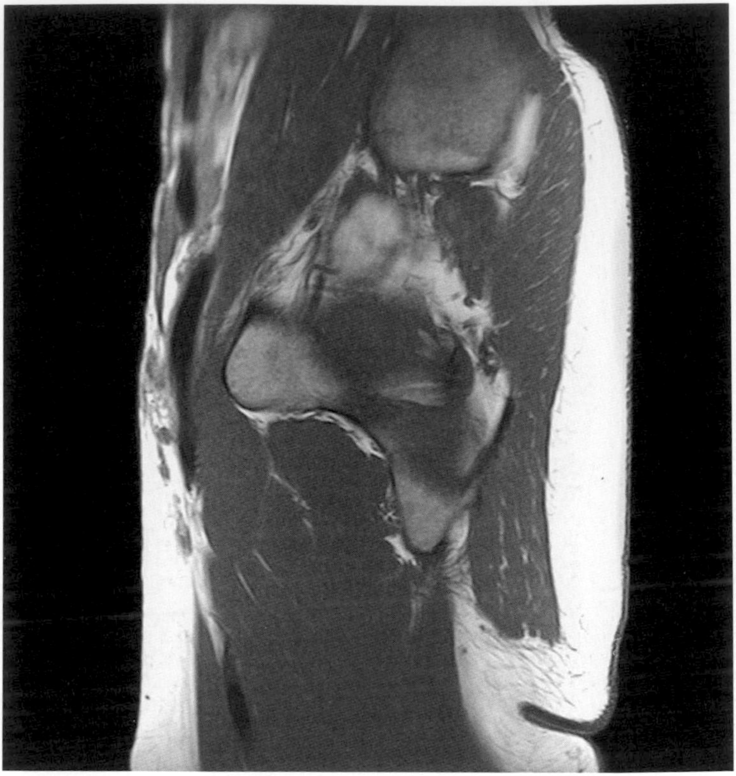

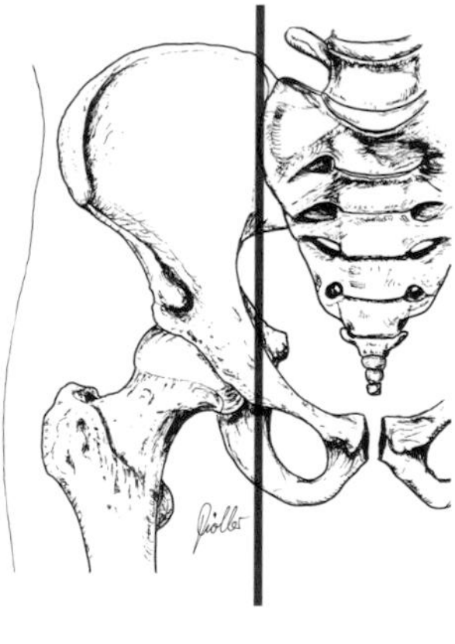

Proximal

Ventral Dorsal

Distal

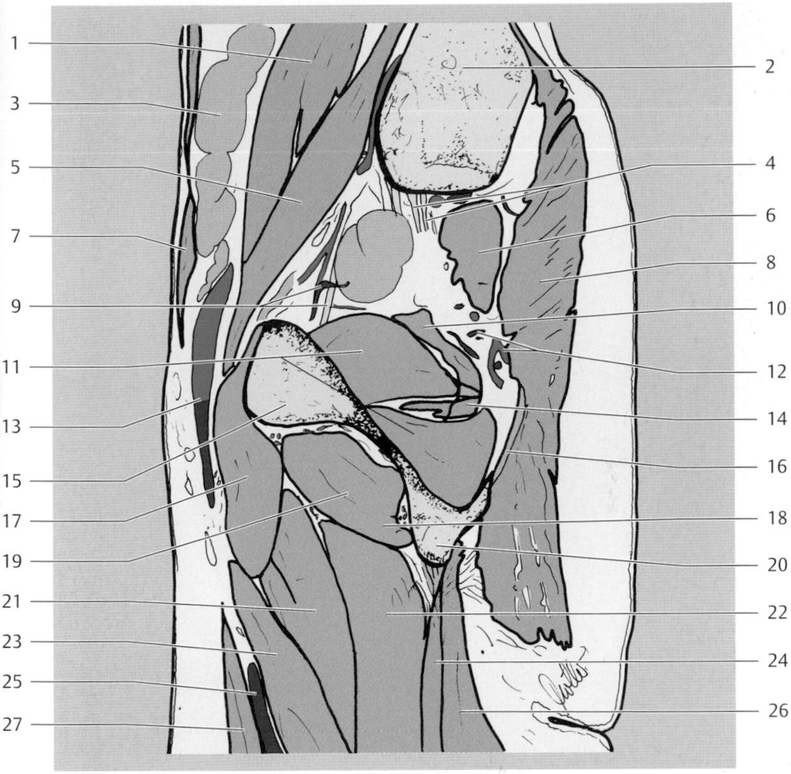

1 Psoas muscle
2 Ilium (wing)
3 Small intestine (ileum)
4 Sacral plexus
5 Iliacus muscle
6 Piriformis muscle
7 Rectus abdominis muscle
8 Gluteus maximus muscle
9 Obturator artery and nerve
10 Gemellus superior muscle
11 Obturator internus muscle
12 Superior gluteal artery and vein and inferior gluteal nerve
13 Femoral artery and vein
14 Gemellus inferior muscle
15 Pubis
16 Sacrotuberous ligament
17 Pectineus muscle
18 Adductor minimus muscle
19 Obturator externus muscle
20 Ischial tuberosity
21 Adductor brevis muscle
22 Adductor magnus muscle
23 Adductor longus muscle
24 Semimembranosus muscle
25 (Superficial) Femoral artery
26 Semitendinosus muscle
27 Sartorius muscle

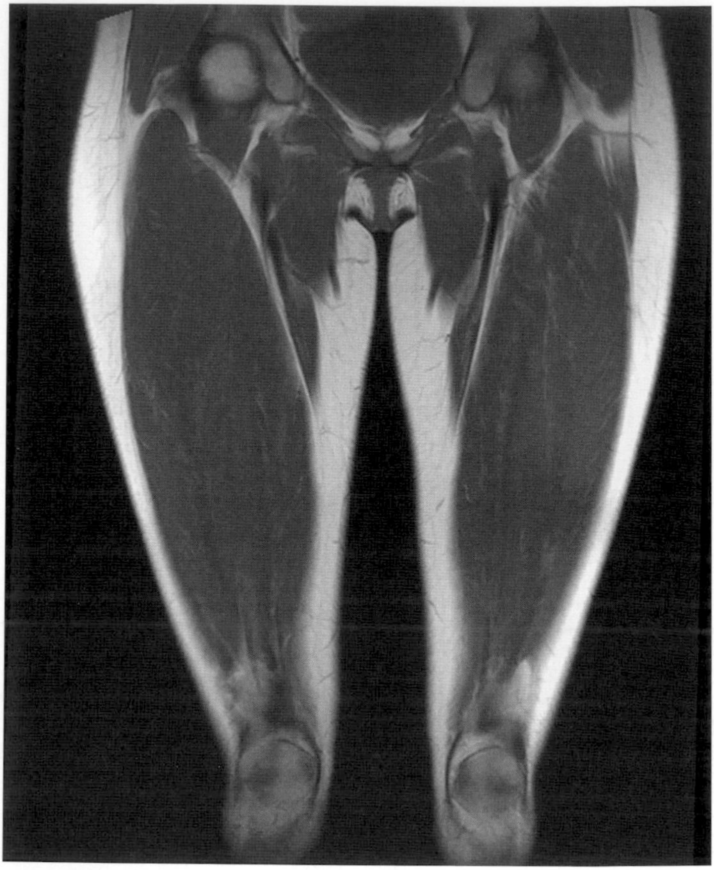

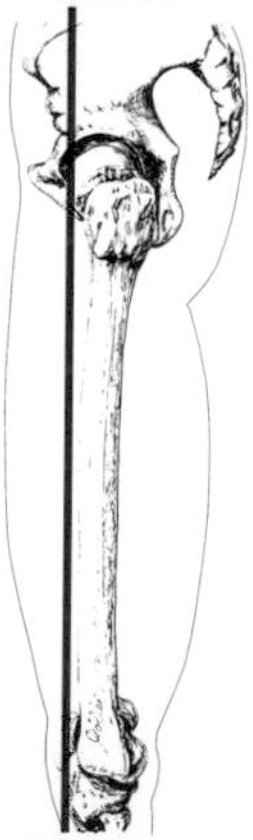

Cranial

Distal

1 Gluteus minimus muscle
2 Gluteus medius muscle
3 Roof of acetabulum
4 Iliofemoral ligament
5 Superior glenoid labrum

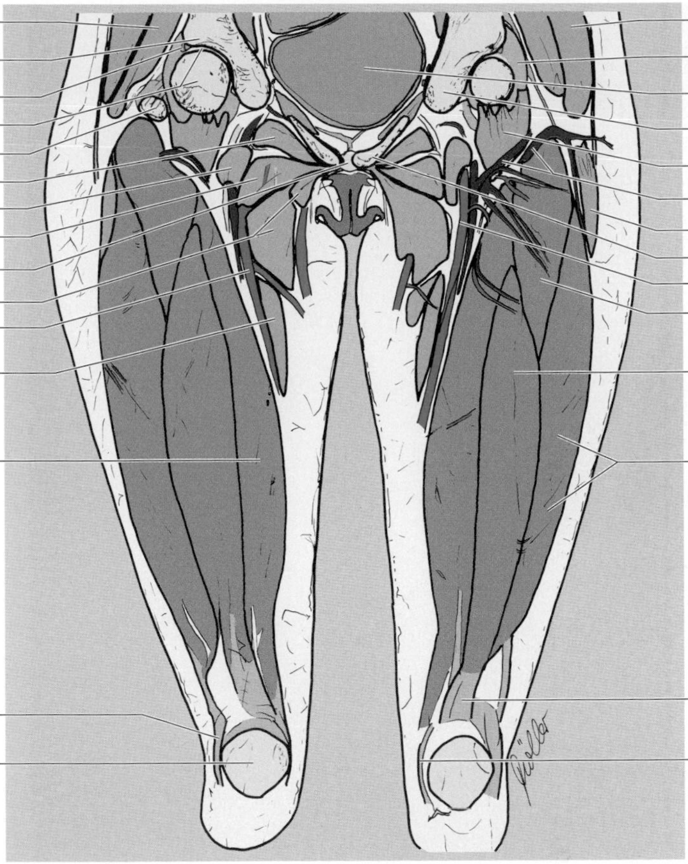

6 Urinary bladder
7 Hip joint + head of femur
8 Pubis (body)
9 Greater trochanter
10 Iliopsoas muscle
11 Obturatorius externus muscle
12 Lateral circumflex femoral artery and vein
13 Pectineus muscle
14 Tensor fasciae latae muscle
15 Adductor brevis muscle
16 Pubis (superior ramus)
17 Symphysis
18 Femoral artery and vein
19 Adductor longus muscle
20 Rectus femoris muscle
21 Great saphenous vein
22 Vastus intermedius muscle
23 Sartorius muscle
24 Vastus lateralis muscle
25 Vastus medialis muscle
26 Quadriceps tendon
27 Lateral patellar retinaculum
28 Medial patellar retinaculum
29 Patella

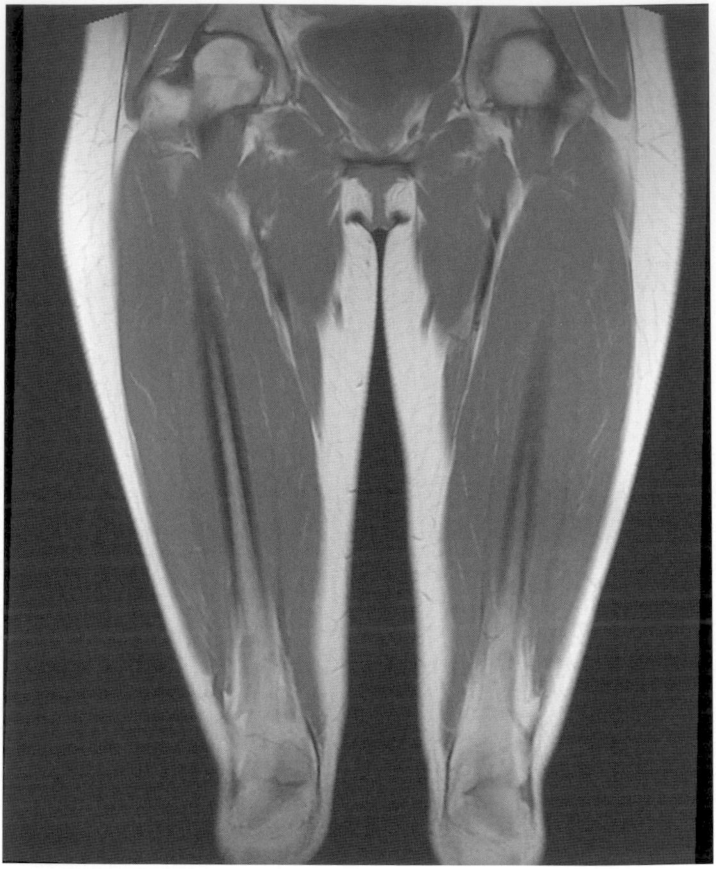

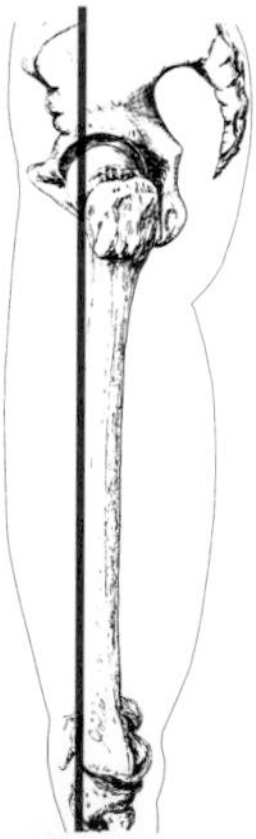

Cranial

Distal

1 Gluteus medius muscle
2 Gluteus minimus muscle
3 Roof of acetabulum
4 Urinary bladder
5 Hip joint
6 Head of femur

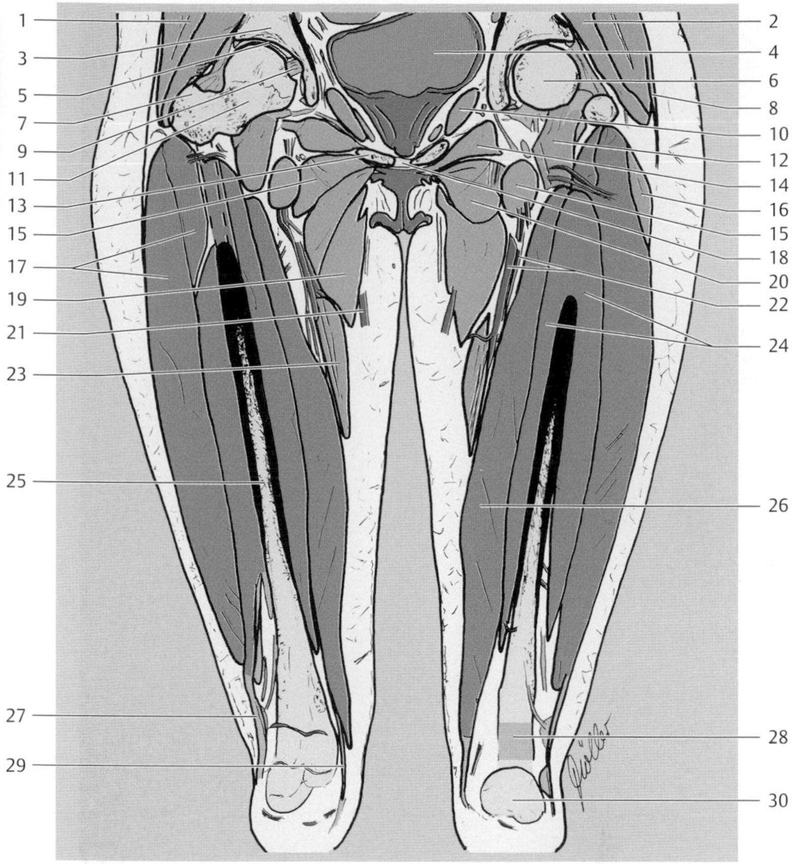

7 Greater trochanter
8 Iliotibial tract
9 Ligament of head of femur
10 Obturator internus muscle
11 Femur (neck)
12 Iliopsoas muscle
13 Pubis (inferior ramus)
14 Obturatorius externus muscle
15 Pectineus muscle
16 Tensor fasciae latae muscle
17 Vastus lateralis muscle
18 Symphysis
19 Adductor longus muscle
20 Adductor brevis muscle
21 Great saphenous vein
22 Femoral artery and vein
23 Sartorius muscle
24 Vastus intermedius muscle
25 Femur (shaft)
26 Vastus medialis muscle
27 Lateral patellar retinaculum
28 Quadriceps tendon
29 Medial patellar retinaculum
30 Patella

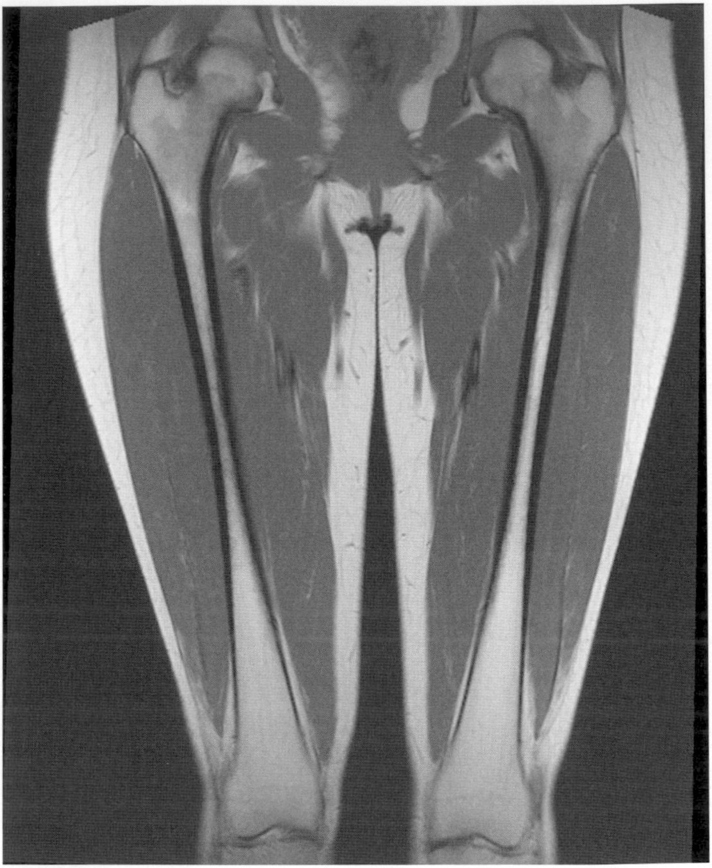

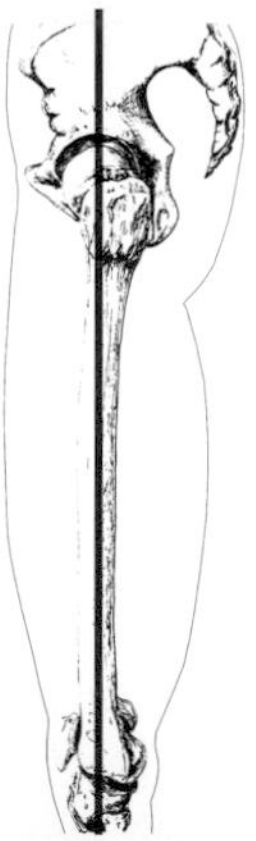

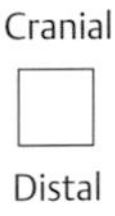

1 Gluteus medius muscle
2 Gluteus minimus muscle
3 Roof of acetabulum
4 Hip joint
5 Head of femur
6 Ligament of head of femur

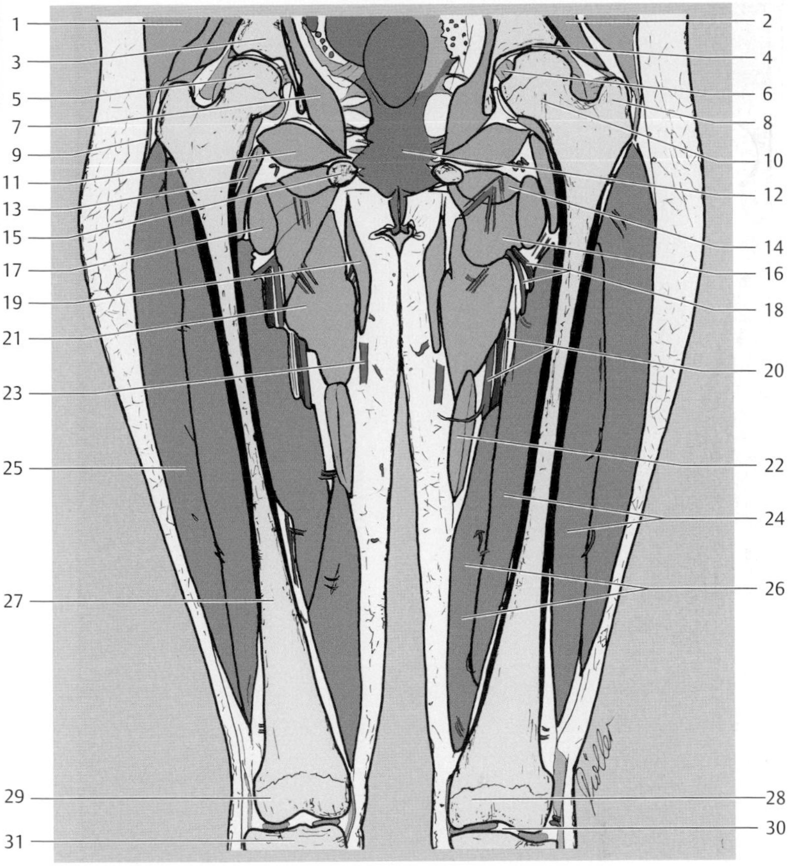

7 Obturator internus muscle
8 Greater trochanter
9 Iliotibial tract
10 Femur (neck)
11 Obturator externus muscle
12 Vagina
13 Iliopsoas muscle (tendon)
14 Adductor minimus muscle
15 Pubis (inferior ramus)
16 Adductor brevis muscle
17 Pectineus muscle
18 Deep femoral artery and vein
19 Gracilis muscle
20 Femoral artery and vein and saphenous nerve
21 Adductor longus muscle
22 Sartorius muscle
23 Great saphenous vein
24 Vastus intermedius muscle
25 Vastus lateralis muscle
26 Vastus medialis muscle
27 Femur (shaft)
28 Medial femoral condyle
29 Lateral femoral condyle
30 Knee joint
31 Head of tibia

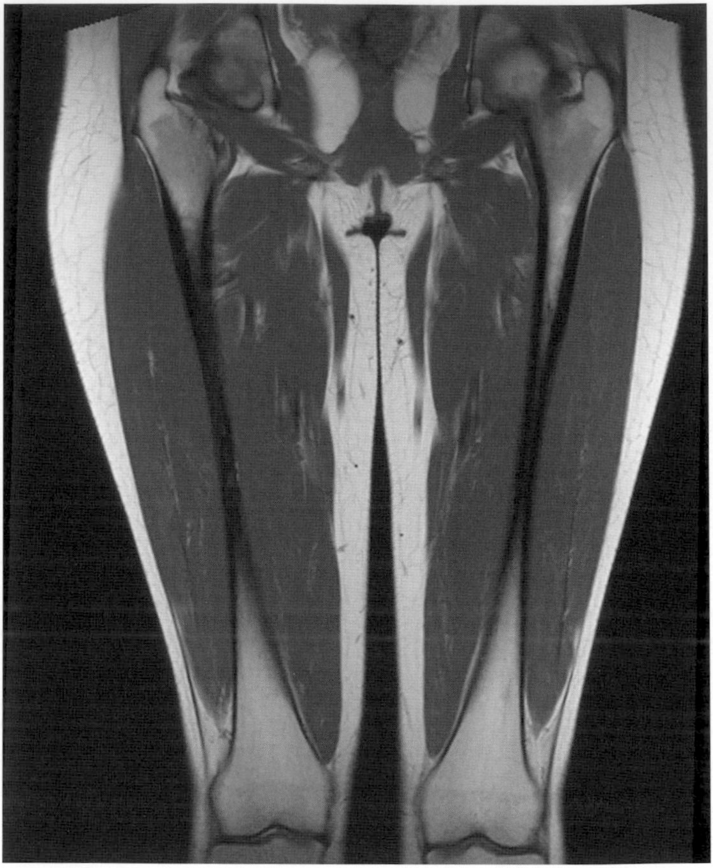

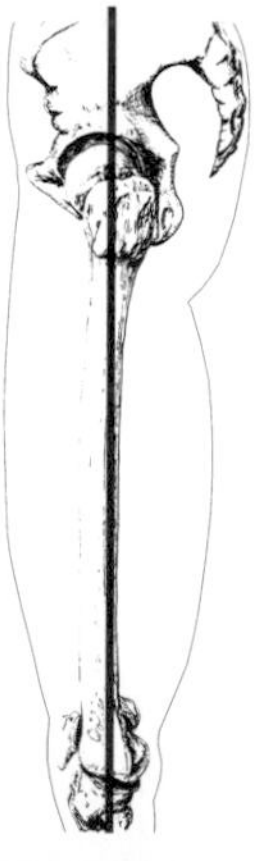

1 Gluteus medius muscle
2 Gluteus minimus muscle
3 Iliacus muscle
4 Roof of acetabulum
5 Piriformis muscle
6 Head of femur
7 Gemellus superior + inferior muscles
8 Greater trochanter
9 Obturator internus muscle
10 Femur (neck)
11 Iliotibial tract
12 Obturator externus muscle

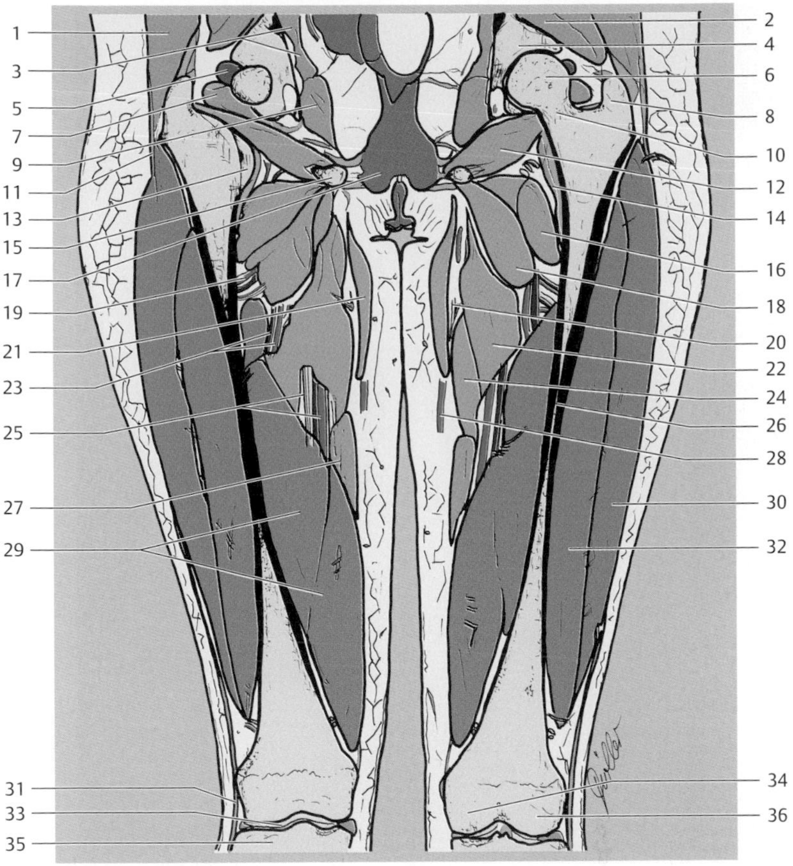

13 Lesser trochanter
14 Iliopsoas muscle
15 Pubis (inferior ramus)
16 Adductor minimus muscle
17 Vagina
18 Adductor brevis muscle
19 Lateral femoral circumflex artery and vein
20 Obturator nerve
21 Gracilis muscle
22 Adductor magnus muscle
23 Deep femoral artery and vein
24 Adductor longus muscle
25 Femoral artery and vein and saphenous nerve
26 Femur (shaft)
27 Sartorius muscle
28 Great saphenous vein
29 Vastus medialis muscle
30 Vastus lateralis muscle
31 Iliotibial tract
32 Vastus intermedius muscle
33 Knee joint
34 Medial femoral condyle
35 Head of tibia
36 Lateral femoral condyle

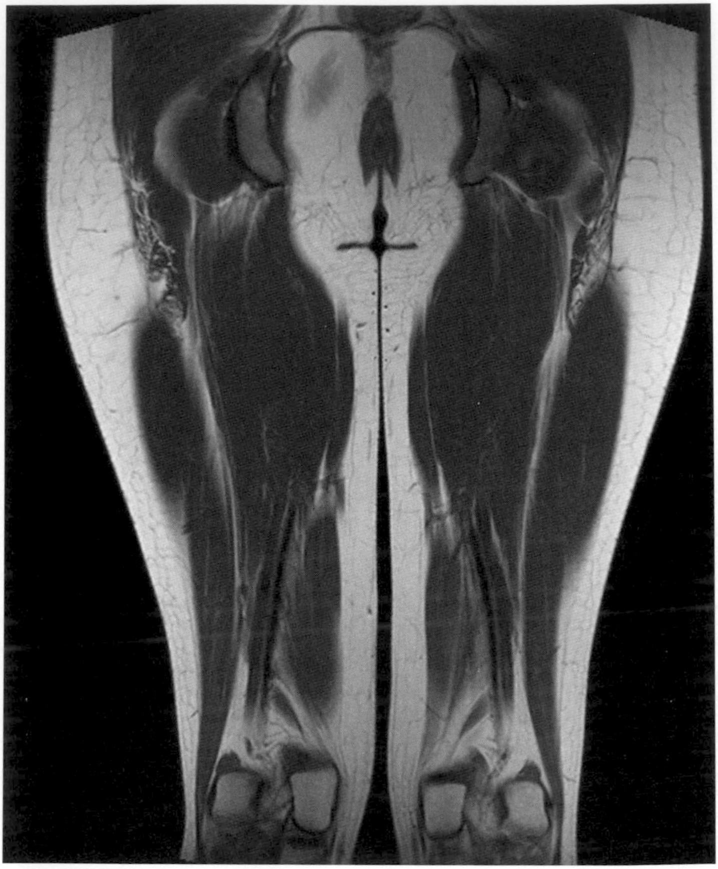

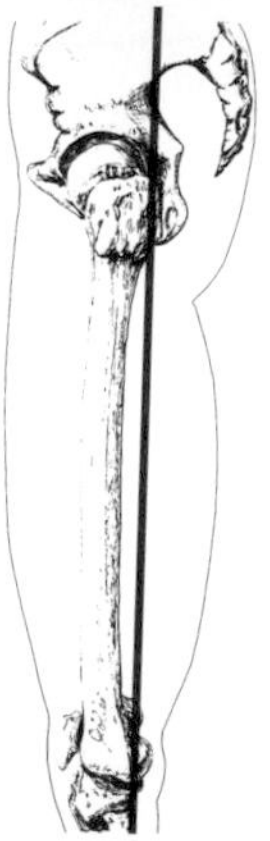

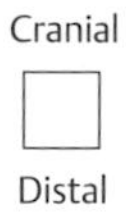

1 Gluteus maximus muscle
2 Levator ani muscle
3 Obturator internus muscle
4 Piriformis muscle
5 Ischium
6 Gemellus superior + inferior muscles
7 Anus and external anal sphincter muscle
8 Ischioanal fossa
9 Sciatic nerve

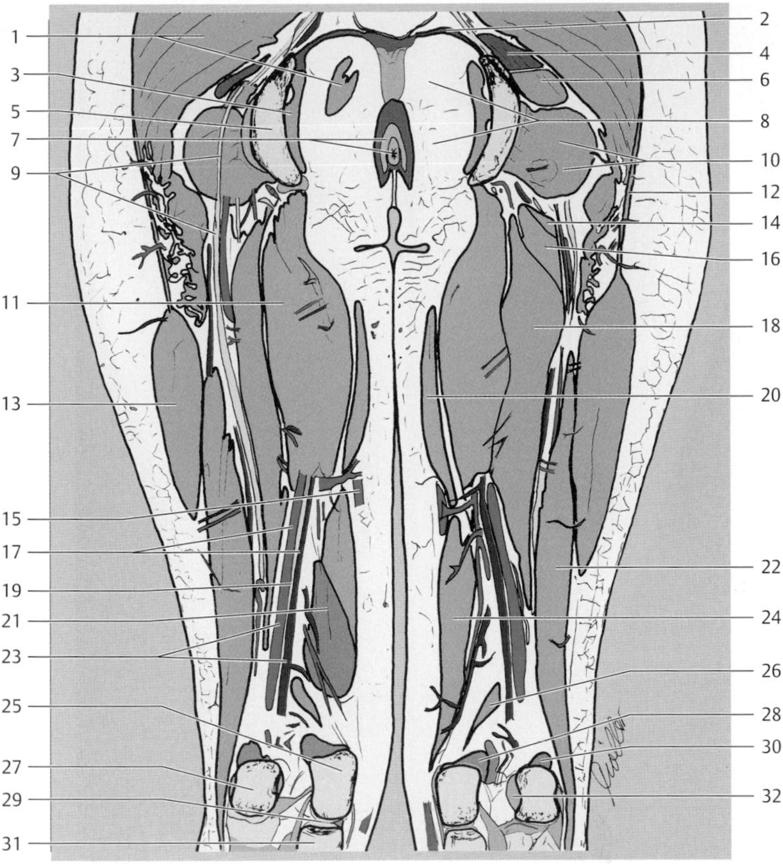

10 Quadratus femoris muscle
11 Adductor magnus muscle
12 Iliotibial tract
13 Vastus lateralis muscle
14 Adductor minimus muscle
15 Great saphenous vein
16 Adductor brevis muscle
17 Femoral artery and vein
18 Semitendinosus muscle
19 Tibial nerve
20 Gracilis muscle
21 Vastus medialis muscle
22 Biceps femoris muscle (long head)
23 Popliteal artery and vein
24 Sartorius muscle
25 Medial femoral condyle
26 Semimembranosus muscle
27 Lateral femoral condyle
28 Gastrocnemius muscle (medial head, attachment)
29 Knee joint
30 Gastrocnemius muscle (lateral head, attachment)
31 Head of tibia
32 Anterior cruciate ligament

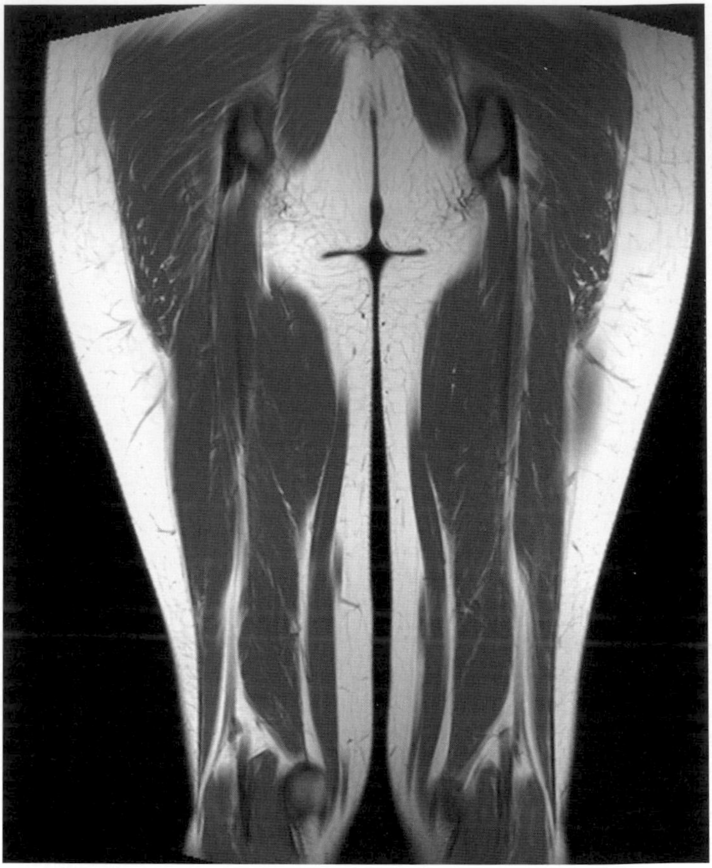

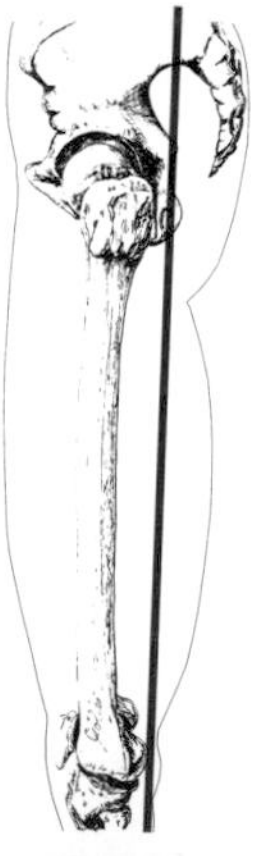

Cranial
Distal

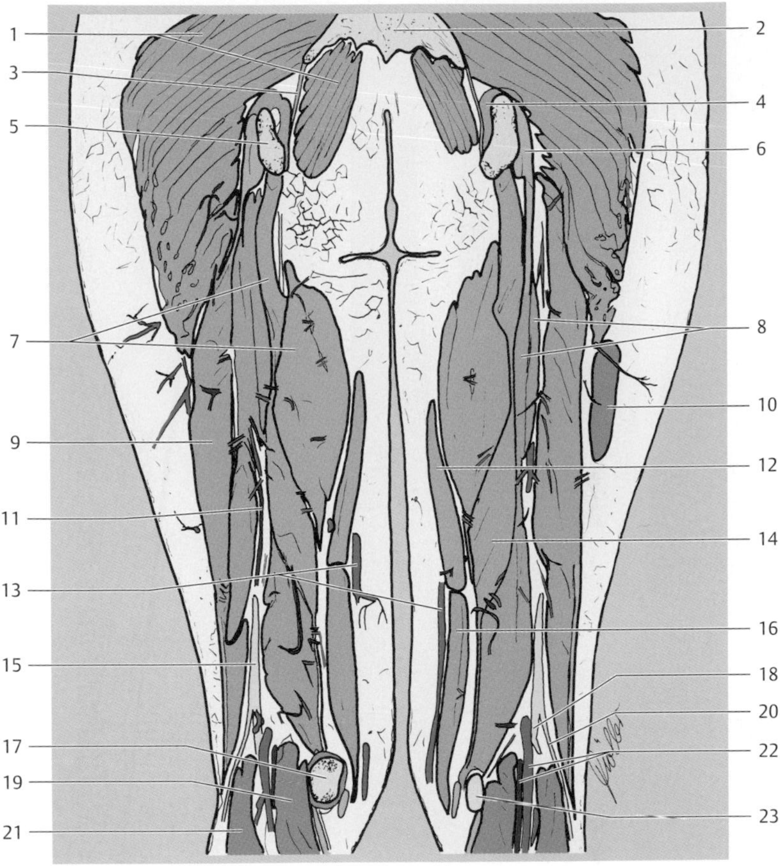

1 Gluteus maximus muscle
2 Sacrum
3 Sacrotuberal ligament
4 Obturator internus muscle
5 Ischium
6 Semitendinosus muscle + biceps femoris muscle (common attachment)
7 Adductor magnus muscle
8 Semitendinosus muscle
9 Biceps femoris muscle (long head)
10 Vastus lateralis muscle
11 Perforating artery
12 Gracilis muscle
13 Great saphenous vein
14 Semimembranosus muscle
15 Sciatic nerve
16 Sartorius muscle
17 Medial femoral condyle
18 Tibial nerve
19 Gastrocnemius muscle (medial head)
20 Common fibular nerve
21 Gastrocnemius muscle (lateral head)
22 Popliteal artery and vein
23 Joint capsule and semimembranosus bursa

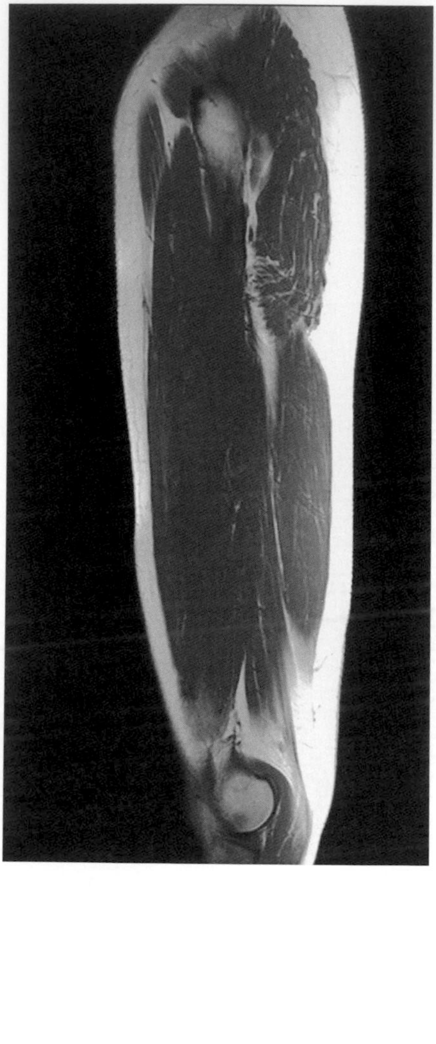

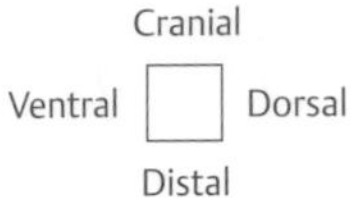
Cranial
Ventral
Dorsal
Distal

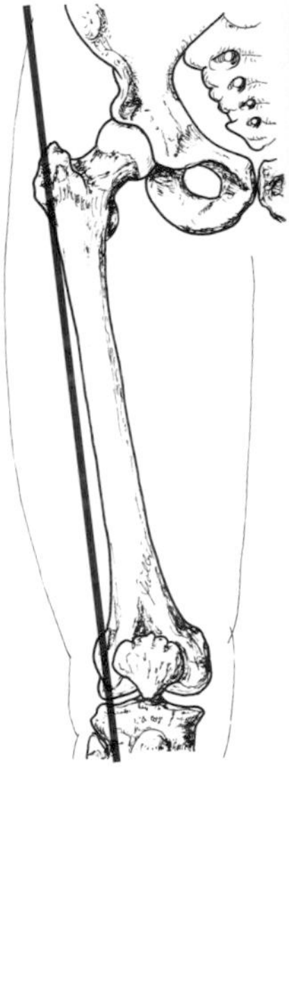

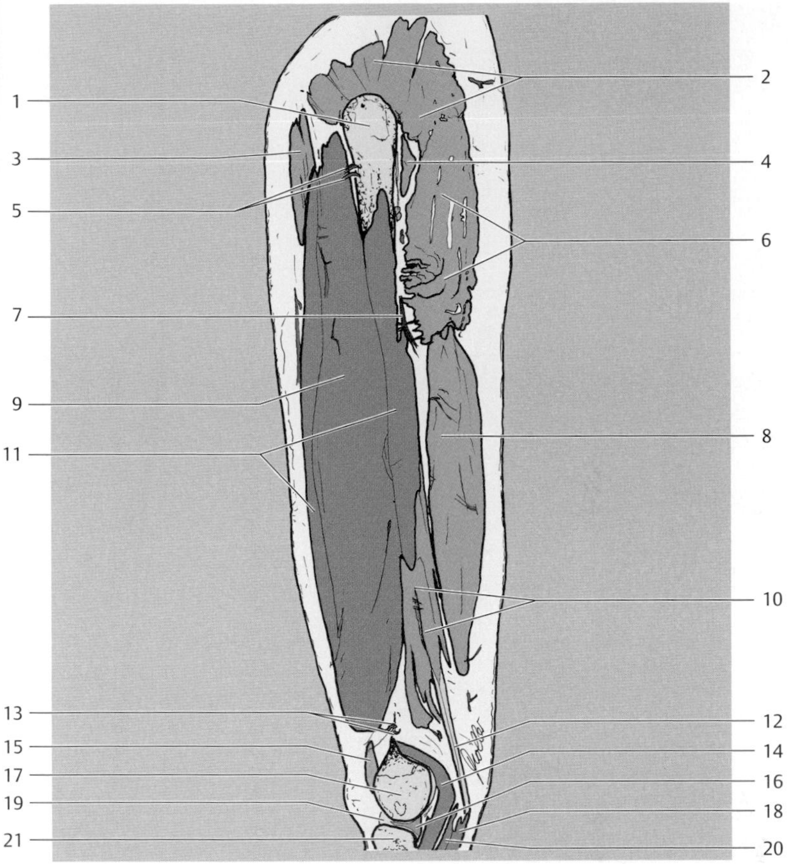

1 Greater trochanter
2 Gluteus medius muscle
3 Tensor fasciae latae muscle
4 Quadratus femoris muscle
5 Lateral circumflex femoral artery and vein
6 Gluteus maximus muscle
7 Perforating arteries
8 Biceps femoris muscle (long head)
9 Vastus intermedius muscle
10 Biceps femoris muscle (short head)
11 Vastus lateralis muscle
12 Common fibular (peroneal) nerve
13 Superior lateral genicular artery and vein
14 Gastrocnemius muscle (lateral head)
15 Quadriceps tendon
16 Lateral meniscus
17 Lateral femoral condyle
18 Soleus muscle
19 Knee joint
20 Plantaris muscle
21 Lateral condyle of tibia

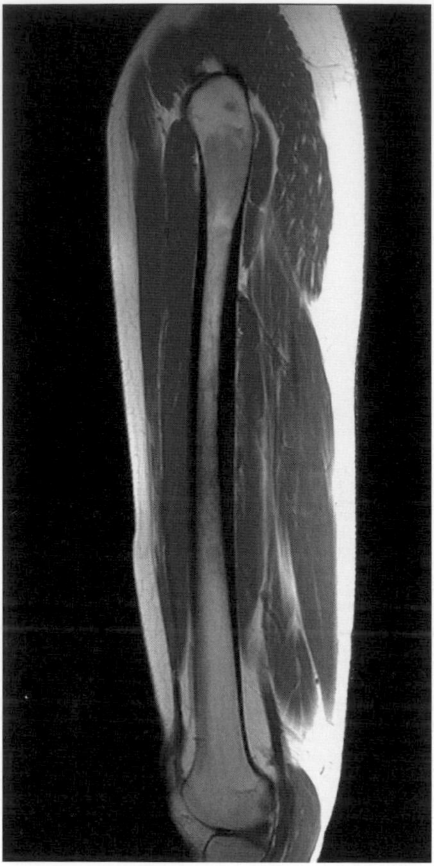

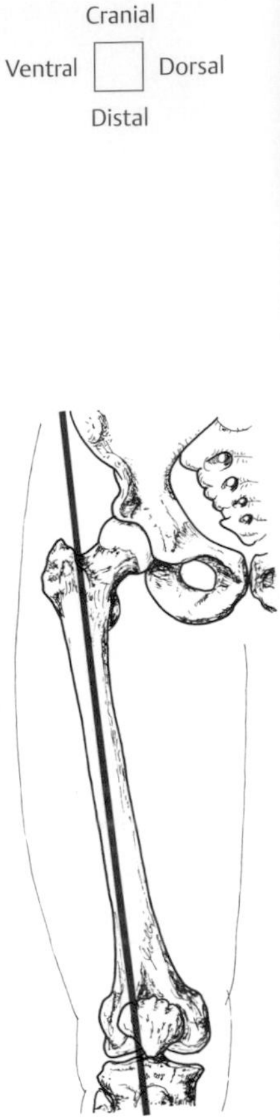
Cranial
Ventral
Dorsal
Distal

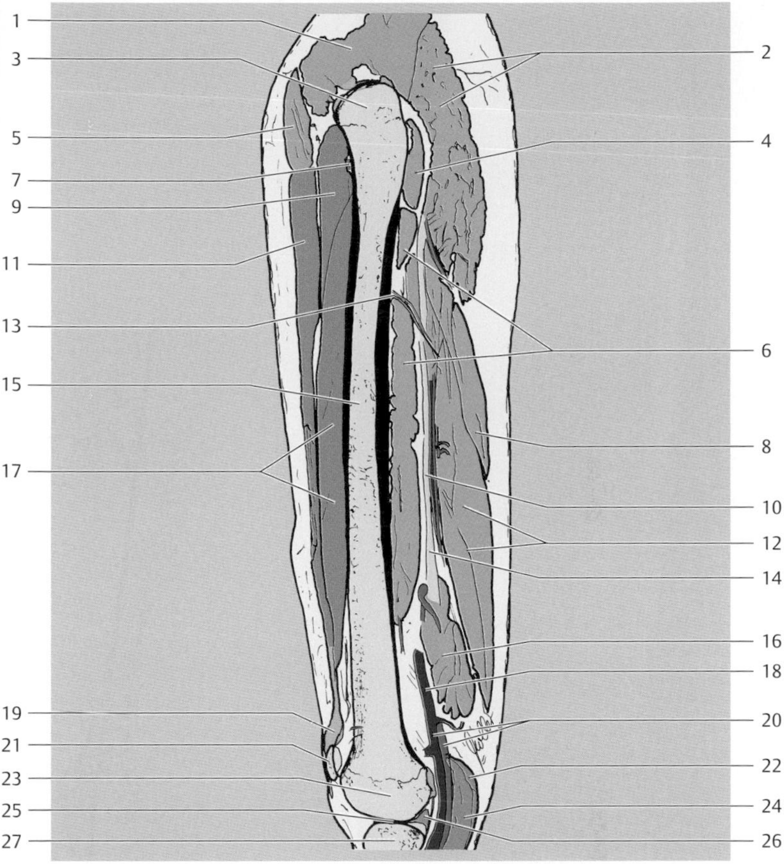

1 Gluteus medius muscle
2 Gluteus maximus muscle
3 Greater trochanter
4 Quadratus femoris muscle
5 Tensor fasciae latae muscle
6 Adductor magnus muscle
7 Lateral circumflex femoral artery and vein
8 Biceps femoris muscle (long head)
9 Vastus lateralis muscle
10 Sciatic nerve
11 Rectus femoris muscle
12 Semitendinosus muscle
13 Perforating arteries
14 Tibial nerve/common peroneal nerve
15 Femur (shaft)
16 Semimembranosus muscle
17 Vastus intermedius muscle
18 Femoral artery and vein
19 Quadriceps tendon
20 Popliteal artery and vein
21 Patella
22 Gastrocnemius muscle (lateral head)
23 Lateral femoral condyle
24 Soleus muscle
25 Knee joint
26 Lateral meniscus, posterior horn
27 Lateral condyle of tibia

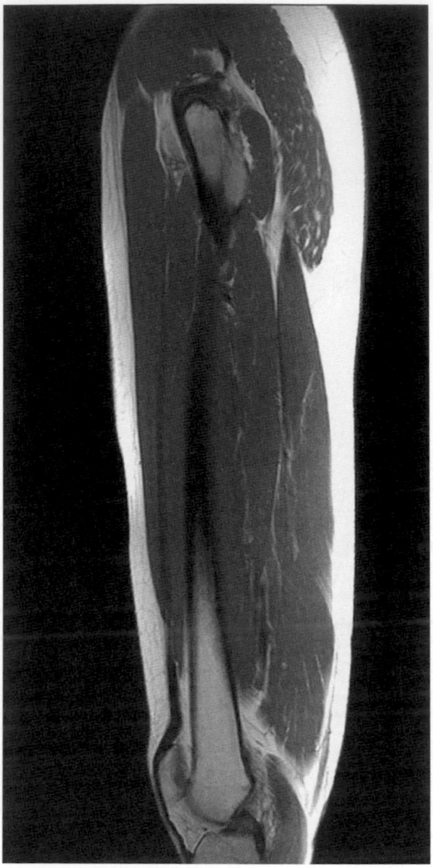

Cranial

Ventral Dorsal

Distal

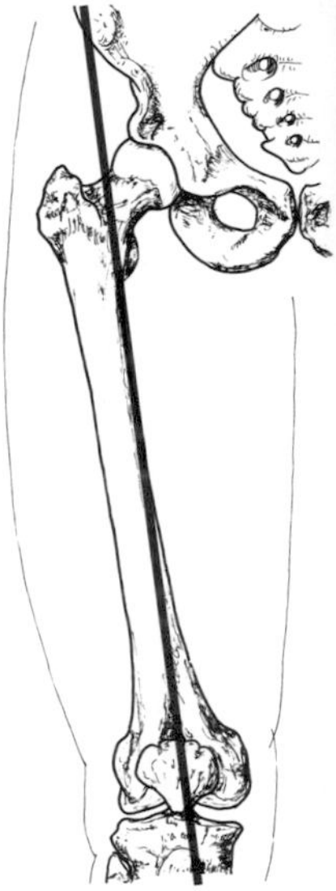

1 Gluteus medius muscle
2 Gluteus maximus muscle
3 Tensor fasciae latae muscle
4 Quadratus femoris muscle
5 Iliofemoral ligament
6 Lesser trochanter

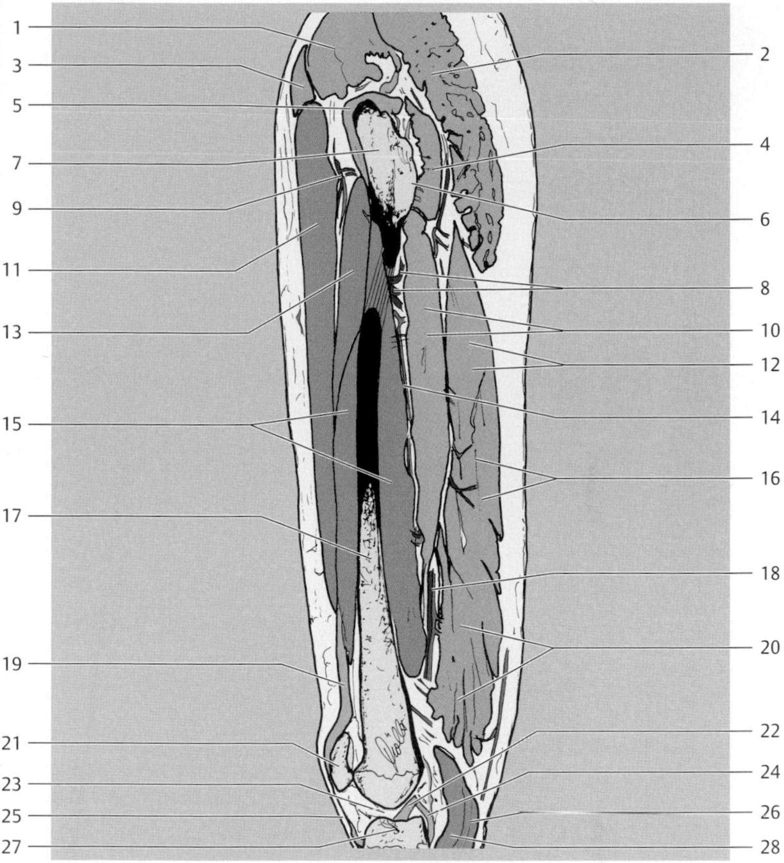

7 Femur (neck)
8 Perforating arteries
9 Lateral circumflex femoral artery and vein
10 Adductor magnus muscle
11 Rectus femoris muscle
12 Biceps femoris muscle (long head)
13 Vastus medialis muscle
14 Deep artery and vein of thigh
15 Vastus intermedius muscle
16 Semitendinosus muscle (tendon)
17 Femur (shaft)
18 Femoral artery and vein
19 Rectus femoris muscle (tendon)
20 Semimembranosus muscle
21 Patella
22 Anterior cruciate ligament
23 Knee joint
24 Posterior cruciate ligament
25 Patellar ligament
26 Gastrocnemius muscle (lateral head)
27 Tibia (head)
28 Soleus muscle

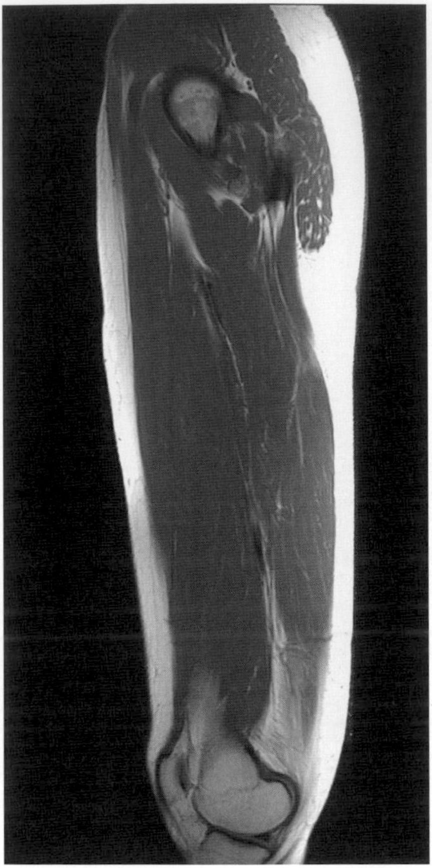

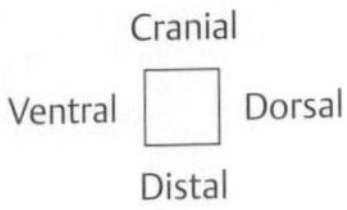

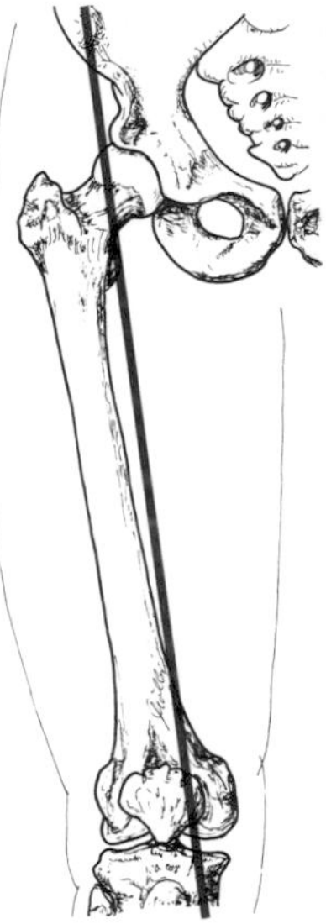

1 Gluteus medius muscle
2 Gluteus maximus muscle
3 Tensor fasciae latae muscle
4 Piriformis muscle
5 Sartorius muscle
6 Obturator internus muscle + gemellus muscles
7 Femur (head)
8 Ischium
9 Obturator externus muscle
10 Quadratus femoris muscle

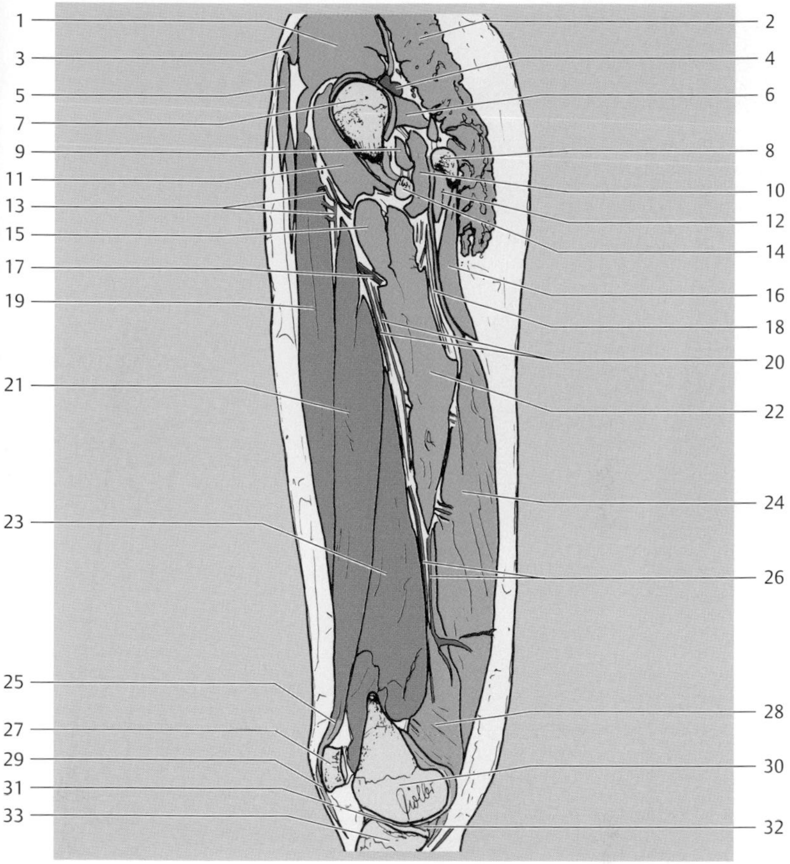

11 Iliopsoas muscle
12 Semitendinosus and semimembranosus muscles (common tendon attachment)
13 Lateral circumflex femoral artery and vein
14 Lesser trochanter
15 Pectineus muscle
16 Biceps femoris muscle (long head)
17 Perforating arteries
18 Sciatic nerve
19 Rectus femoris muscle
20 Deep femoral artery and vein
21 Vastus intermedius muscle
22 Adductor magnus muscle
23 Vastus medialis muscle
24 Semitendinosus muscle
25 Quadriceps tendon
26 Femoral artery and vein
27 Patella
28 Semimembranosus muscle
29 Patellar ligament
30 Medial femoral condyle
31 Knee joint
32 Medial meniscus (posterior horn)
33 Medial tibial condyle

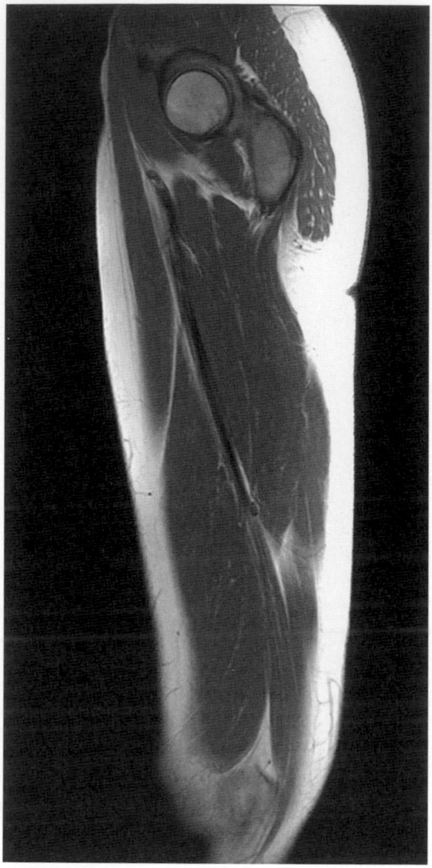

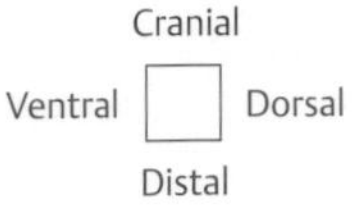

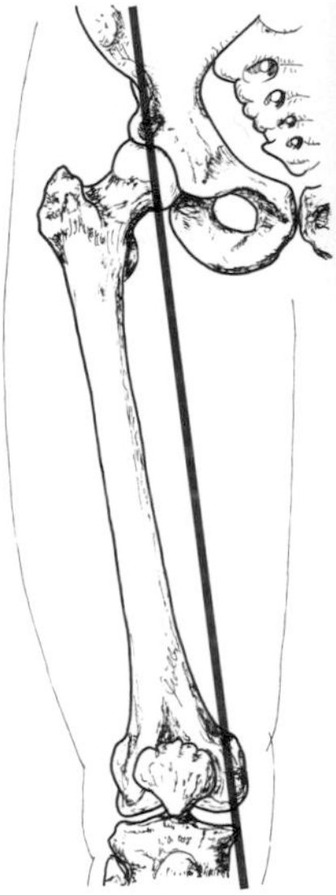

1 Gluteus medius muscle
2 Gluteus minimus muscle
3 Ilium
4 Gluteus maximus muscle
5 Iliopsoas muscle

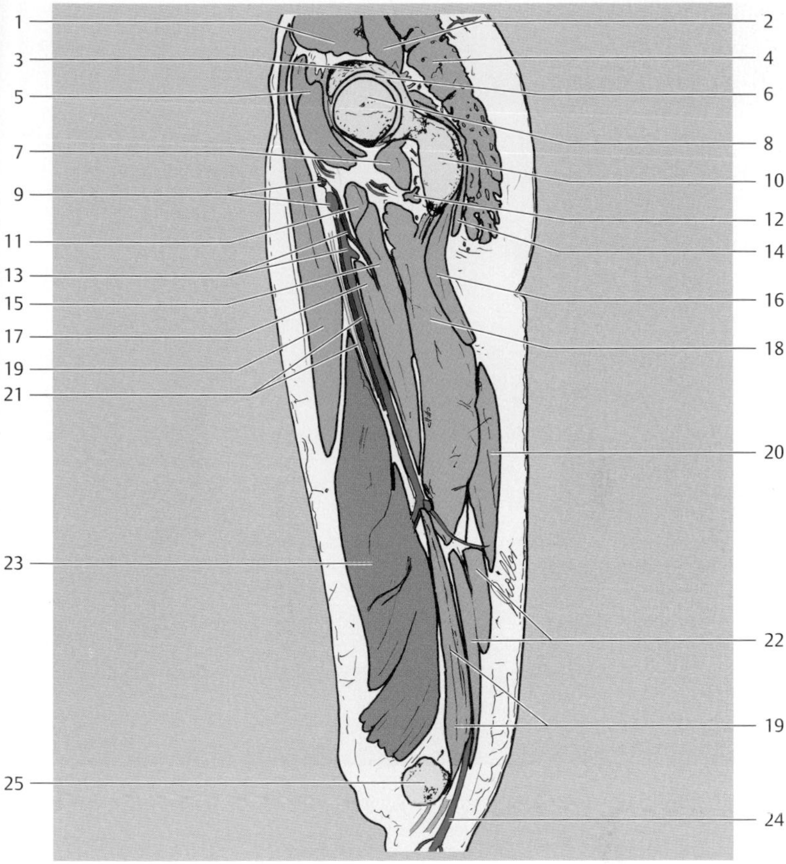

6 Hip joint
7 Obturator externus muscle
8 Femur (head)
9 Lateral circumflex femoral artery and vein
10 Ischium
11 Pectineus muscle
12 Quadratus femoris muscle
13 Deep artery of thigh
14 Biceps femoris muscle (long head, attachment)
15 Adductor brevis muscle
16 Semitendinosus muscle
17 Adductor longus muscle
18 Adductor magnus muscle
19 Sartorius muscle
20 Semimembranosus muscle
21 Femoral artery and vein + saphenous nerve
22 Gracilis muscle
23 Vastus medialis muscle
24 Great saphenous vein
25 Medial femoral condyle

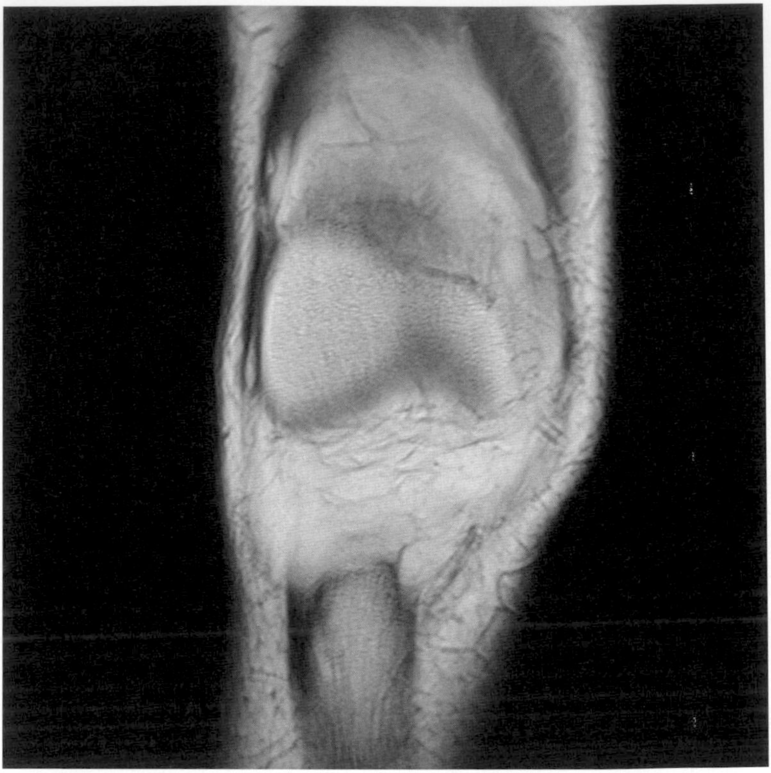

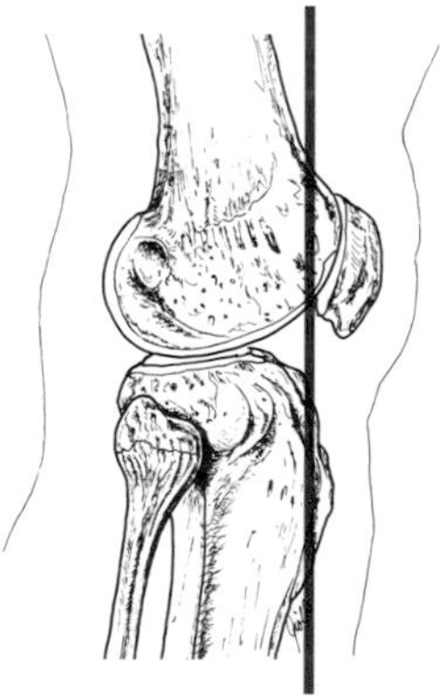

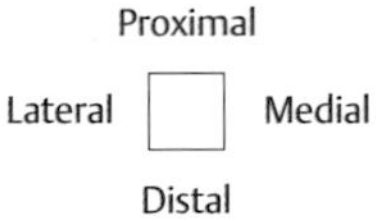
Proximal
Lateral
Medial
Distal

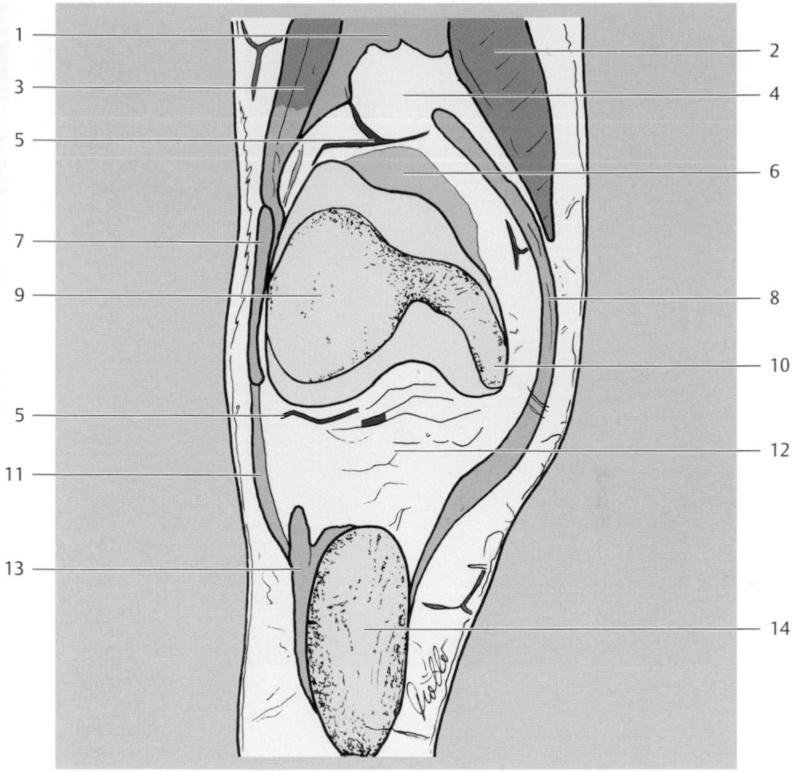

1 Quadriceps tendon
2 Vastus medialis muscle
3 Vastus lateralis muscle
4 Suprapatellar fat pad
5 Genicular anastomosis
6 Suprapatellar bursa
7 Iliotibial tract
8 Medial patellar retinaculum
9 Lateral femoral condyle
10 Medial femoral condyle
11 Lateral patellar retinaculum
12 Infrapatellar fat pad
13 Patellar ligament
14 Tibia (tuberosity)

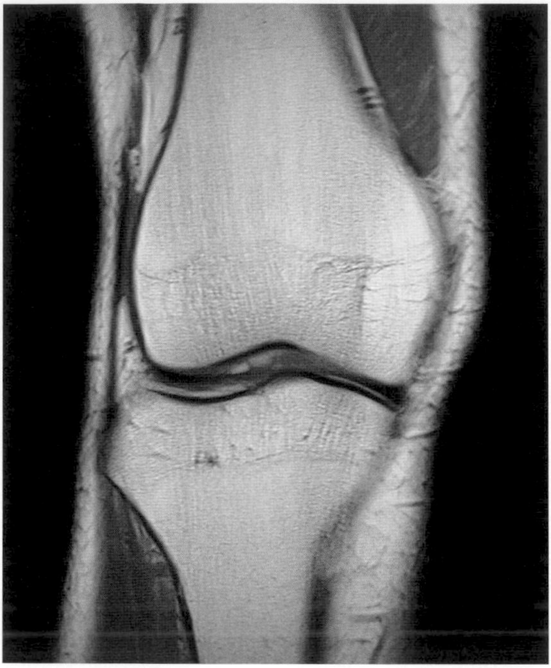

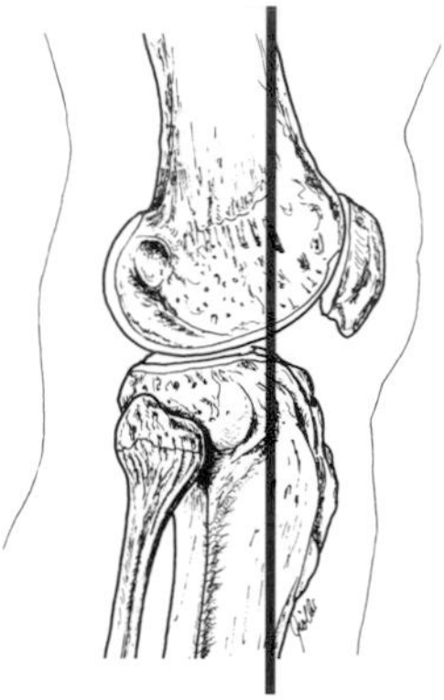

Proximal

Lateral Medial

Distal

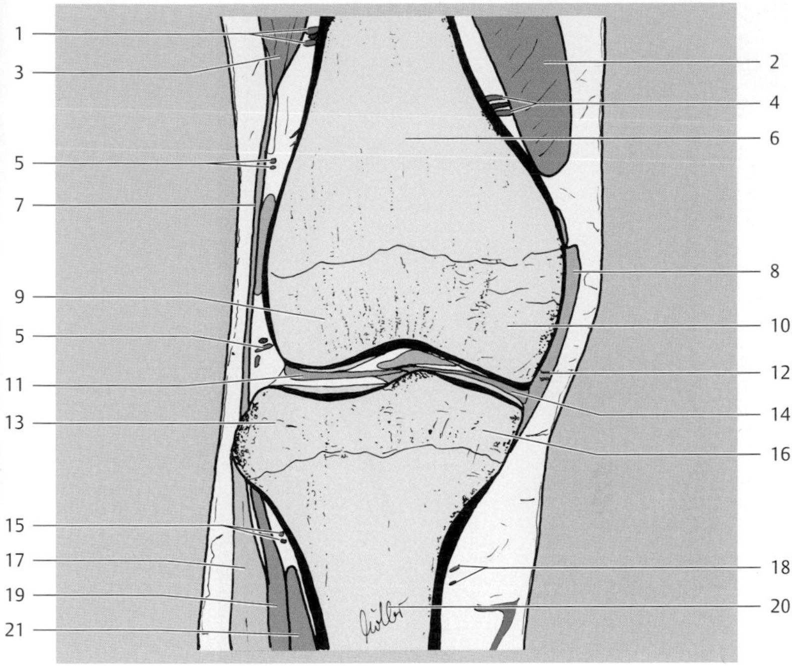

1 Superior lateral genicular artery and vein
2 Vastus medialis muscle
3 Vastus lateralis muscle
4 Superior medial genicular artery and vein
5 Genicular anastomosis
6 Femur (shaft)
7 Iliotibial tract
8 Medial collateral ligament
9 Lateral femoral condyle
10 Medial femoral condyle
11 Lateral meniscus (anterior horn)
12 Descending genicular artery and vein (articular branches)
13 Lateral tibial condyle
14 Medial meniscus (anterior horn)
15 Inferior lateral genicular artery and vein
16 Medial tibial condyle
17 Peroneus (fibularis) longus muscle
18 Inferior medial genicular artery and vein
19 Extensor digitorum longus muscle
20 Tibia (shaft)
21 Tibialis anterior muscle

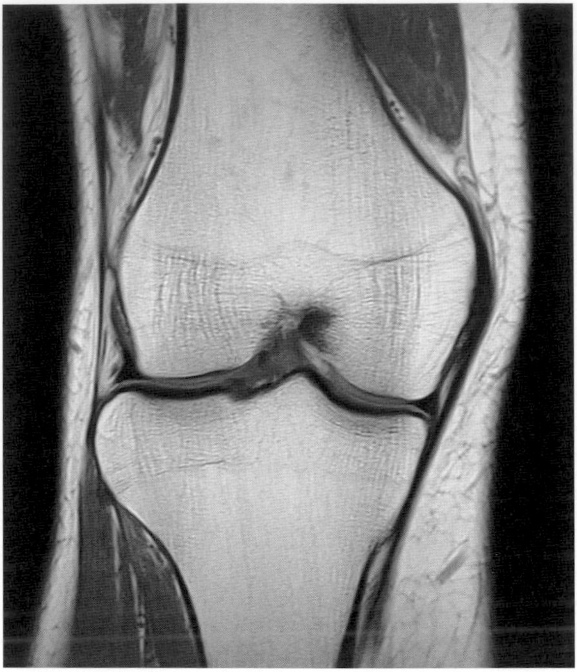

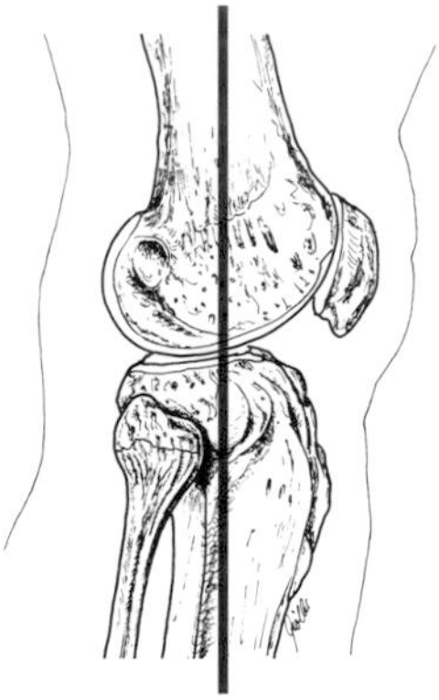

Proximal

Lateral | Medial

Distal

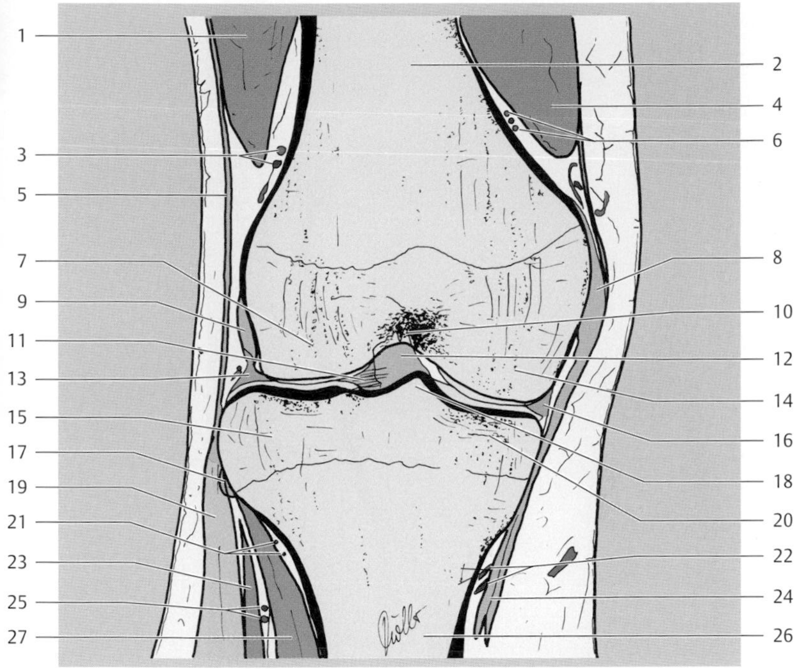

1 Vastus lateralis muscle
2 Femur (shaft)
3 Superior lateral genicular artery and vein
4 Vastus medialis muscle
5 Iliotibial tract
6 Superior medial genicular artery and vein
7 Lateral femoral condyle
8 Medial collateral ligament
9 Popliteus muscle (tendon)
10 Intercondylar fossa
11 Transverse ligament of knee
12 Anterior cruciate ligament
13 Lateral meniscus (intermediate portion)
14 Medial femoral condyle
15 Lateral tibial condyle
16 Medial meniscus (intermediate portion)
17 Anterior ligament of fibular head
18 Medial intercondylar tubercle
19 Peroneus (fibularis) longus muscle
20 Medial tibial condyle
21 Inferior lateral genicular artery and vein
22 Inferior medial genicular artery and vein
23 Extensor digitorum longus muscle
24 Pes anserinus (superficial)
25 Anterior tibial recurrent artery and vein
26 Tibia (shaft)
27 Tibialis anterior muscle

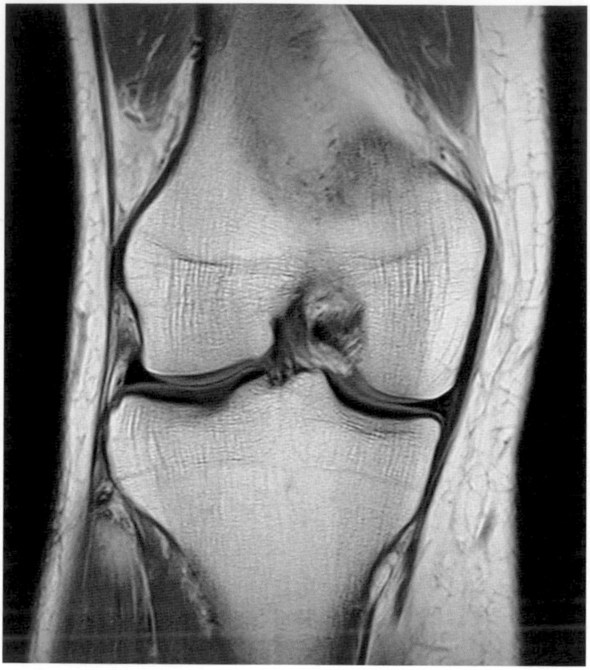

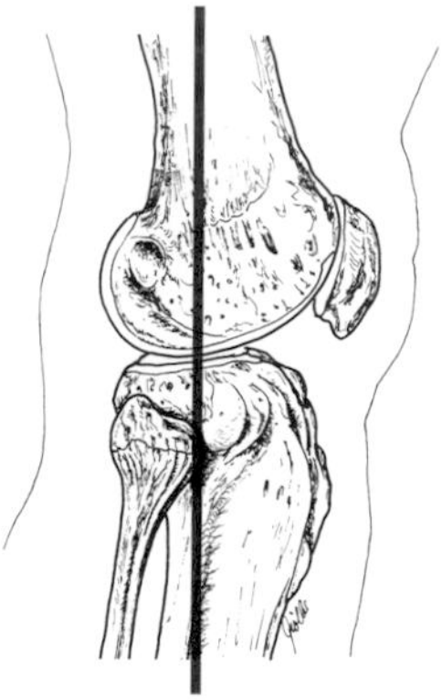

Proximal

Lateral ☐ Medial

Distal

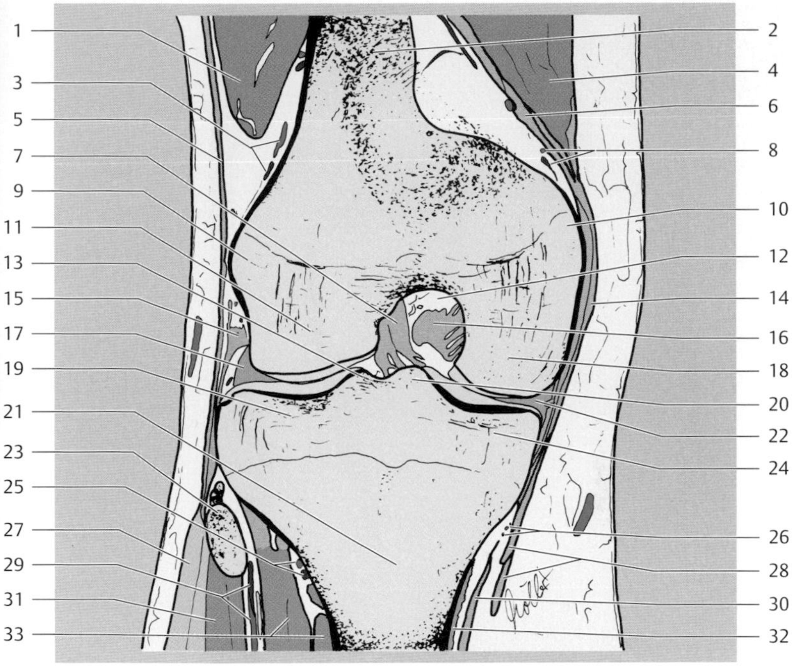

1 Vastus lateralis muscle
2 Femur (shaft)
3 Superior lateral genicular artery and vein
4 Vastus medialis muscle
5 Iliotibial tract
6 Adductor magnus muscle (tendon)
7 Anterior cruciate ligament
8 Superior medial genicular artery and vein
9 Lateral epicondyle
10 Medial epicondyle
11 Lateral femoral condyle
12 Intercondylar fossa
13 Lateral intercondylar tubercle
14 Medial collateral ligament
15 Popliteus muscle (tendon)
16 Posterior cruciate ligament
17 Lateral meniscus (intermediate portion)
18 Medial femoral condyle
19 Lateral tibial condyle
20 Medial intercondylar tubercle
21 Tibia (shaft)
22 Medial meniscus (intermediate portion)
23 Fibula (head)
24 Medial tibial condyle
25 Inferior lateral genicular artery and vein
26 Inferior medial genicular artery and vein
27 Peroneus (fibularis) longus muscle
28 Pes anserinus (superficial)
29 Anterior tibial recurrent artery and vein
30 Semimembranosus muscle (tibial attachment, deep pes anserinus)
31 Extensor digitorum longus muscle
32 Popliteus muscle (tibial attachment)
33 Tibialis anterior muscle

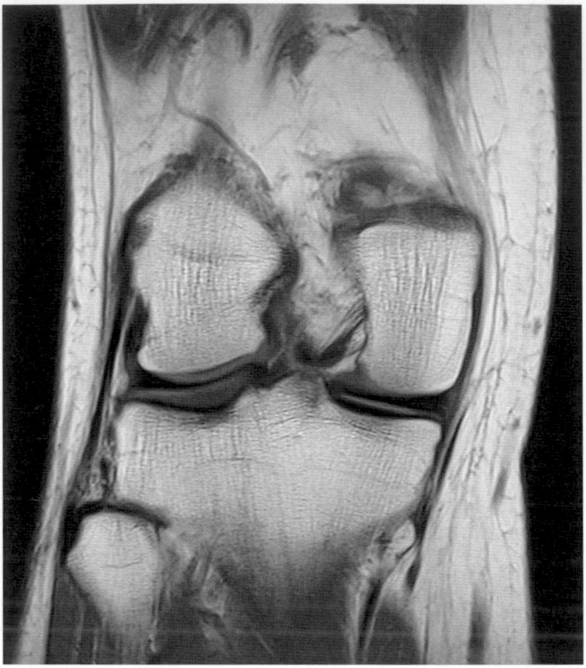

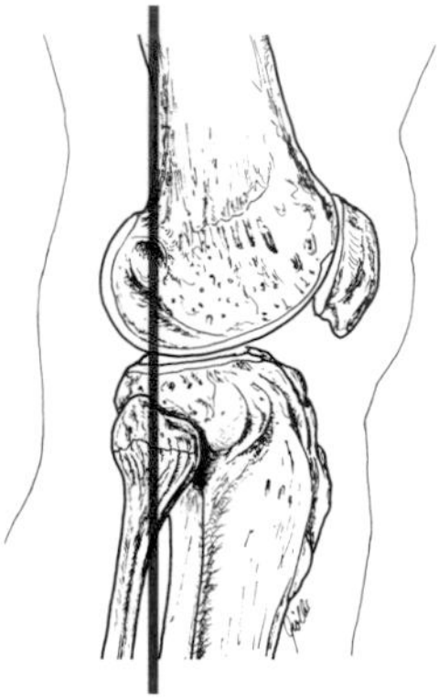

Proximal

Lateral ☐ Medial

Distal

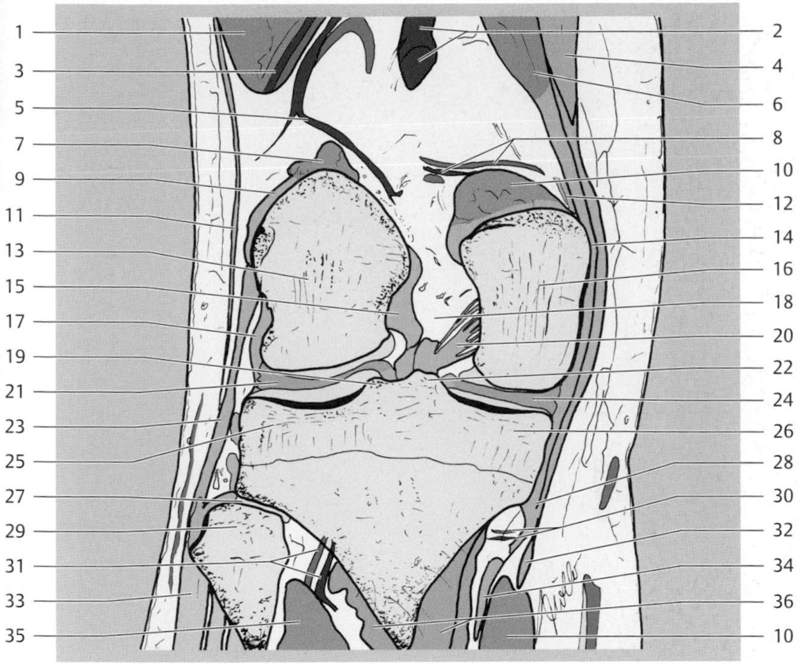

1 Vastus lateralis muscle
2 Popliteal artery
3 Superior lateral genicular artery
4 Sartorius muscle
5 Medial genicular artery
6 Vastus medialis muscle
7 Gastrocnemius muscle (lateral head, femoral attachment)
8 Superior medial genicular artery and vein
9 Plantaris muscle (tendon)
10 Gastrocnemius muscle (medial head)
11 Iliotibial tract
12 Adductor magnus muscle (tendon attachment)
13 Lateral femoral condyle
14 Medial collateral ligament
15 Anterior cruciate ligament
16 Medial femoral condyle
17 Popliteus muscle (tendon)
18 Intercondylar fossa
19 Lateral intercondylar tubercle
20 Posterior cruciate ligament
21 Lateral meniscus (posterior horn)
22 Medial intercondylar tubercle
23 Fibular collateral ligament
24 Medial meniscus (posterior horn)
25 Lateral tibial condyle
26 Medial tibial condyle
27 Tibiofibular joint
28 Pes anserinus (superficial)
29 Fibula (head)
30 Inferior medial genicular artery and vein
31 Inferior lateral genicular artery and vein
32 Semitendinosus muscle (tendon)
33 Peroneus (fibularis) longus muscle
34 Semimembranosus muscle (tibial attachment, deep pes anserinus)
35 Tibialis posterior muscle
36 Popliteus muscle

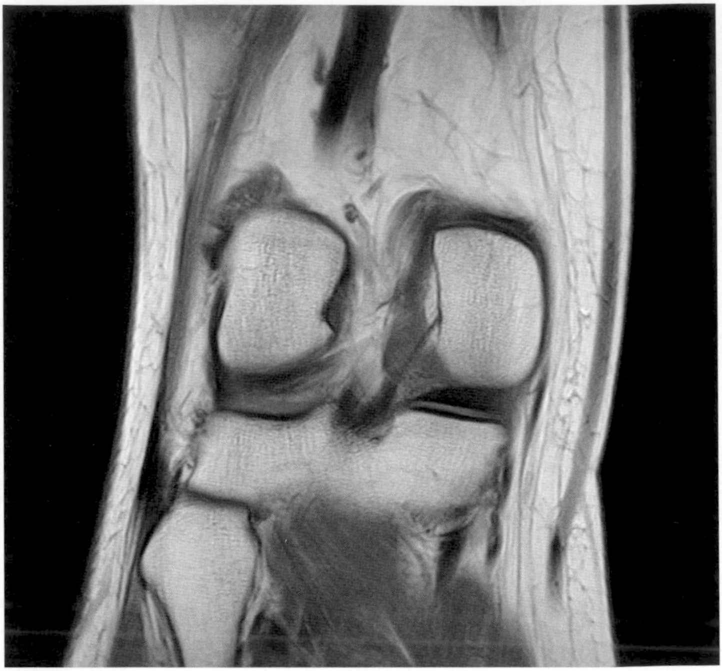

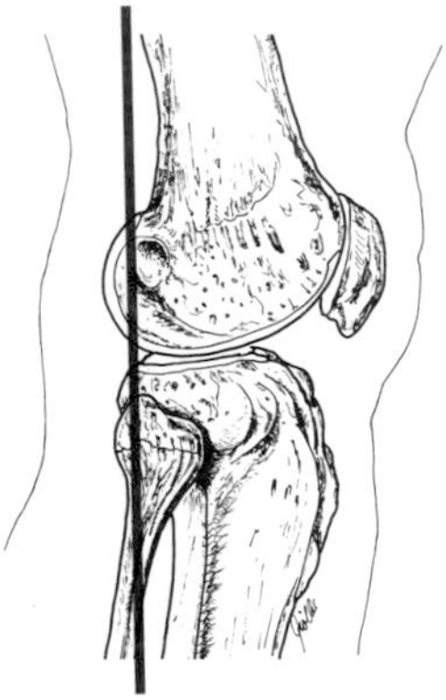

Proximal

Lateral ☐ Medial

Distal

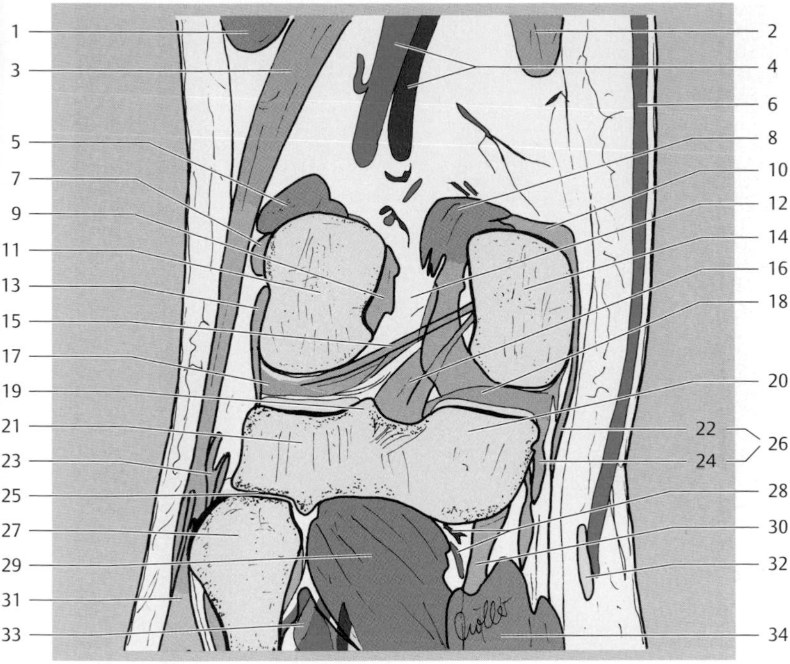

1 Vastus lateralis muscle
2 Sartorius muscle
3 Biceps femoris muscle
4 Popliteal artery and vein
5 Gastrocnemius muscle (lateral head, femoral attachment)
6 Great saphenous vein
7 Plantaris muscle (tendon attachment)
8 Gastrocnemius muscle (medial head, femoral attachment)
9 Anterior cruciate ligament
10 Joint capsule
11 Lateral femoral condyle
12 Intercondylar fossa
13 Popliteus muscle (tendon)
14 Medial femoral condyle
15 Posterior meniscofemoral ligament (Wrisberg ligament)
16 Posterior cruciate ligament
17 Lateral meniscus (posterior horn)
18 Medial meniscus (posterior horn)
19 Lateral intercondylar tuberosity
20 Tibia (medial head)
21 Tibia (lateral head)
22 Gracilis muscle (tendon)
23 Collateral fibular ligament
24 Semitendinosus muscle (tendon)
25 Tibiofibular joint (proximal)
26 Pes anserinus (superficial)
27 Fibula (head)
28 Inferior medial genicular artery and vein
29 Popliteus muscle
30 Semimembranosus muscle (tibial attachment, deep pes anserinus)
31 Peroneus (fibularis) longus muscle
32 Saphenous nerve
33 Tibialis posterior muscle
34 Gastrocnemius muscle (medial head)

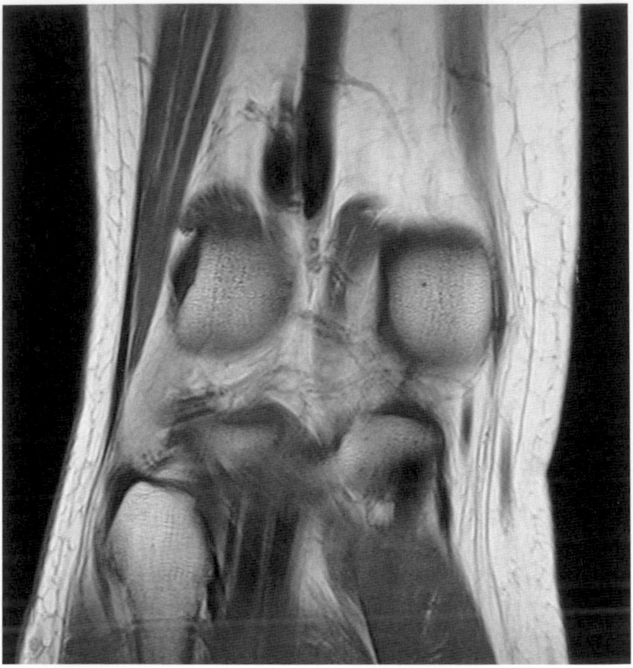

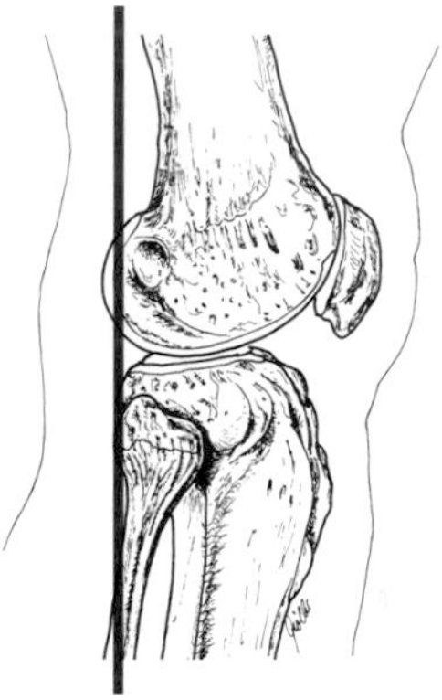

Proximal

Lateral ☐ Medial

Distal

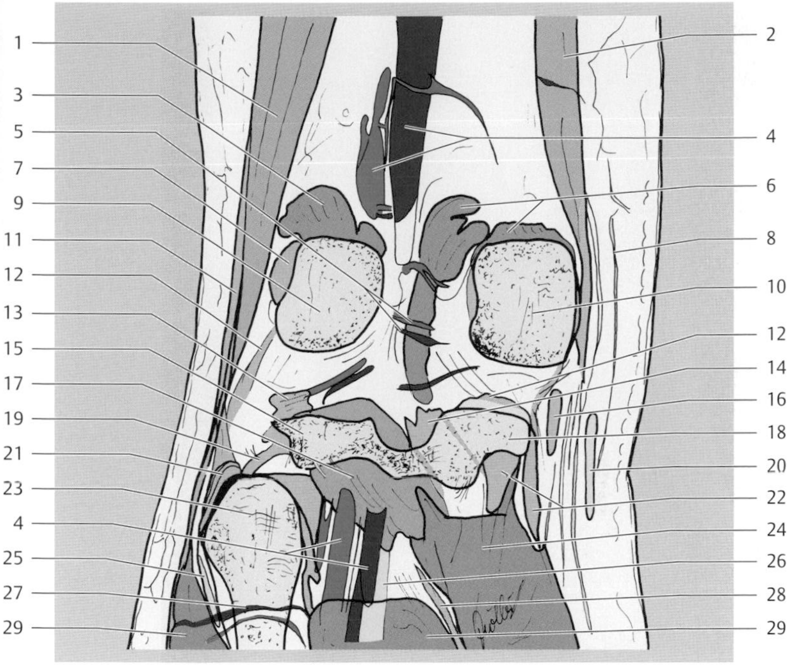

1 Biceps femoris muscle
2 Gracilis muscle
3 Gastrocnemius muscle (lateral head)
4 Popliteal artery and vein
5 Sural arteries and veins
6 Gastrocnemius muscle (medial head, femoral attachment)
7 Plantaris muscle (tendon)
8 Saphenous nerve (branch)
9 Lateral femoral condyle
10 Medial femoral condyle
11 Iliotibial tract
12 Joint capsule
13 Arcuate popliteal ligament
14 Oblique popliteal ligament
15 Lateral tibial condyle
16 Semitendinosus muscle (tendon)
17 Popliteus muscle
18 Medial tibial condyle
19 Fibular collateral ligament
20 Saphenous nerve
21 Posterior ligament of fibular head
22 Semimembranosus muscle (tibial attachment, deep pes anserinus)
23 Fibula (head)
24 Gastrocnemius muscle (medial head)
25 Common fibular (peroneal) nerve
26 Tibial nerve
27 Posterior tibial artery (circumflex fibular branch)
28 Plantaris muscle (tendon)
29 Soleus muscle

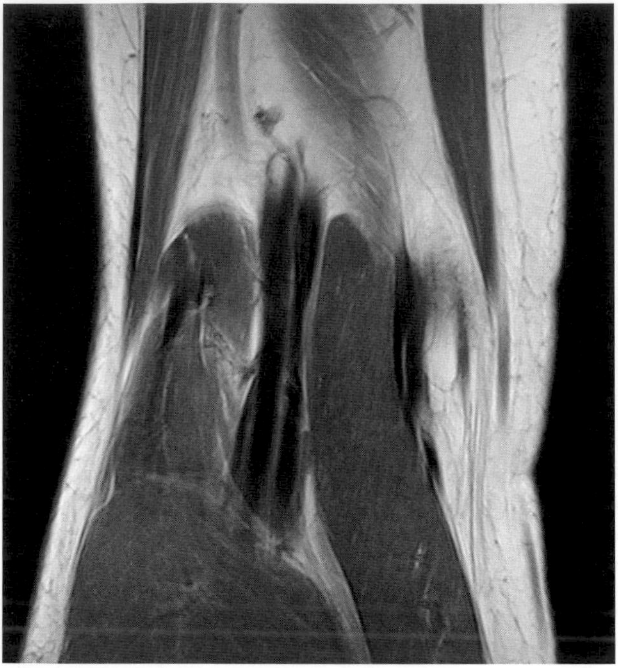

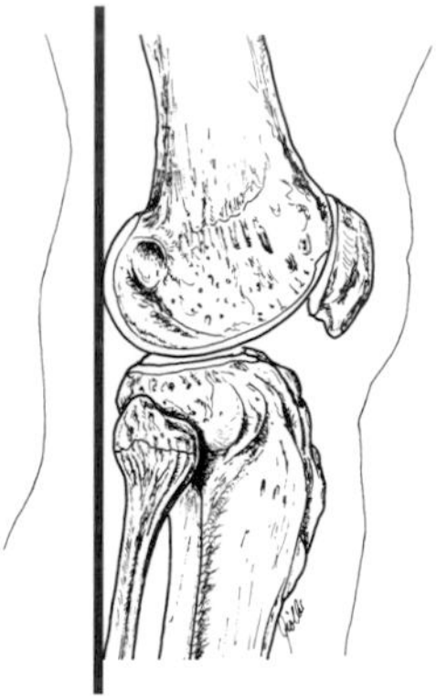

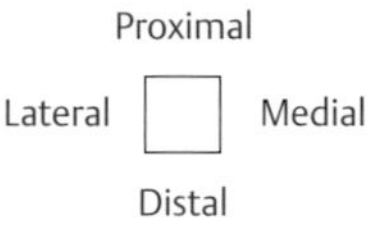
Proximal
Lateral
Medial
Distal

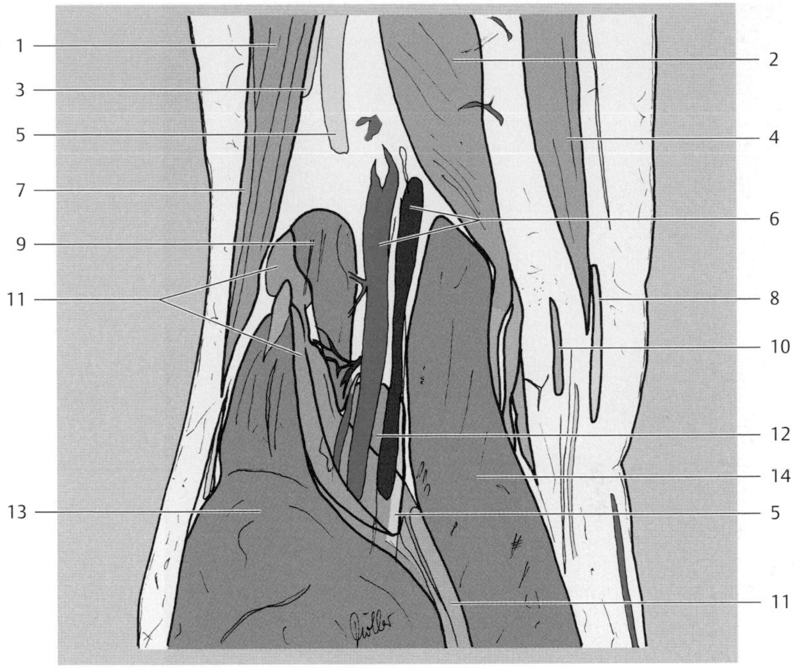

1 Biceps femoris muscle
2 Semimembranosus muscle
3 Common fibular (peroneal) nerve
4 Gracilis muscle
5 Tibial nerve
6 Popliteal artery and vein
7 Iliotibial tract
8 Saphenous nerve
9 Gastrocnemius muscle (lateral head)
10 Semitendinosus muscle (tendon)
11 Plantaris muscle (+ tendon)
12 Popliteus muscle
13 Soleus muscle
14 Gastrocnemius muscle (medial head)

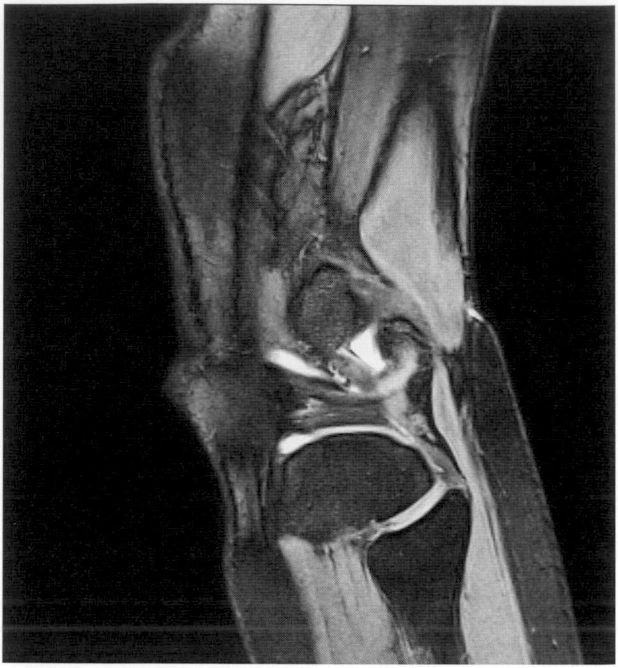

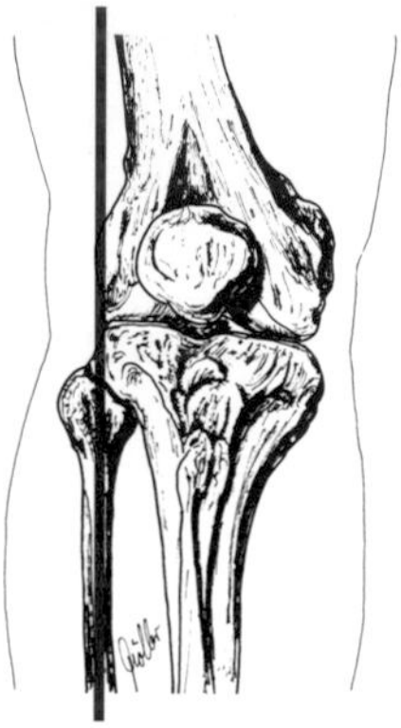

Proximal
Ventral
Dorsal
Distal

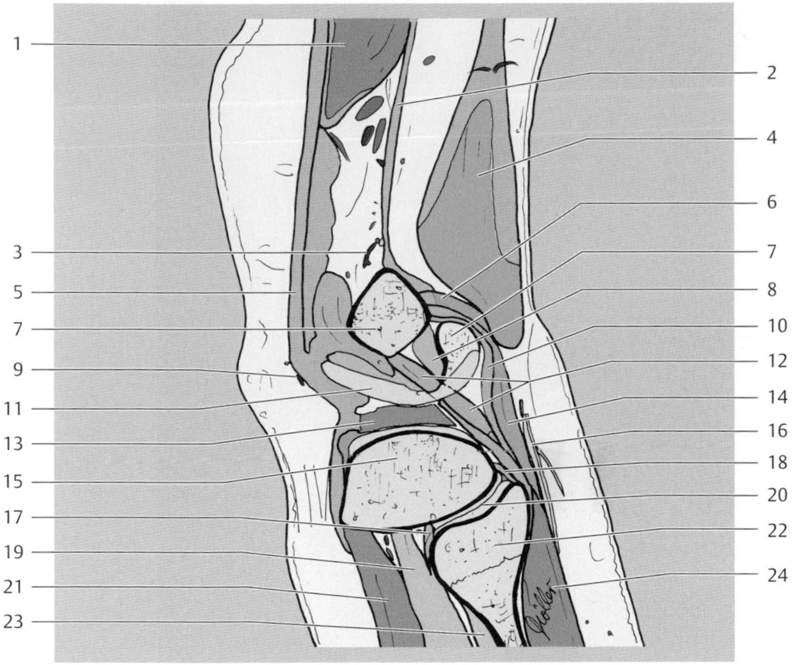

1 Vastus lateralis muscle
2 Iliotibial tract
3 Blood vessels to genicular anastomosis
4 Biceps femoris muscle
5 Lateral patellar retinaculum
6 Gastrocnemius muscle (lateral head)
7 Lateral femoral condyle
8 Lateral joint recess
9 Inferior lateral genicular artery
10 Joint capsule
11 Femur (lateral condyle, joint cartilage)
12 Popliteus muscle (tendon)
13 Lateral meniscus (intermediate portion)
14 Plantaris muscle (+ tendon attachment)
15 Lateral tibial condyle
16 Common fibular (peroneal) nerve
17 Anterior ligament of fibular head
18 Posterior ligament of fibular head
19 Tibialis posterior muscle
20 Tibiofibular joint
21 Tibialis anterior muscle
22 Fibula (head)
23 Peroneus (fibularis) longus muscle
24 Soleus muscle

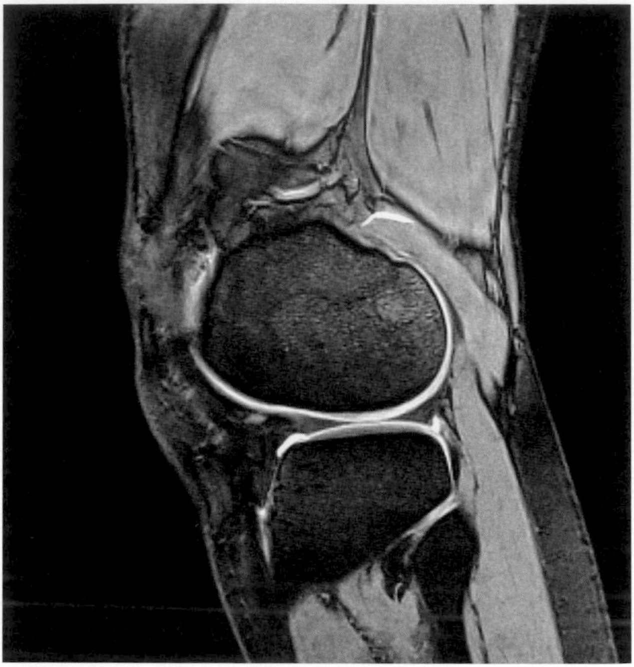

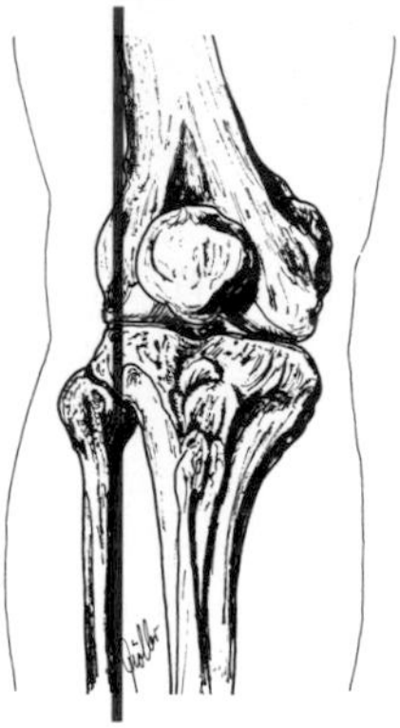

Proximal

Ventral ☐ Dorsal

Distal

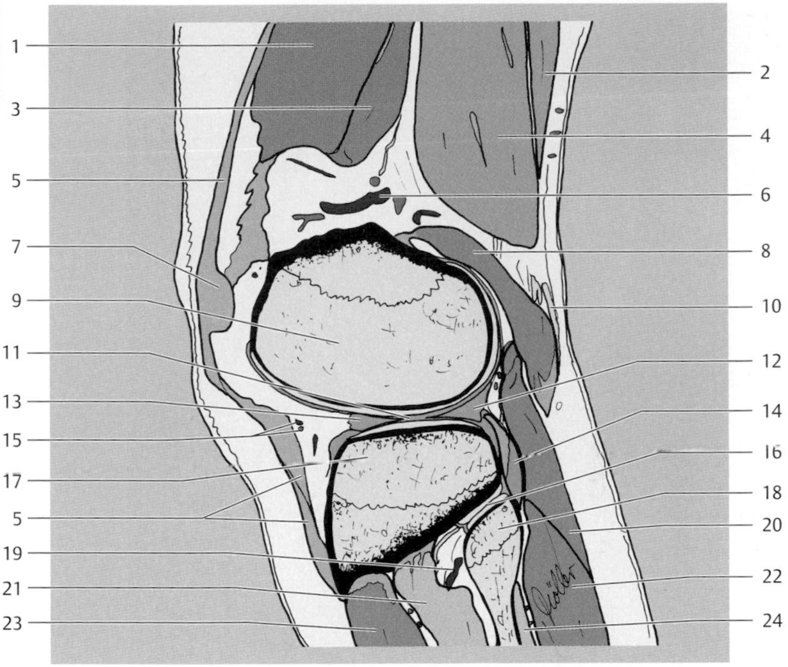

1 Vastus lateralis muscle
2 Biceps femoris muscle (long head)
3 Vastus intermedius muscle
4 Biceps femoris muscle (short head)
5 Lateral patellar retinaculum (longitudinal)
6 Superior lateral genicular artery and vein
7 Lateral patellar retinaculum (transverse)
8 Gastrocnemius muscle (lateral head)
9 Lateral femoral condyle
10 Common fibular (peroneal) nerve
11 Knee joint
12 Lateral meniscus (posterior horn)
13 Lateral meniscus (anterior horn)
14 Popliteus muscle (with tendon)
15 Inferior lateral genicular artery and vein
16 Tibiofibular joint (proximal)
17 Lateral tibial condyle
18 Fibula (head)
19 Anterior tibial artery
20 Plantaris muscle
21 Tibialis posterior muscle
22 Soleus muscle
23 Tibialis anterior muscle
24 Peroneus (fibularis) longus muscle

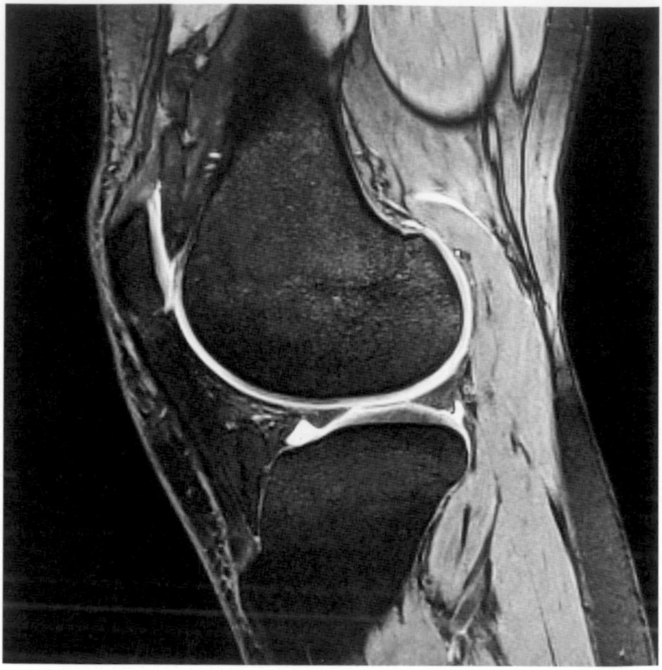

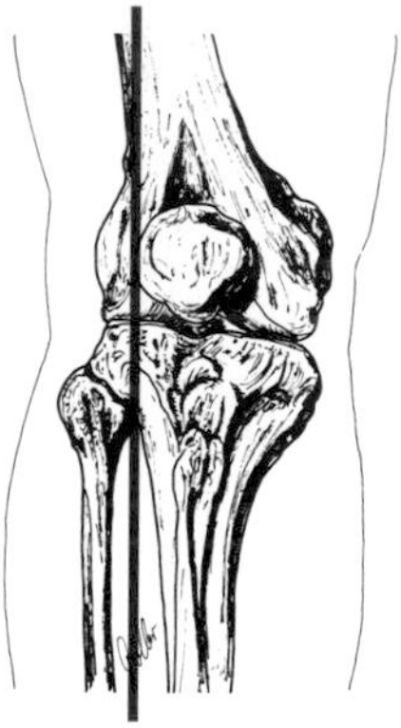

Proximal

Ventral Dorsal

Distal

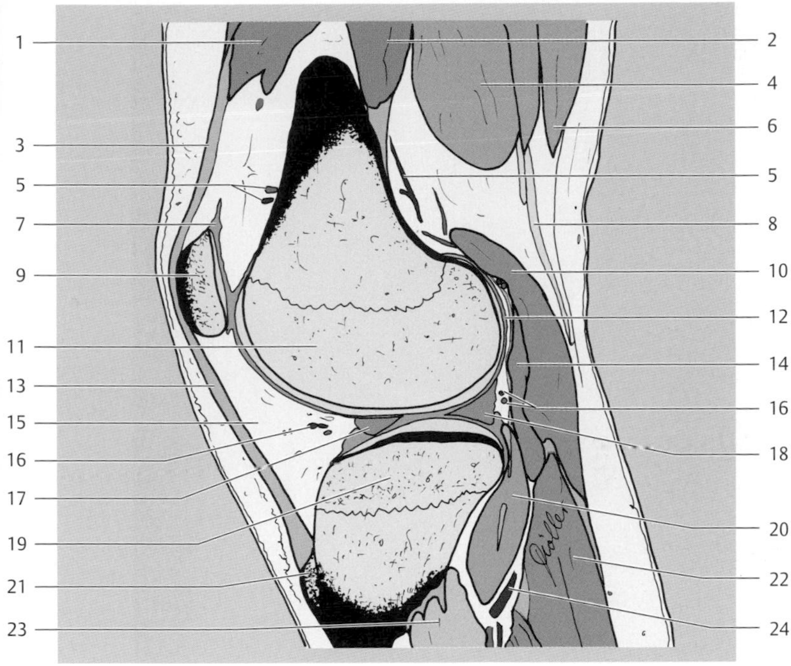

1 Vastus lateralis muscle
2 Vastus intermedius muscle
3 Quadriceps tendon
4 Biceps femoris muscle (short head)
5 Superior lateral genicular artery and vein
6 Biceps femoris muscle (long head)
7 Suprapatellar bursa
8 Common fibular (peroneal) nerve
9 Patella
10 Gastrocnemius muscle (lateral head)
11 Lateral femoral condyle
12 Joint capsule
13 Patellar ligament
14 Plantaris muscle
15 Infrapatellar fat pad
16 Inferior lateral genicular artery and vein
17 Lateral meniscus (anterior horn)
18 Lateral meniscus (posterior horn)
19 Lateral condyle of tibia
20 Popliteus muscle
21 Tibial tuberosity
22 Soleus muscle
23 Tibialis posterior muscle
24 Anterior tibial artery

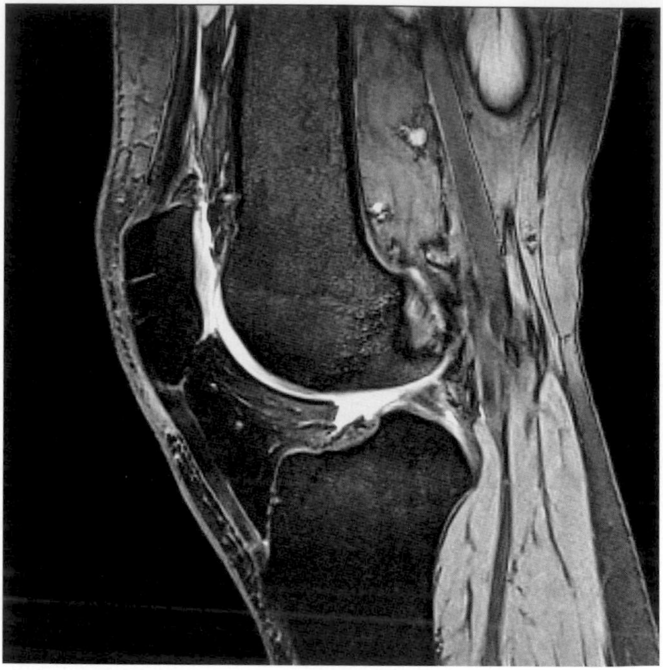

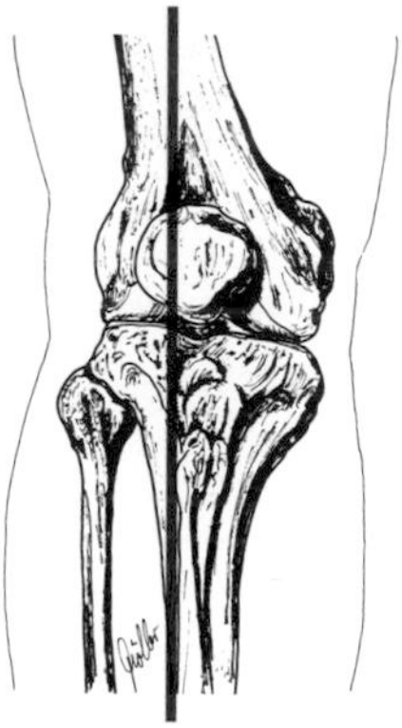

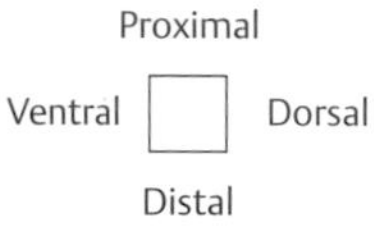
Proximal
Ventral
Dorsal
Distal

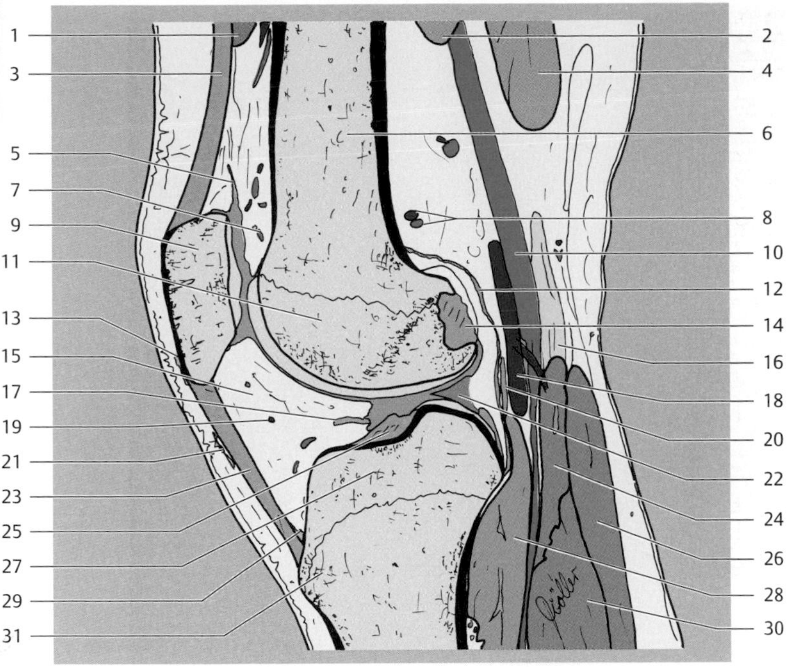

1 Vastus medialis muscle
2 Biceps femoris muscle
3 Quadriceps tendon
4 Semimembranosus muscle
5 Suprapatellar bursa
6 Femur (shaft)
7 Patellar anastomosis
8 Superior lateral genicular artery and vein
9 Patella
10 Popliteal vein
11 Lateral femoral condyle
12 Joint capsule
13 Subcutaneous prepatellar bursa
14 Anterior cruciate ligament (femoral attachment)
15 Infrapatellar fat pad
16 Tibial nerve
17 Transverse ligament of knee
18 Popliteal artery
19 Inferior lateral genicular artery and vein
20 Oblique popliteal ligament
21 Subcutaneous infrapatellar bursa
22 Lateral meniscus (posterior horn, inner attachment)
23 Patellar ligament
24 Plantaris muscle
25 Posterior cruciate ligament (tibial origin)
26 Gastrocnemius muscle (lateral head)
27 Head of tibia
28 Popliteus muscle
29 Deep infrapatellar bursa
30 Soleus muscle
31 Tibial tuberosity

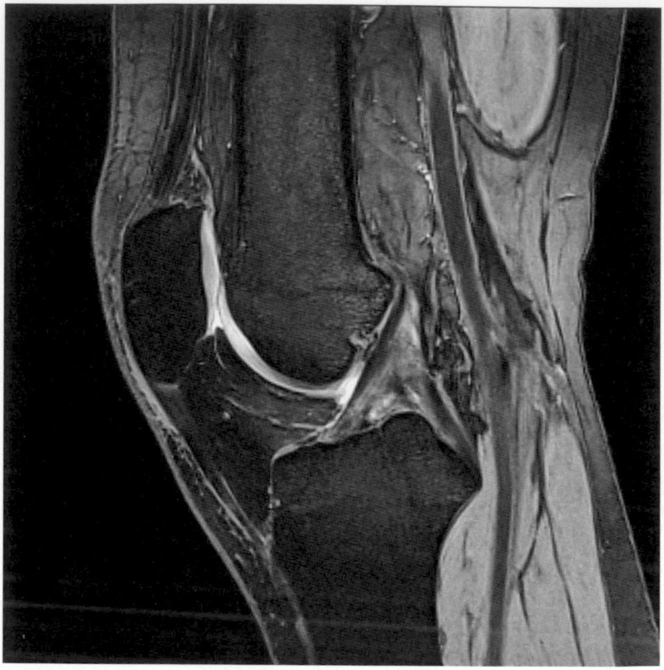

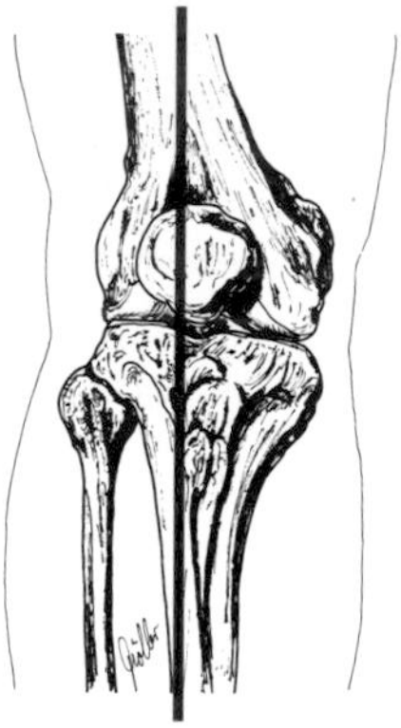

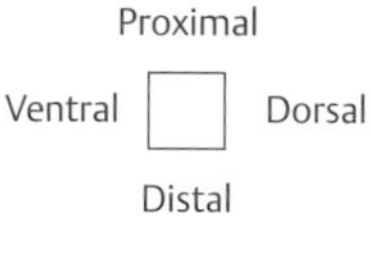
Proximal
Ventral
Dorsal
Distal

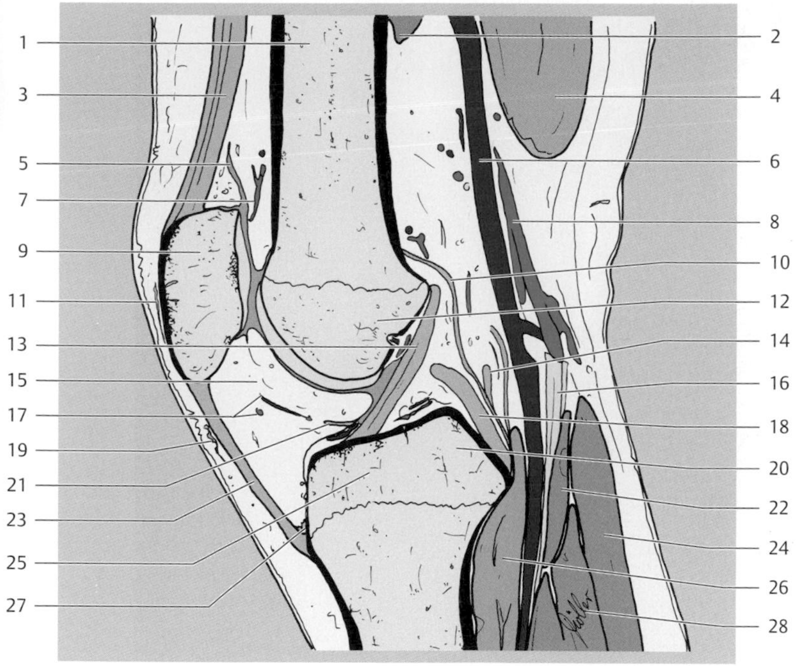

1 Femur (shaft)
2 Vastus medialis muscle
3 Quadriceps tendon
4 Semimembranosus muscle
5 Suprapatellar bursa
6 Popliteal artery
7 Patellar anastomosis
8 Popliteal vein
9 Patella
10 Joint capsule
11 Subcutaneous prepatellar bursa
12 Femur (intercondylar part)
13 Anterior cruciate ligament
14 Oblique popliteal ligament
15 Infrapatellar fat pad
16 Tibial nerve
17 Inferior lateral genicular artery and vein
18 Posterior cruciate ligament
19 Subcutaneous infrapatellar bursa
20 Medial intercondylar tubercle
21 Transverse ligament of knee
22 Plantaris muscle
23 Patellar ligament
24 Gastrocnemius muscle (lateral head)
25 Head of tibia
26 Popliteus muscle
27 Deep infrapatellar bursa
28 Soleus muscle

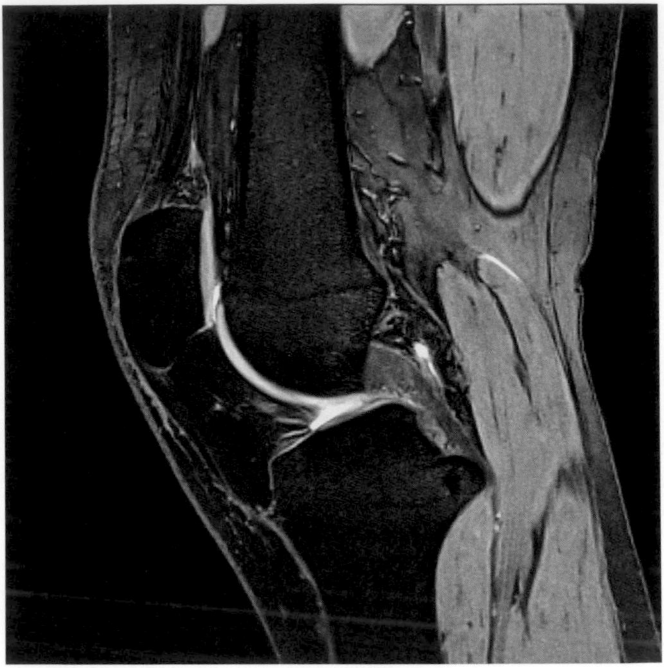

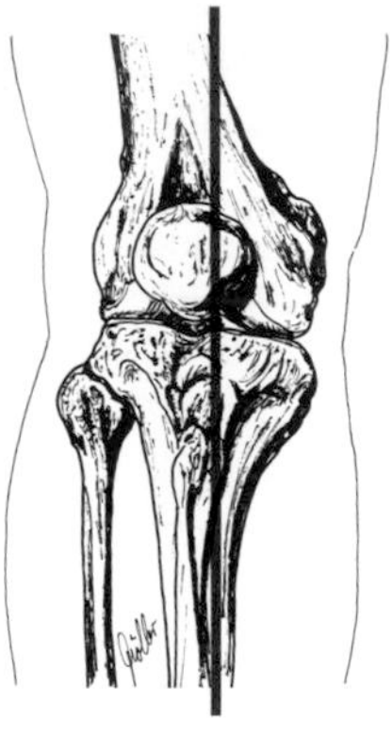

Proximal

Ventral ☐ Dorsal

Distal

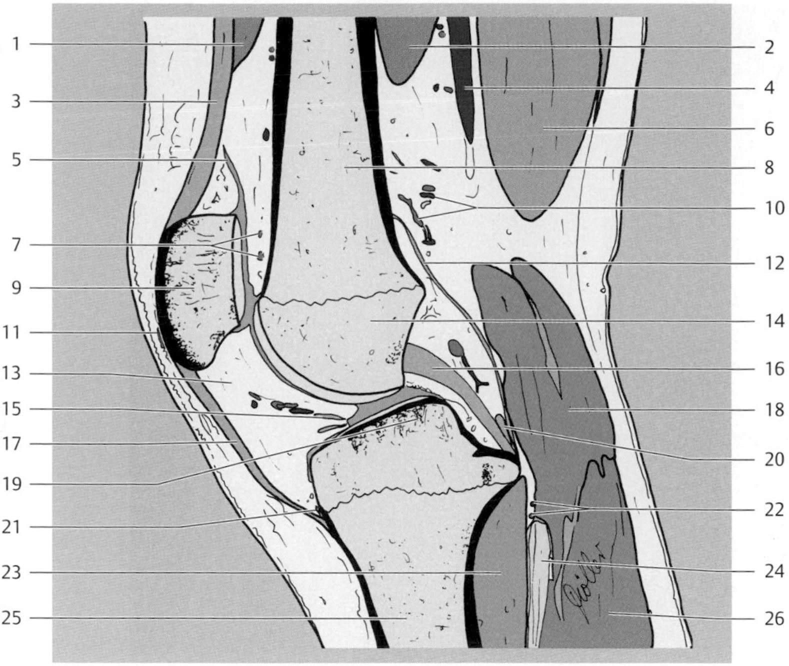

1 Rectus femoris muscle
2 Vastus medialis muscle
3 Quadriceps tendon
4 Superficial femoral artery
5 Suprapatellar bursa
6 Semimembranosus muscle
7 Patellar anastomosis
8 Femur (shaft)
9 Patella
10 Superior medial genicular artery and vein
11 Subcutaneous prepatellar bursa
12 Joint capsule
13 Infrapatellar fat pad
14 Medial femoral condyle
15 Transverse ligament of knee
16 Posterior cruciate ligament
17 Patellar ligament
18 Gastrocnemius muscle (medial head)
19 Medial intercondylar tubercle of tibial condyle
20 Posterior meniscofemoral ligament (Wrisberg ligament)
21 Deep infrapatellar bursa
22 Inferior medial genicular artery and vein
23 Popliteus muscle
24 Tibial nerve
25 Tibia (shaft)
26 Gastrocnemius muscle (lateral head)

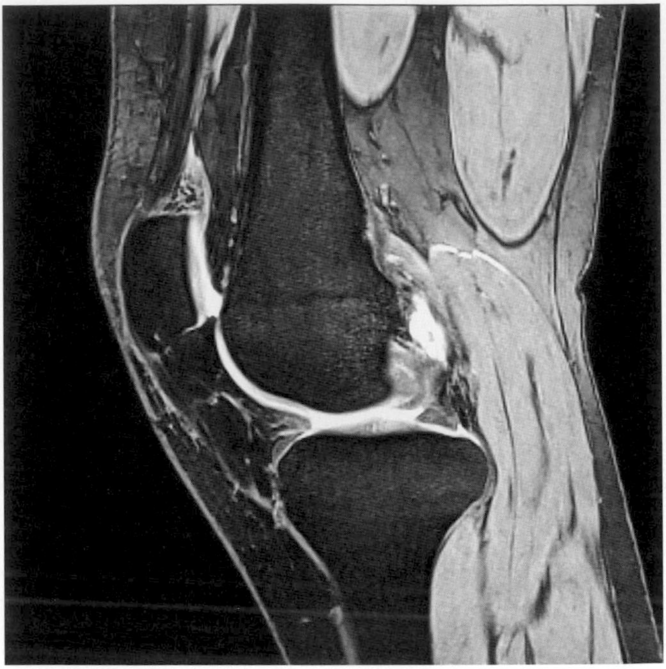

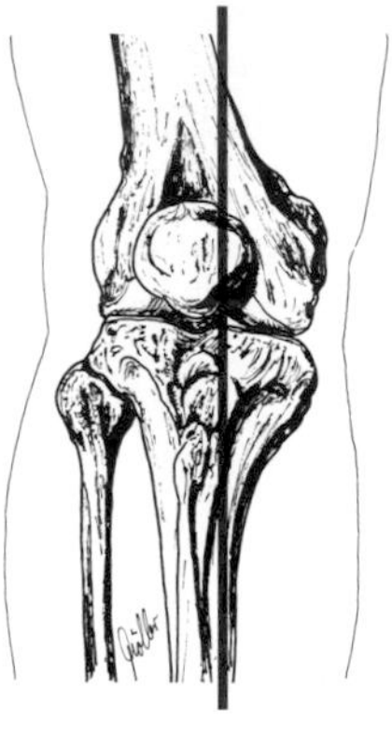

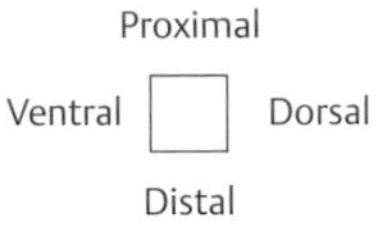
Proximal
Ventral
Dorsal
Distal

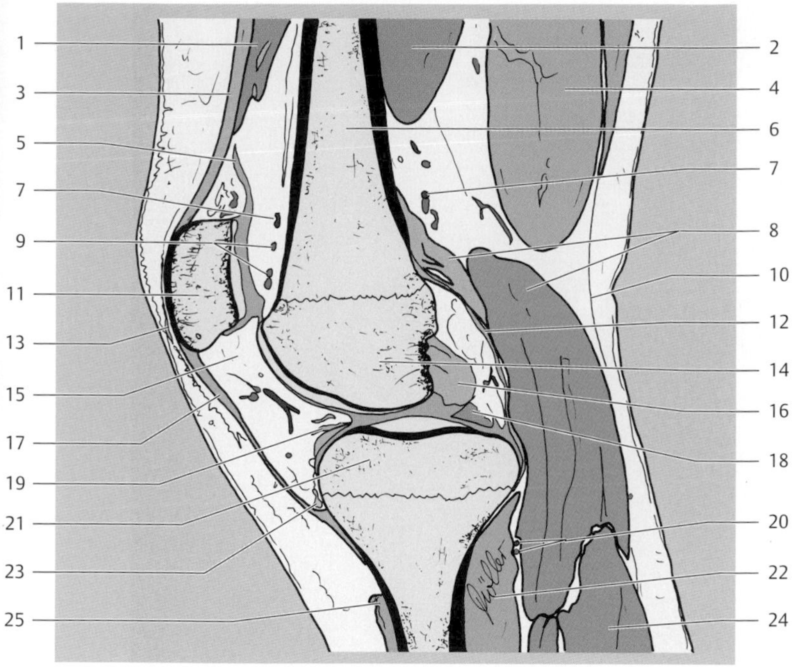

1 Rectus femoris muscle
2 Vastus medialis muscle
3 Quadriceps tendon
4 Semimembranosus muscle
5 Suprapatellar bursa
6 Femur (shaft)
7 Superior medial genicular artery and vein
8 Gastrocnemius muscle (medial head + muscle attachment)
9 Patellar anastomosis
10 Deep fascia of leg
11 Patella
12 Joint capsule
13 Subcutaneous prepatellar bursa
14 Medial femoral condyle
15 Infrapatellar fat pad
16 Posterior cruciate ligament (attachment)
17 Patellar ligament
18 Medial meniscus (posterior horn, inner attachment)
19 Transverse ligament of knee
20 Inferior medial genicular artery and vein
21 Medial tibial condyle
22 Popliteus muscle
23 Deep infrapatellar bursa
24 Gastrocnemius muscle (lateral head)
25 Sartorius muscle (attachment, part of superficial pes anserinus)

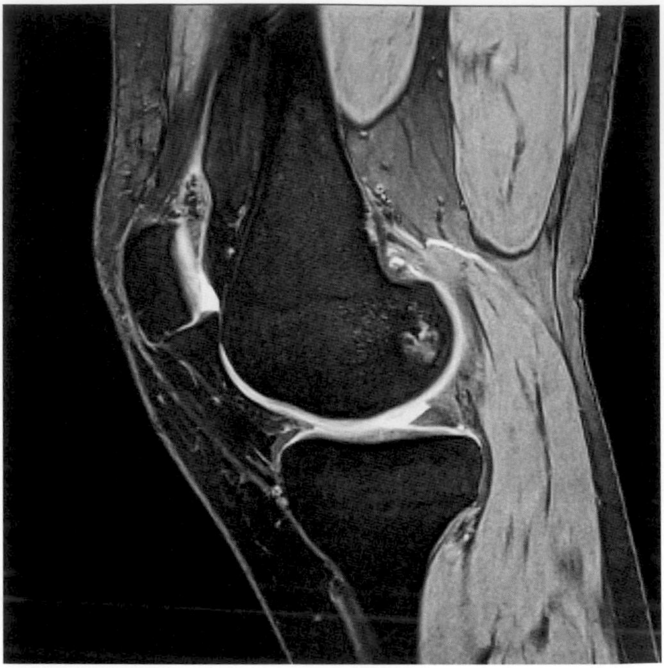

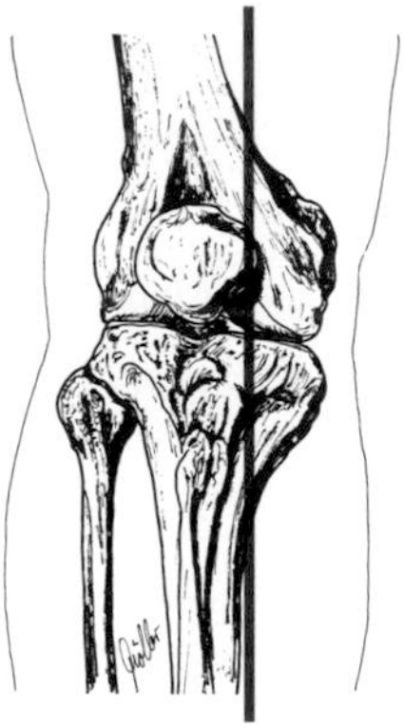

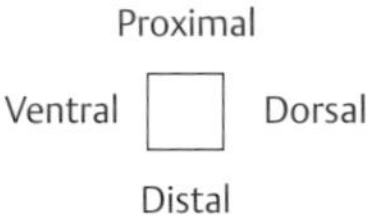
Proximal
Ventral
Dorsal
Distal

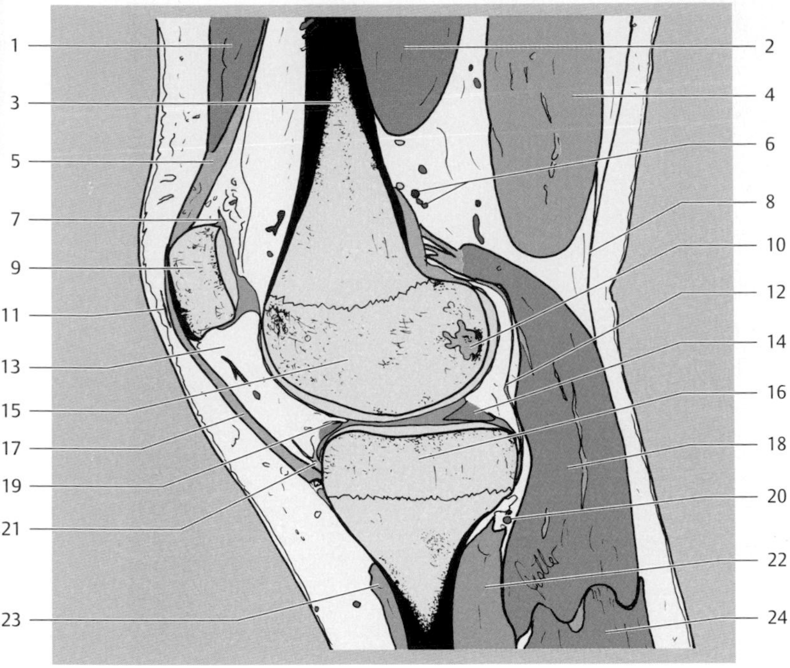

1 Rectus femoris muscle
2 Vastus medialis muscle
3 Femur (shaft)
4 Semimembranosus muscle
5 Quadriceps tendon
6 Superior medial genicular artery and vein
7 Suprapatellar bursa
8 Deep fascia of leg
9 Patella
10 Posterior cruciate ligament (attachment)
11 Subcutaneous prepatellar bursa
12 Joint capsule
13 Infrapatellar fat pad
14 Medial meniscus (posterior horn)
15 Medial femoral condyle
16 Medial condyle of tibia
17 Patellar ligament
18 Gastrocnemius muscle (medial head)
19 Transverse ligament of knee
20 Inferior medial genicular artery and vein
21 Deep infrapatellar bursa
22 Popliteus muscle
23 Sartorius muscle (attachment, part of superficial pes anserinus)
24 Gastrocnemius muscle (lateral head)

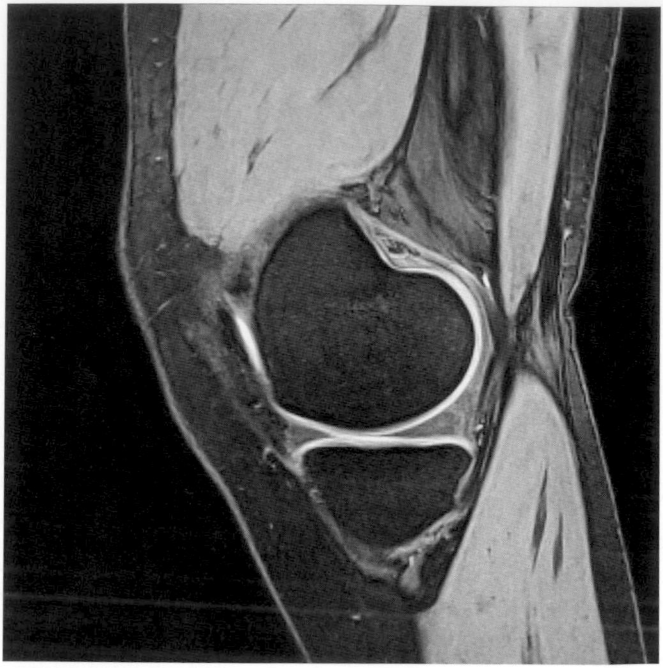

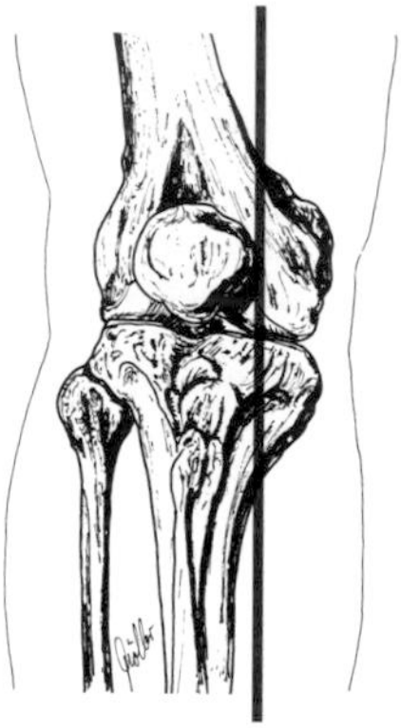

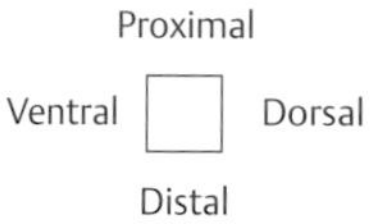
Proximal
Ventral
Dorsal
Distal

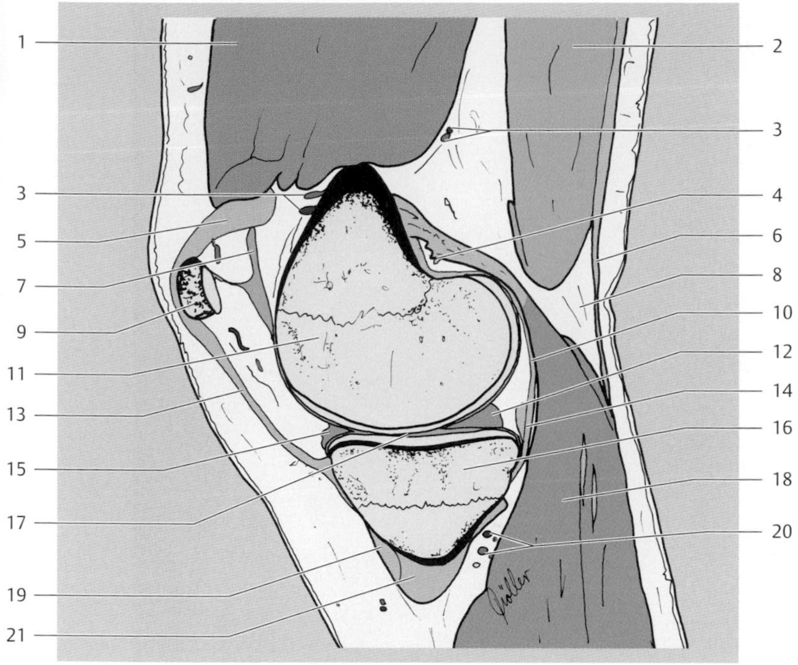

1 Vastus medialis muscle
2 Semimembranosus muscle
3 Superior medial genicular artery and vein
4 Medial subtendinous bursa of gastrocnemius
5 Medial patellar retinaculum
6 Deep fascia of leg
7 Suprapatellar bursa
8 Popliteal fossa
9 Patella
10 Joint capsule
11 Medial femoral condyle
12 Medial meniscus (posterior horn)
13 Medial patellar retinaculum
14 Oblique popliteal ligament
15 Medial meniscus (anterior horn)
16 Medial tibial condyle
17 Knee joint
18 Gastrocnemius muscle (medial head)
19 Sartorius muscle (attachment, part of superficial pes anserinus)
20 Inferior medial genicular artery and vein
21 Pes anserinus (superficial part)

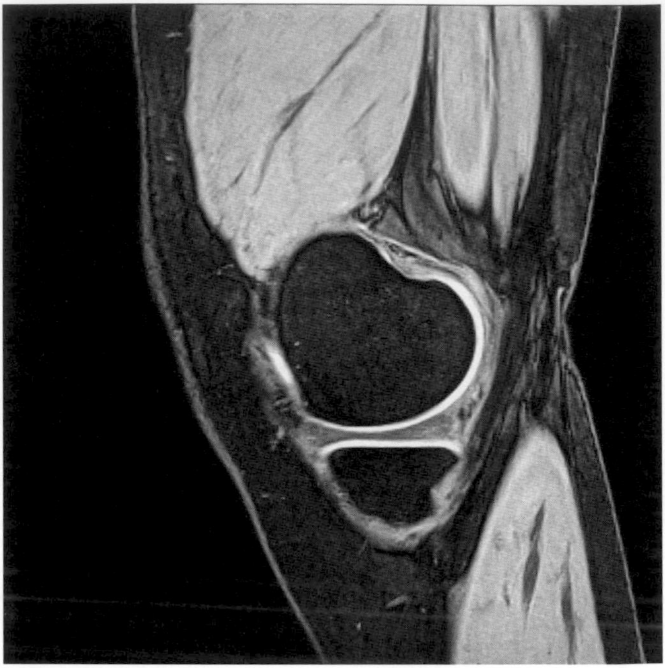

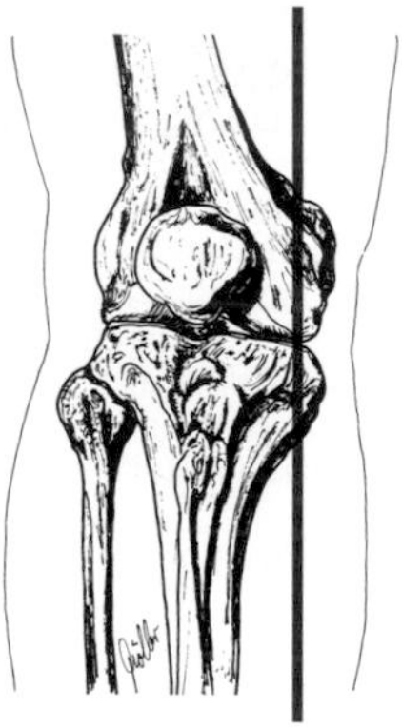

Proximal

Ventral ☐ Dorsal

Distal

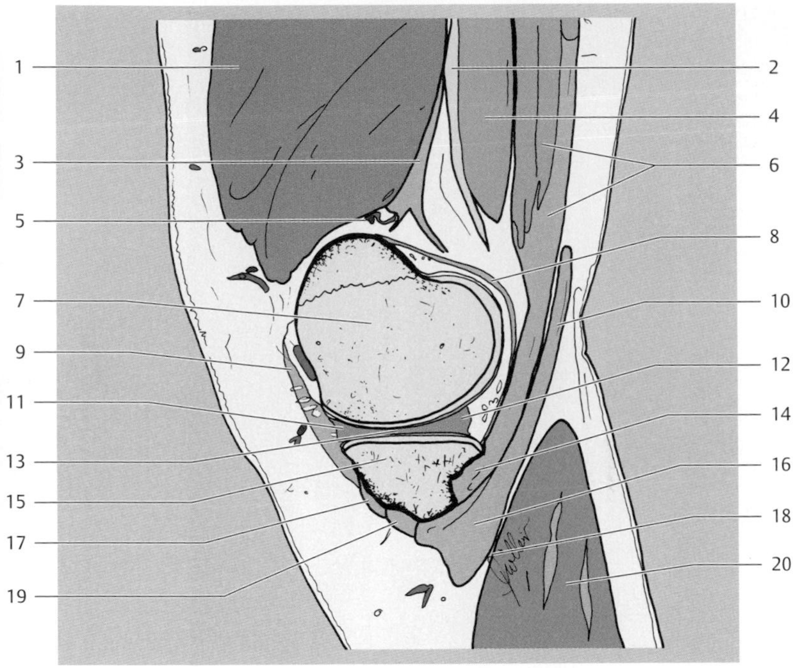

1 Vastus medialis muscle
2 Saphenous nerve
3 Adductor magnus muscle (tendon)
4 Sartorius muscle
5 Superior medial genicular artery and vein
6 Semimembranosus muscle (+ tendon)
7 Medial femoral condyle
8 Joint capsule
9 Medial patellar retinaculum
10 Semitendinosus muscle (tendon)
11 Medial meniscus (anterior horn)
12 Medial meniscus (posterior horn)
13 Medial meniscus (intermediate portion)
14 Pes anserinus (deep part)
15 Medial tibial condyle
16 Pes anserinus (superficial part)
17 Sartorius muscle (attachment, part of superficial pes anserinus)
18 Anserine bursa
19 Gracilis muscle (attachment, part of superficial pes anserinus)
20 Gastrocnemius muscle (medial head)

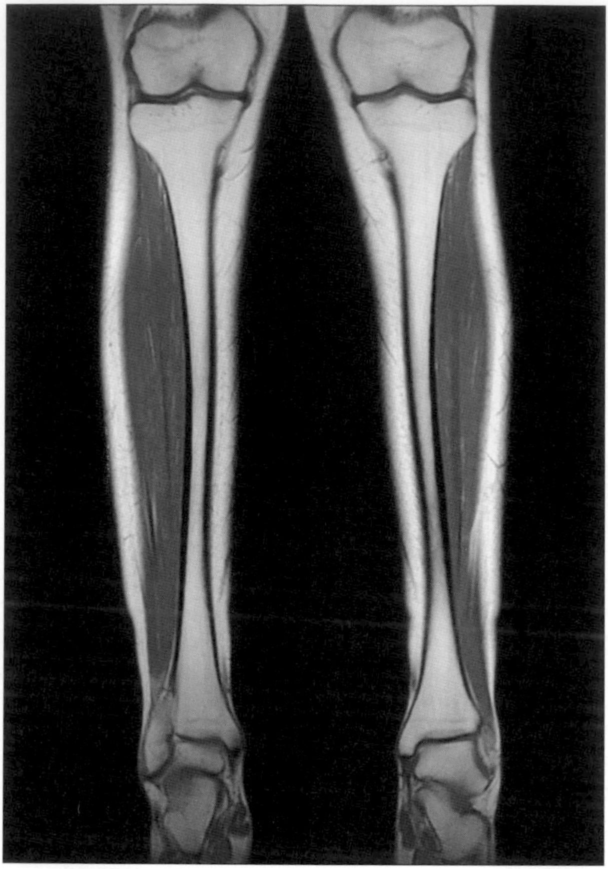

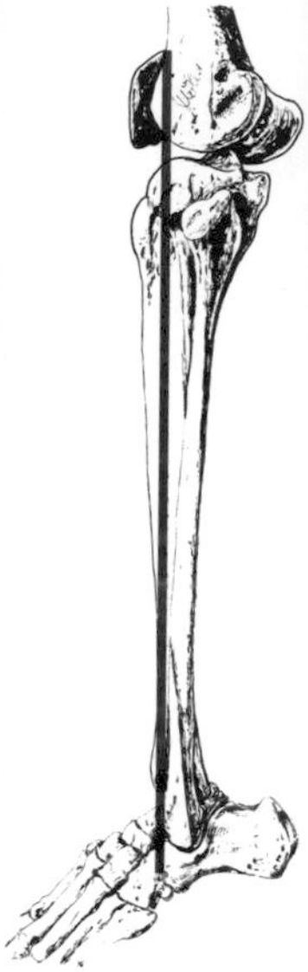

1 Gastrocnemius muscle (medial head, femoral attachment)
2 Gastrocnemius muscle (lateral head, femoral attachment)
3 Plantaris muscle (tendon)
4 Medial collateral ligament
5 Fibular collateral ligament
6 Medial femoral condyle
7 Popliteus muscle (tendon)
8 Lateral femoral condyle
9 Lateral meniscus (intermediate portion)
10 Iliotibial tract

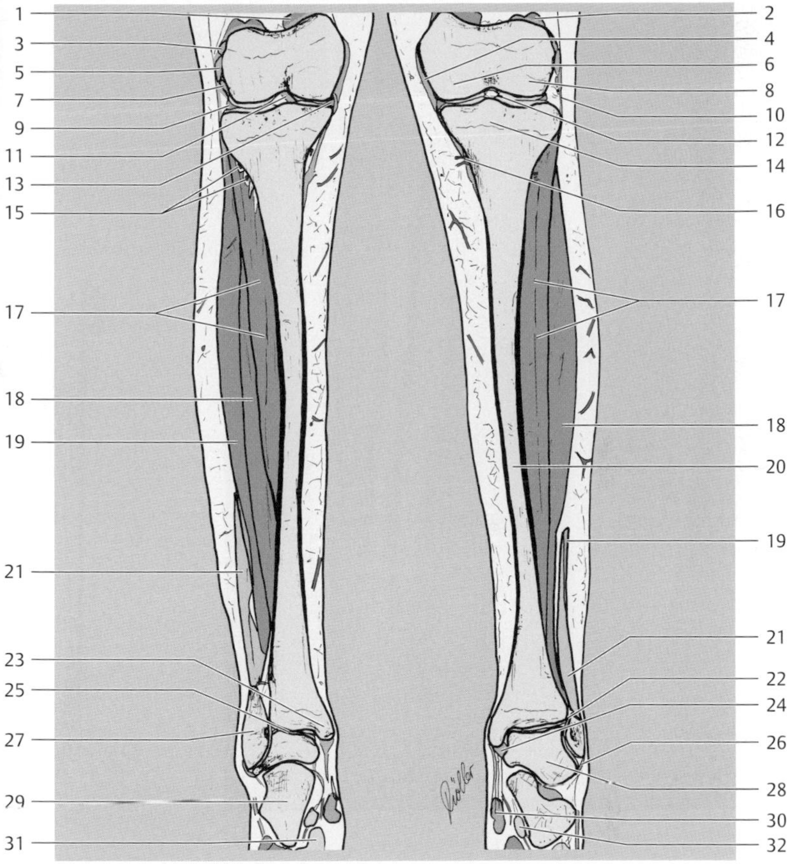

11 Anterior cruciate ligament
12 Knee joint
13 Medial meniscus (intermediate portion)
14 Tibia (head)
15 Inferior lateral genicular artery and vein
16 Inferior medial genicular artery and vein
17 Tibialis anterior muscle
18 Extensor digitorum longus muscle
19 Extensor hallucis longus muscle (tendon)
20 Tibia (shaft)
21 Peroneus (fibularis) brevis muscle
22 Talofibular joint
23 Medial malleolus
24 Deltoid ligament
25 Ankle joint
26 Anterior talofibular ligament
27 Fibula
28 Talus
29 Calcaneus
30 Abductor hallucis muscle
31 Flexor digitorum brevis muscle
32 Quadratus plantae muscle

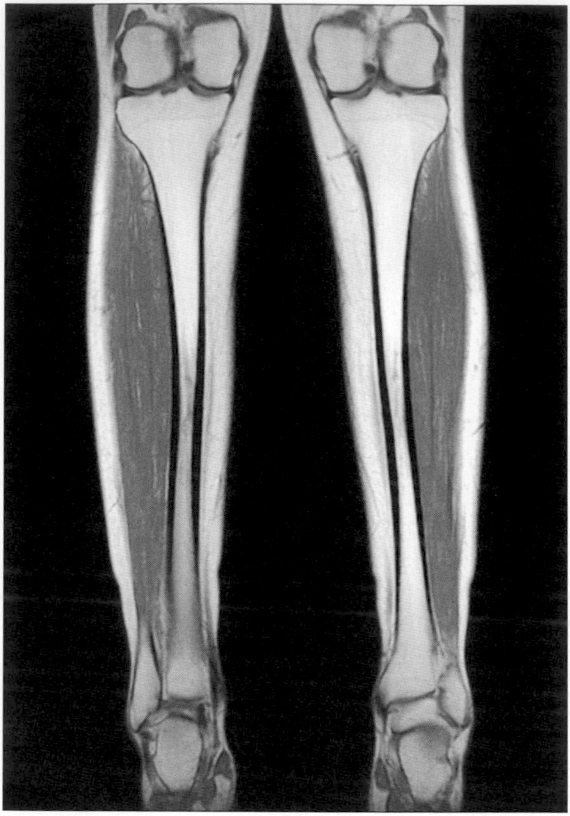

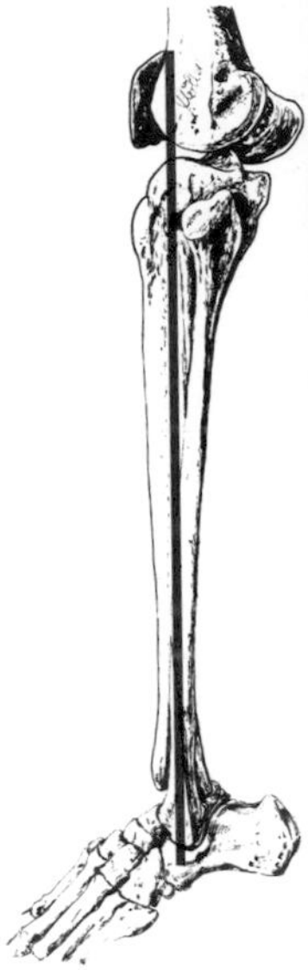

1 Biceps femoris muscle
2 Medial collateral ligament
3 Gastrocnemius muscle (lateral head, femoral attachment)
4 Medial femoral condyle
5 Gastrocnemius muscle (medial head, femoral attachment)
6 Intercondylar fossa
7 Popliteus muscle (tendon)
8 Lateral femoral condyle
9 Lateral meniscus (intermediate portion)
10 Iliotibial tract
11 Posterior cruciate ligament
12 Knee joint
13 Anterior cruciate ligament
14 Lateral tibial condyle
15 Medial meniscus (intermediate portion)
16 Intercondylar tubercle
17 Popliteus muscle (tibial attachment)
18 Medial tibial condyle
19 Anterior tibial artery and vein, deep peroneal (fibular) nerve
20 Pes anserinus (superficial)

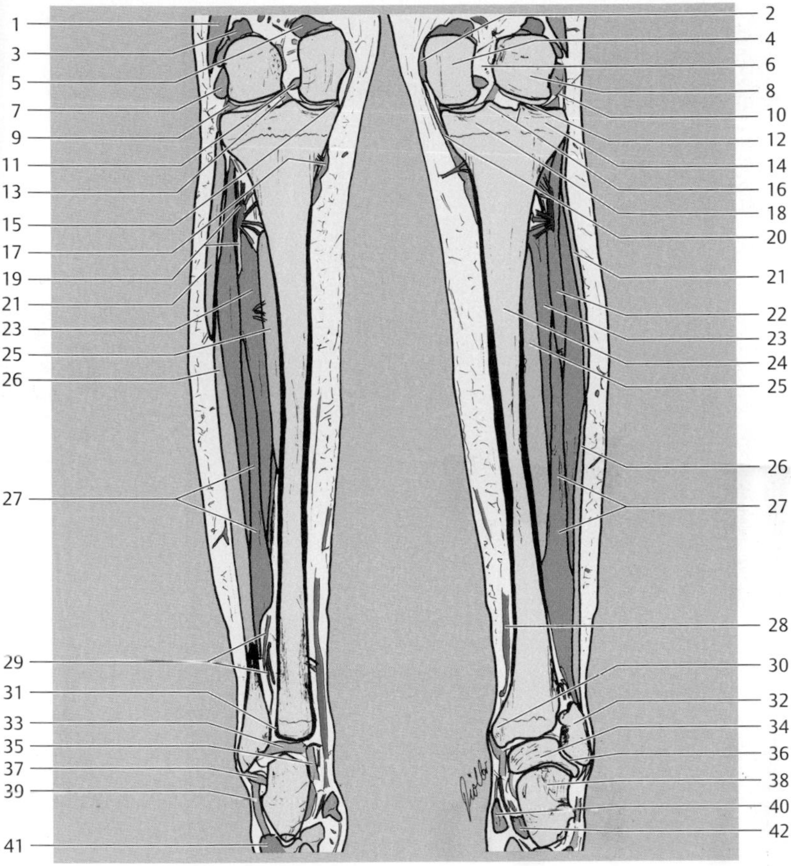

21 Peroneus (fibularis) longus muscle
22 Extensor digitorum longus muscle
23 Tibialis anterior muscle
24 Tibia (shaft)
25 Tibialis posterior muscle
26 Peroneus (fibularis) brevis muscle
27 Extensor hallucis longus muscle
28 Great saphenous vein
29 Fibular artery and vein
30 Medial malleolus
31 Inferior tibiofibular joint (syndesmosis)
32 Lateral malleolus
33 Posterior talofibular ligament
34 Talus
35 Flexor digitorum longus muscle (tendon)
36 Talofibular joint
37 Calcaneofibular ligament
38 Calcaneus
39 Peroneus (fibularis) longus and brevis muscles (tendons)
40 Abductor hallucis muscle
41 Abductor digiti minimi muscle
42 Quadratus plantae muscle

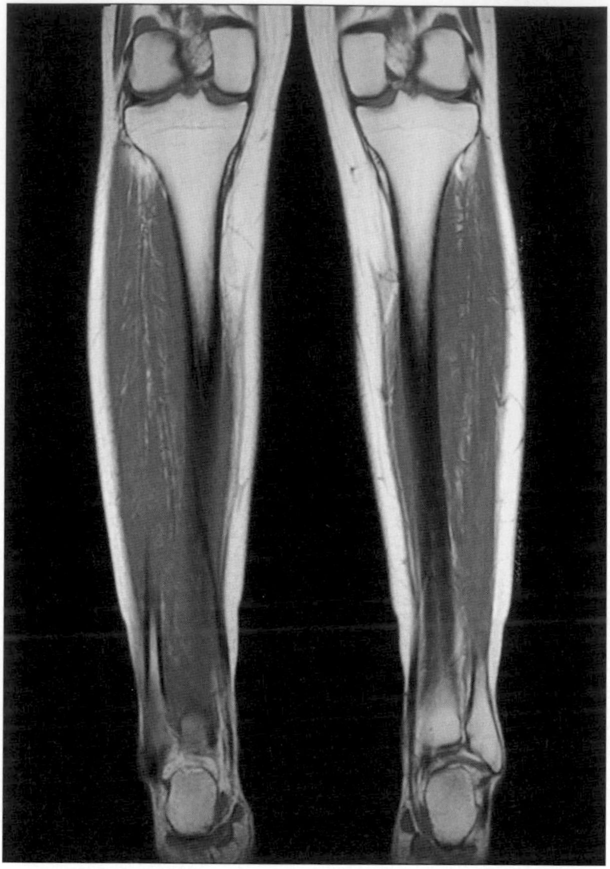

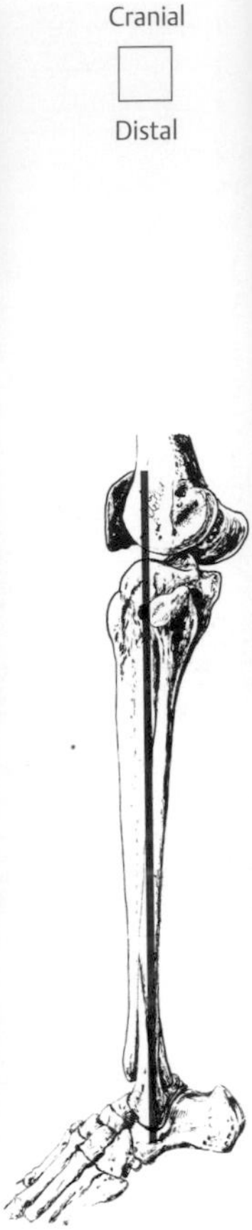

1 Biceps femoris muscle
2 Sartorius and gracilis muscles (tendons)
3 Medial femoral condyle
4 Gastrocnemius muscle (lateral head, femoral attachment)
5 Lateral femoral condyle
6 Gastrocnemius muscle (medial head, femoral attachment)
7 Plantaris muscle (tendon)
8 Lateral collateral ligament
9 Posterior cruciate ligament
10 Medial meniscus (intermediate portion)
11 Popliteus muscle (tendon)
12 Popliteus muscle (tibial attachment)
13 Lateral meniscus (intermediate portion)
14 Peroneus (fibularis) longus muscle
15 Anterior cruciate ligament
16 Tibialis anterior muscle
17 Tibia (head)
18 Soleus muscle

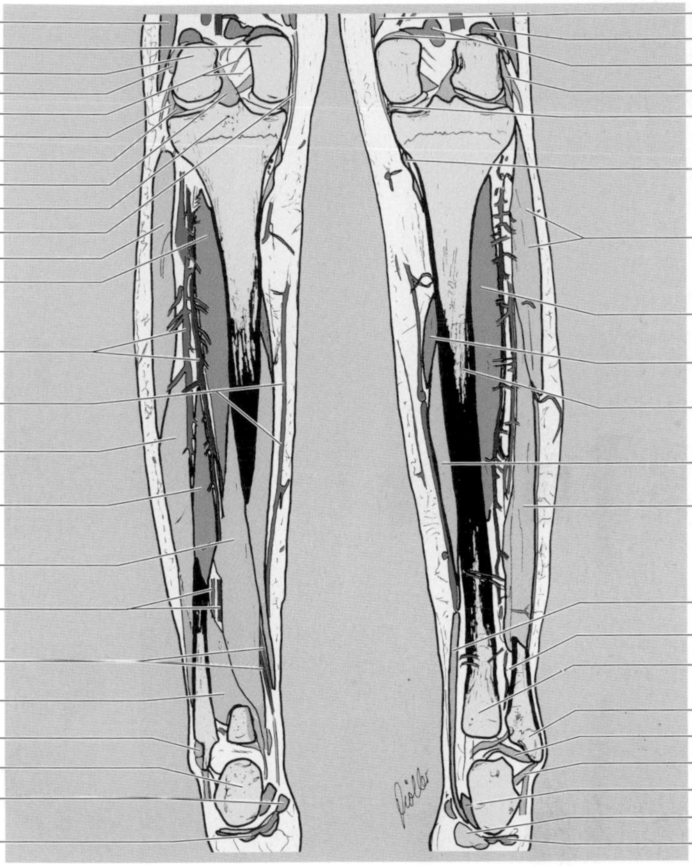

19 Medial collateral ligament
20 Tibia (shaft)
21 Anterior tibial artery and vein and deep peroneal nerve
22 Flexor digitorum longus muscle
23 Great saphenous vein
24 Peroneus (fibularis) brevis muscle
25 Extensor hallucis longus muscle
26 Fibular artery and vein
27 Tibialis posterior muscle
28 Tibia
29 Posterior tibial artery and vein
30 Fibula
31 Flexor hallucis longus muscle
32 Posterior talofibular ligament
33 Peroneus (fibularis) longus and brevis muscles (tendons)
34 Calcaneofibular ligament
35 Calcaneus
36 Quadratus plantae muscle
37 Abductor hallucis muscle
38 Flexor digitorum brevis muscle
39 Flexor digitorum brevis muscle and plantar aponeurosis
40 Abductor digiti minimi muscle

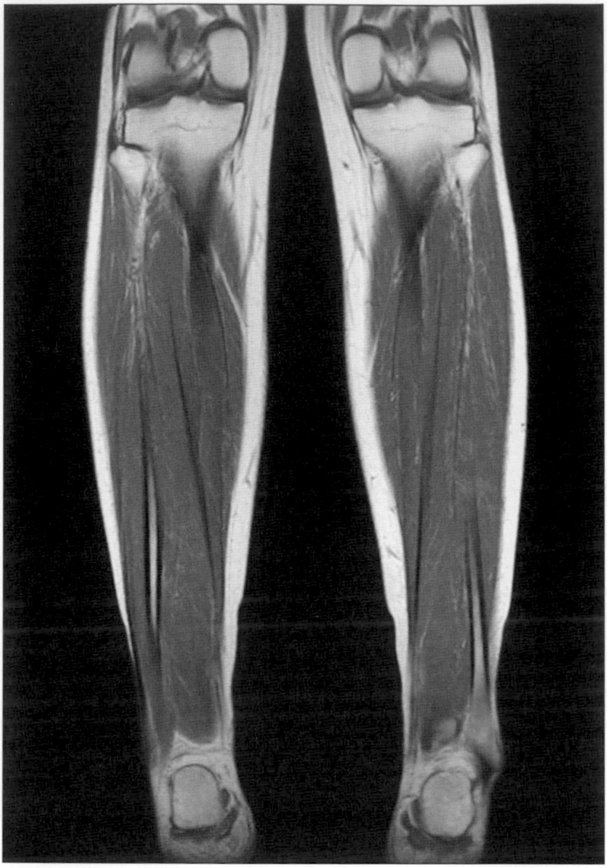

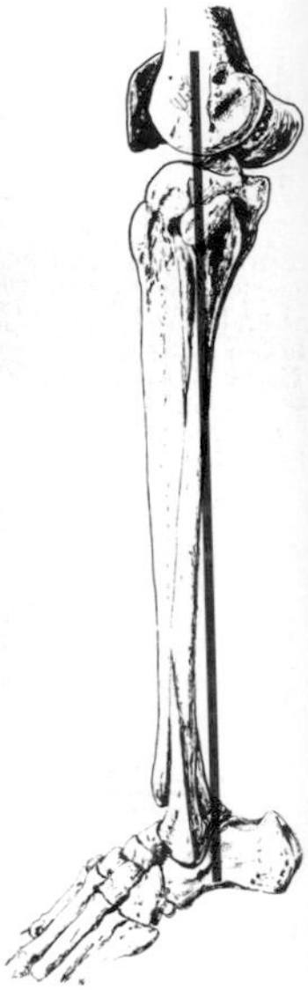

1 Biceps femoris muscle
2 Sartorius and gracilis muscles (tendons)
3 Medial femoral condyle
4 Gastrocnemius muscle (lateral head, femoral attachment)
5 Lateral femoral condyle
6 Gastrocnemius muscle (medial head, femoral attachment)
7 Anterior cruciate ligament
8 Posterior cruciate ligament
9 Tibia (head)
10 Lateral meniscus (intermediate portion)
11 Fibular collateral ligament
12 Medial meniscus (intermediate portion)
13 Tibiofibular joint
14 Fibula (head)
15 Popliteus muscle (tibial attachment)
16 Tibia (shaft)

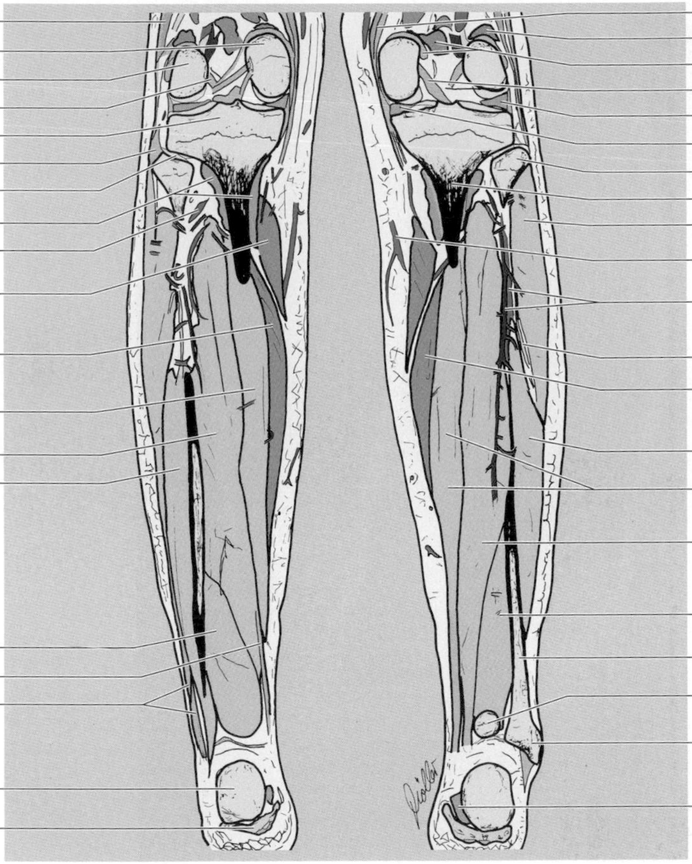

17 Anterior tibial artery and vein and deep peroneal nerve
18 Peroneus (fibularis) longus muscle
19 Gastrocnemius muscle (medial head)
20 Great saphenous vein
21 Soleus muscle
22 Fibular artery and vein
23 Flexor digitorum longus muscle
24 Superficial fibular nerve
25 Tibialis posterior muscle
26 Peroneus (fibularis) brevis muscle
27 Flexor hallucis longus muscle
28 Fibula (shaft)
29 Peroneus (fibularis) longus and brevis muscles (tendons)
30 Tibia
31 Calcaneus
32 Malleolus lateralis
33 Flexor digitorum brevis muscle
34 Quadratus plantae muscle

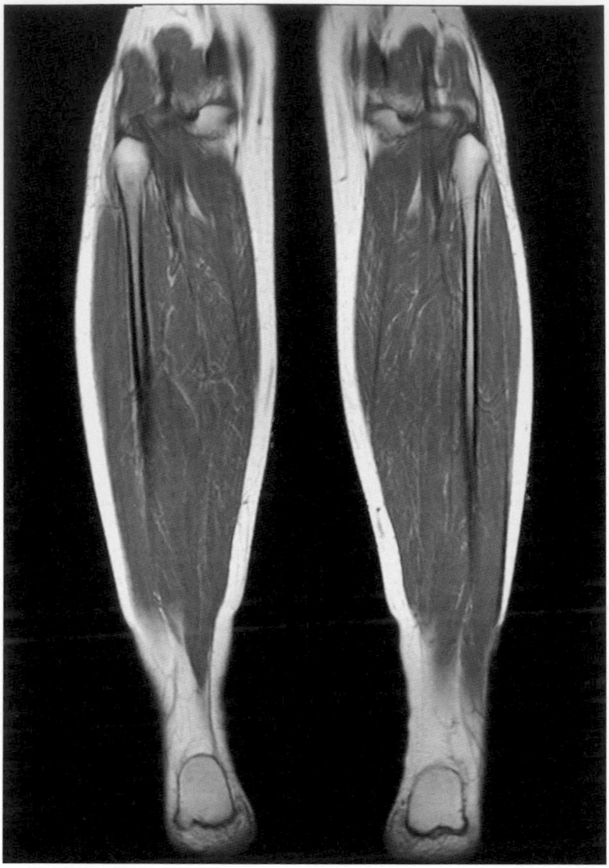

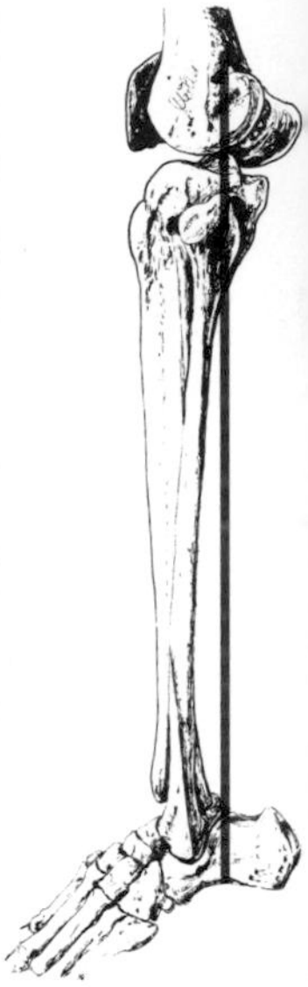

1 Gracilis muscle (tendon)
2 Gastrocnemius muscle (medial head)
3 Sartorius muscle (tendon)
4 Popliteal artery and vein
5 Semimembranosus muscle (tendon)

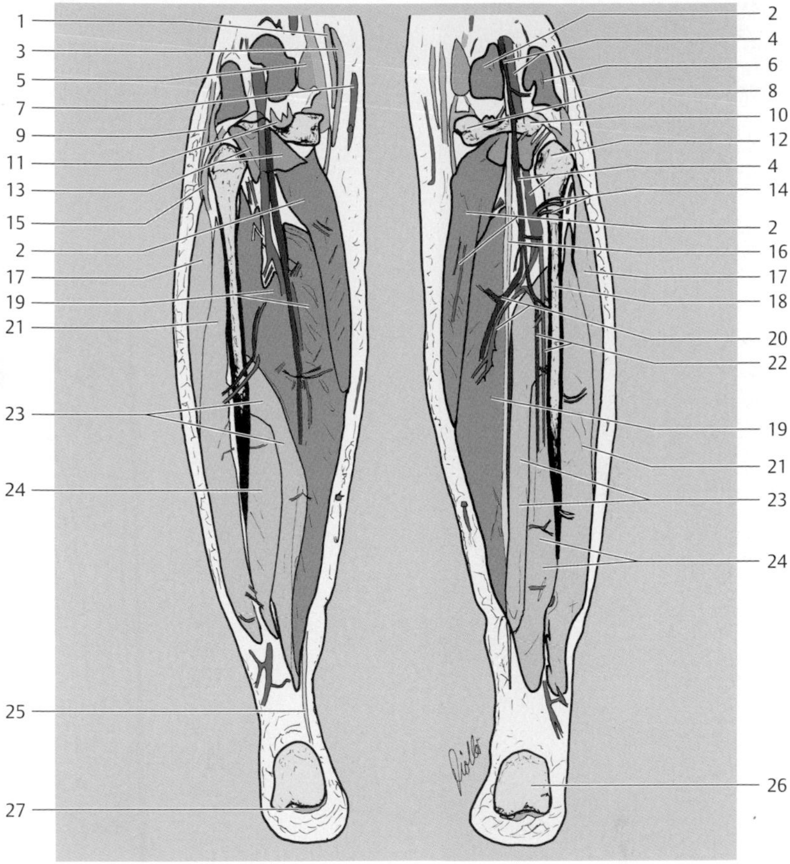

6 Gastrocnemius muscle (lateral head)
7 Great saphenous vein
8 Tibia (medial condyle)
9 Iliotibial tract
10 Tibia (lateral condyle)
11 Anterior cruciate ligament
12 Fibula (head)
13 Popliteus muscle
14 Posterior tibial recurrent artery and vein
15 Fibular collateral ligament
16 Posterior tibial nerve
17 Peroneus (fibularis) longus muscle
18 Fibula (shaft)
19 Soleus muscle
20 Posterior tibial artery and vein
21 Peroneus (fibularis) brevis muscle
22 Fibular artery and vein
23 Tibialis posterior muscle
24 Flexor hallucis longus muscle
25 Tibial nerve
26 Calcaneus
27 Plantar aponeurosis

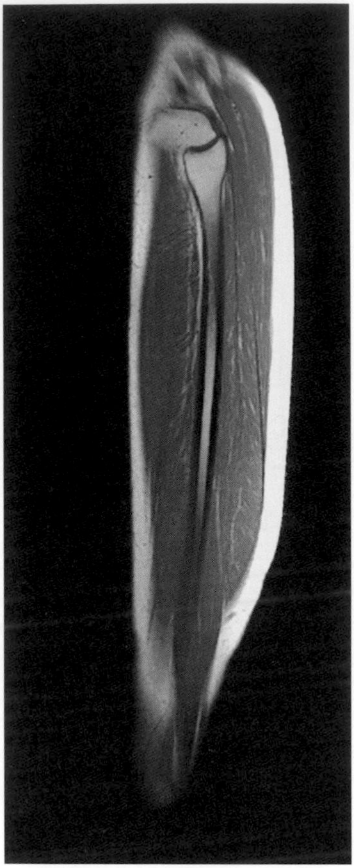

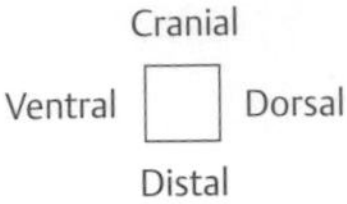
Cranial
Ventral
Dorsal
Distal

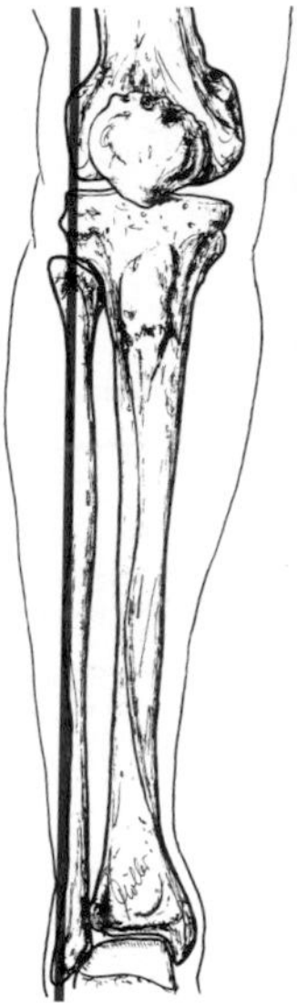

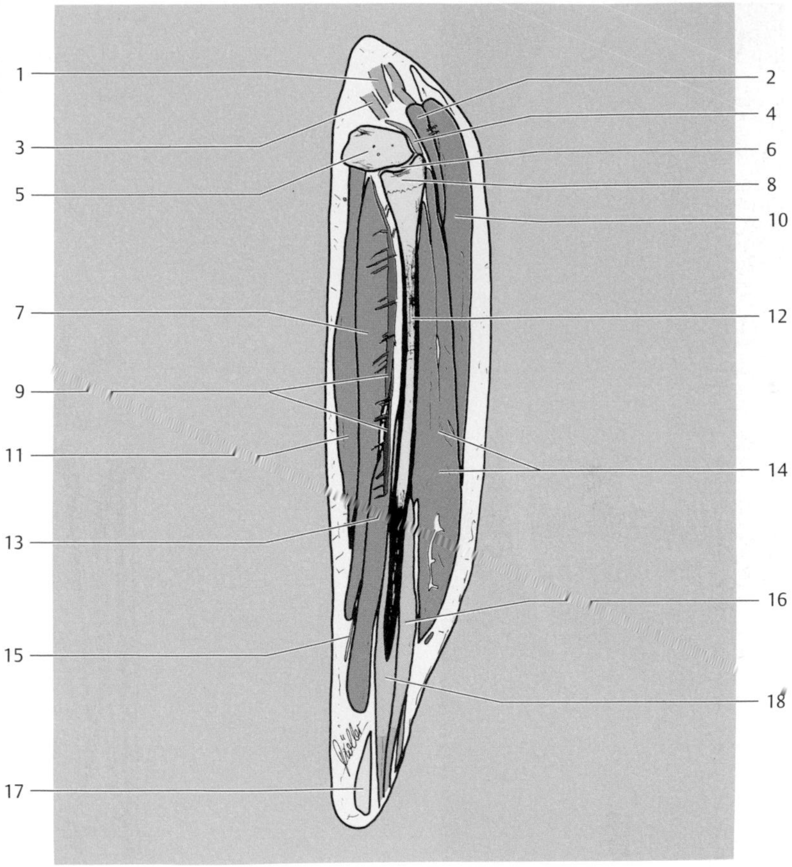

1 Iliotibial tract
2 Plantaris muscle (+ tendon)
3 Lateral patellar retinaculum
4 Popliteus muscle and arcuate popliteal ligament
5 Tibia (head)
6 Tibiofibular joint (superior tibiofibular joint)
7 Extensor digitorum longus muscle
8 Fibula (head)
9 Tibialis anterior artery and vein
10 Gastrocnemius muscle (lateral head)
11 Tibialis anterior muscle
12 Fibula (shaft)
13 Extensor hallucis longus muscle
14 Soleus muscle
15 Superficial fibular nerve
16 Peroneus (fibularis) longus muscle
17 Fibula (lateral malleolus)
18 Peroneus (fibularis) brevis muscle

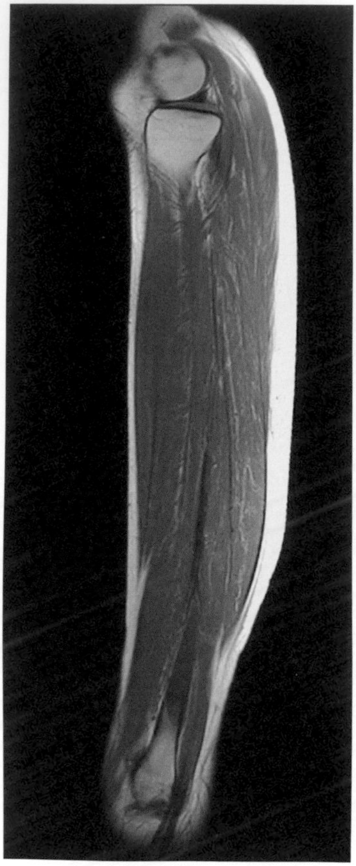

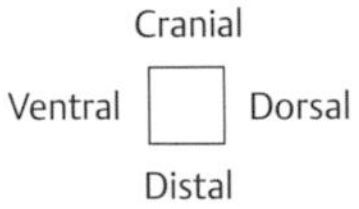

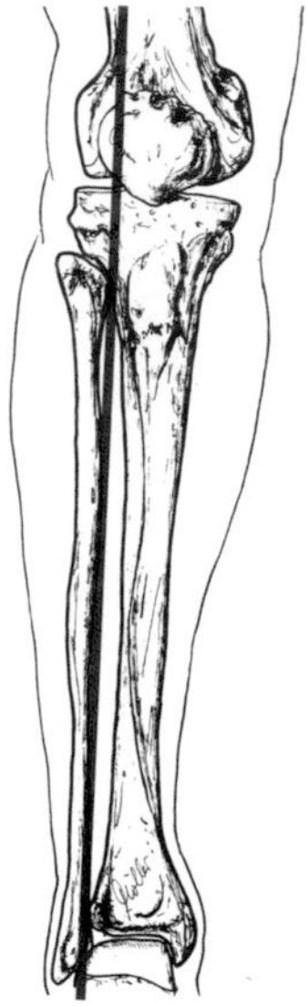

1 Iliotibial tract
2 Biceps femoris muscle (tendon)
3 Lateral patellar retinaculum
4 Gastrocnemius muscle
(lateral head, attachment)
5 Knee joint

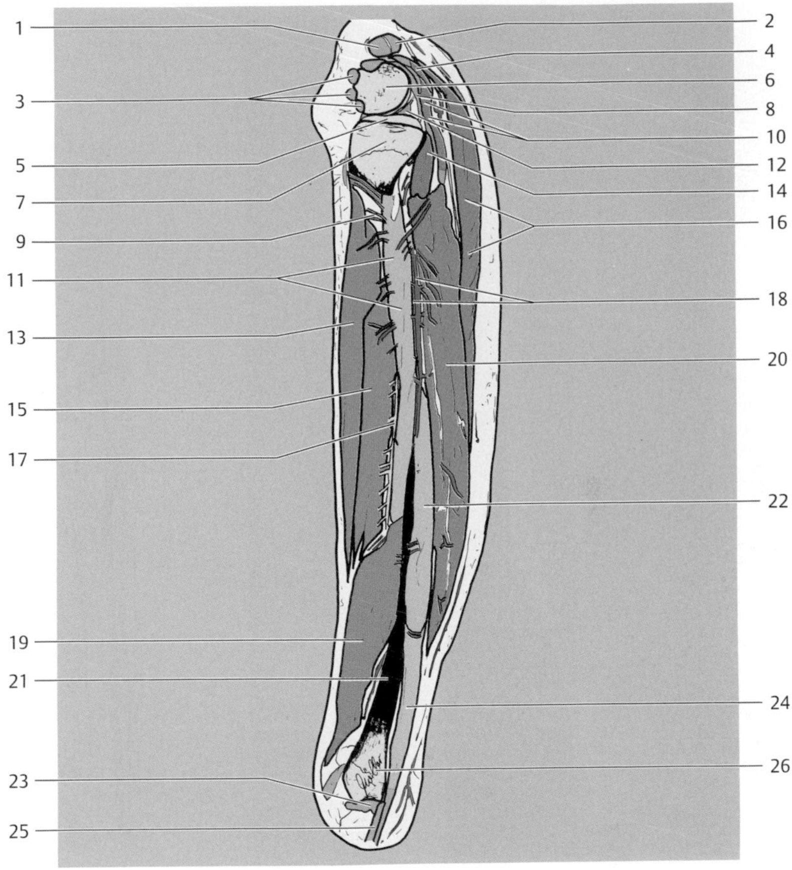

6 Lateral femoral condyle
7 Tibia (head)
8 Joint capsule of knee
9 Tibialis anterior artery and vein
10 Plantaris muscle (+ tendon)
11 Posterior tibialis muscle
12 Lateral meniscus (posterior horn)
13 Tibialis anterior muscle
14 Popliteus muscle
15 Extensor digitorum longus muscle
16 Gastrocnemius muscle (lateral head)
17 Superficial fibular nerve
18 Fibular artery and vein
19 Extensor hallucis longus muscle
20 Soleus muscle
21 Fibula (shaft)
22 Flexor hallucis longus muscle
23 Calcaneofibular ligament
24 Peroneus (fibularis) longus muscle
25 Peroneus (fibularis) brevis muscle (tendon)
26 Fibula (lateral malleolus)

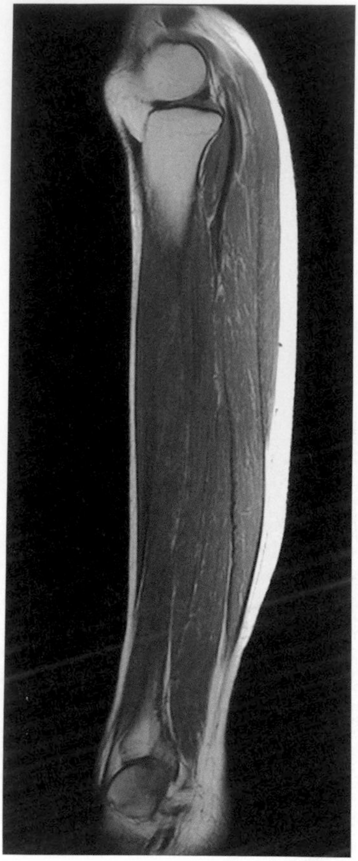

Cranial

Ventral Dorsal

Distal

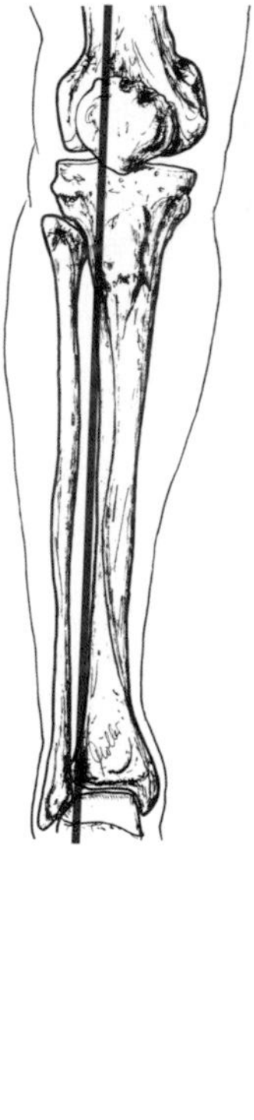

1 Iliotibial tract
2 Biceps femoris muscle (tendon)
3 Lateral patellar retinaculum
4 Gastrocnemius muscle
(lateral head, attachment)

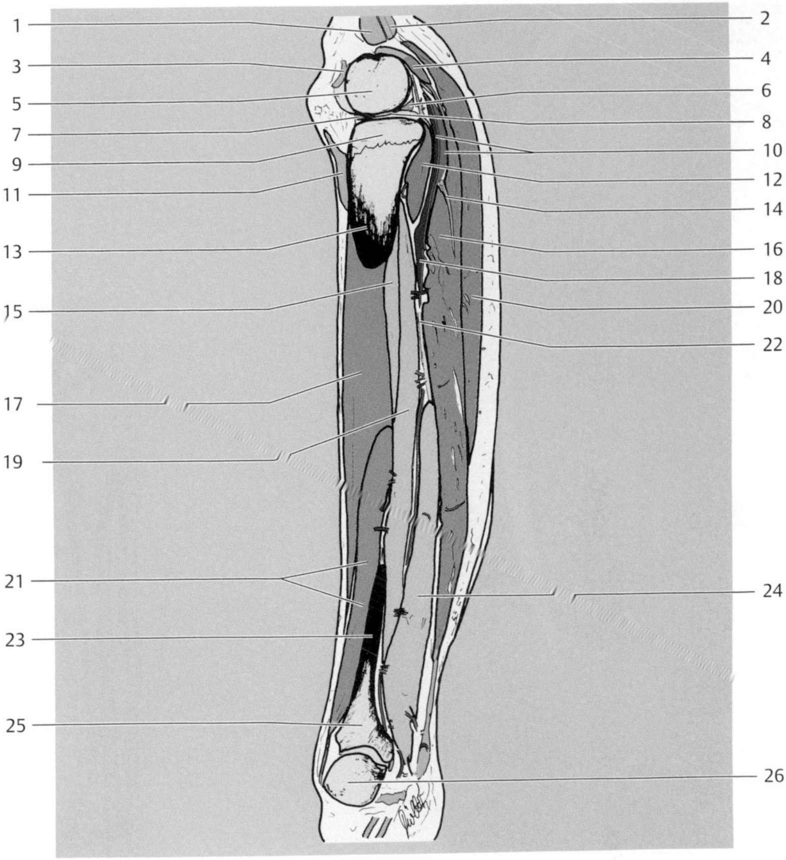

5 Lateral femoral condyle
6 Lateral meniscus (posterior horn)
7 Lateral meniscus (anterior horn)
8 Knee joint
9 Tibia (head)
10 Popliteal artery and vein
11 Patellar ligament
12 Popliteus muscle
13 Tibia (shaft)
14 Plantaris muscle (+ tendon)
15 Flexor digitorum longus muscle
16 Soleus muscle
17 Tibialis anterior muscle
18 Tibiofibular trunk
19 Posterior tibialis muscle
20 Gastrocnemius muscle (lateral head)
21 Extensor hallucis longus muscle
22 Tibialis nerve
23 Tibia (shaft)
24 Flexor hallucis longus muscle
25 Tibia
26 Talus

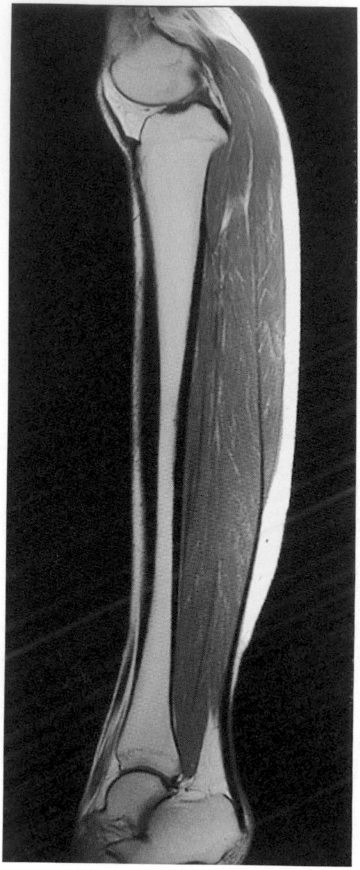

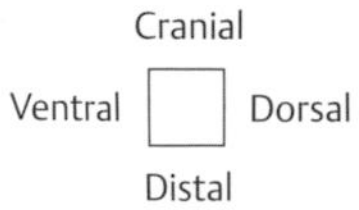

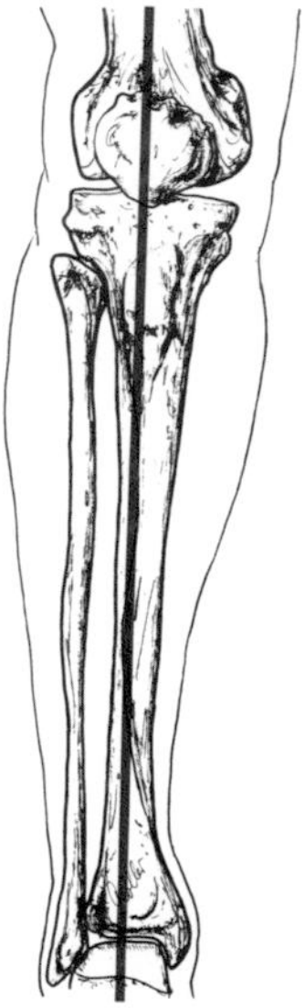

1 Superior lateral genicular artery and vein
2 Tibial nerve
3 Femur
4 Popliteal artery and vein
5 Infrapatellar (Hoffa) fat pad
6 Gastrocnemius muscle (lateral head)
7 Patellar tendon
8 Posterior cruciate ligament
9 Tibial tuberosity
10 Anterior cruciate ligament

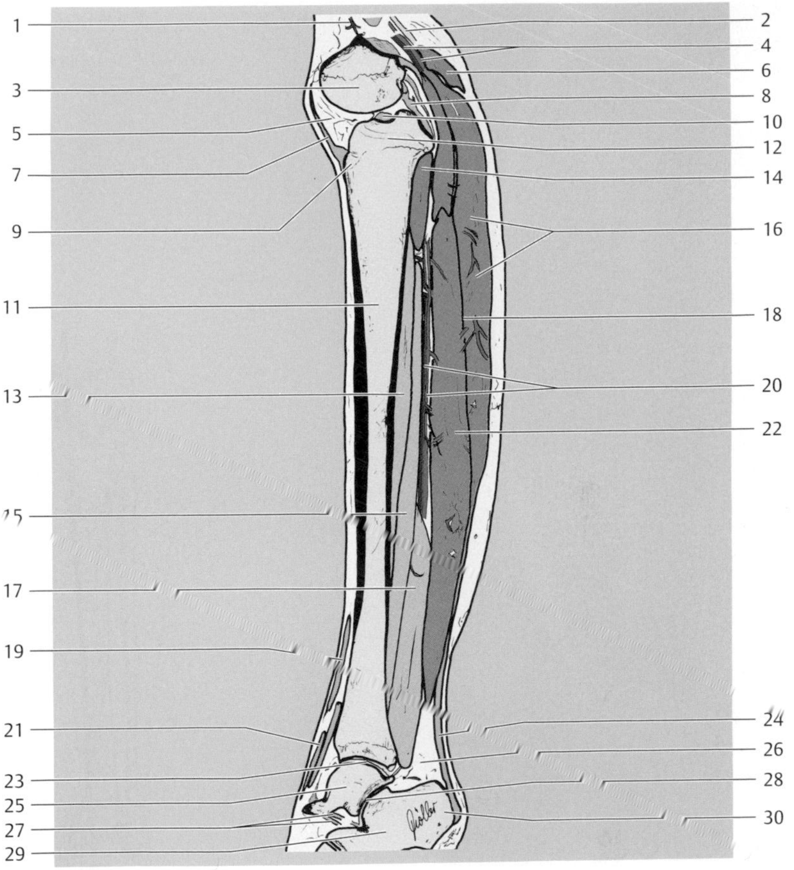

11 Tibia (shaft)
12 Tibia (head)
13 Flexor digitorum longus muscle
14 Popliteus muscle
15 Tibialis posterior muscle
16 Gastrocnemius muscle (medial head)
17 Flexor hallucis longus muscle
18 Plantaris muscle (tendon)
19 Tibialis anterior muscle (tendon)
20 Posterior tibial artery and vein and tibial nerve
21 Extensor digitorum longus muscle and extensor hallucis longus muscle (tendons)
22 Soleus muscle
23 Ankle joint
24 Achilles tendon (calcaneal tendon)
25 Talus
26 Pre-Achilles fat body
27 Talocalcaneal interosseous ligament
28 Subtalar joint
29 Calcaneus
30 Calcaneal tuberosity

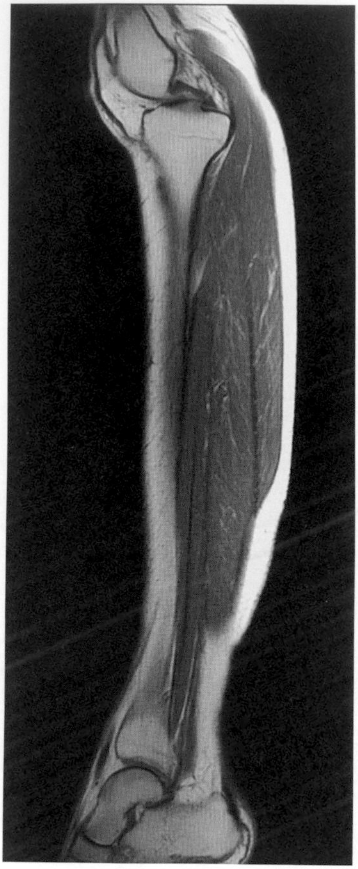

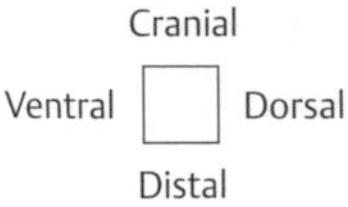

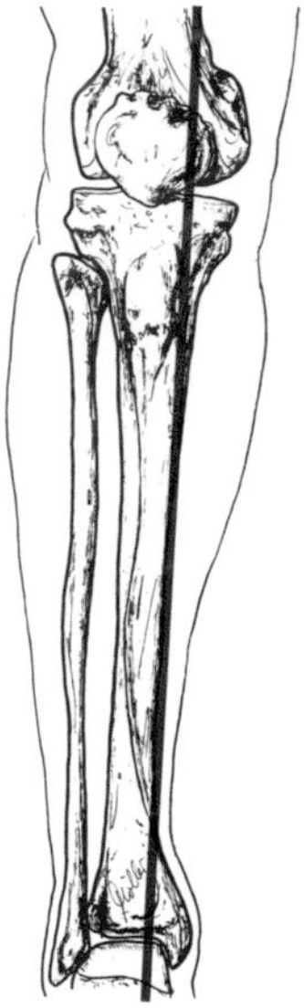

1 Quadriceps tendon
2 Popliteal artery and vein
3 Patella
4 Gastrocnemius muscle (lateral head)
5 Femur
6 Posterior cruciate ligament
7 Infrapatellar (Hoffa) fat pad
8 Medial meniscus (posterior horn)
9 Patellar tendon
10 Anterior cruciate ligament

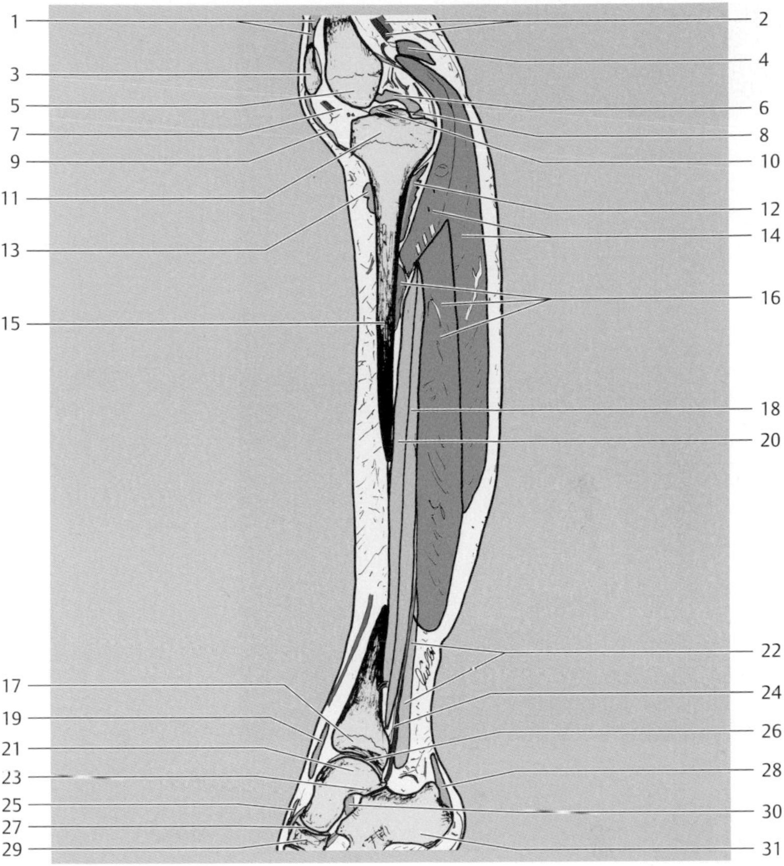

11 Tibia (head)
12 Popliteus muscle
13 Pes anserinus tendon
14 Gastrocnemius muscle (medial head)
15 Tibia (shaft)
16 Soleus muscle
17 Tibia
18 Tibialis posterior muscle
19 Tibialis anterior muscle (tendon)
20 Flexor digitorum longus muscle
21 Talus
22 Flexor hallucis longus muscle
23 Subtalar joint
24 Posterior tibial artery and vein and tibial nerve
25 Extensor digitorum longus muscle (tendon)
26 Ankle joint
27 Talonavicular joint
28 Achilles tendon (calcaneal tendon)
29 Navicular
30 Talocalcaneal interosseous ligament
31 Calcaneus

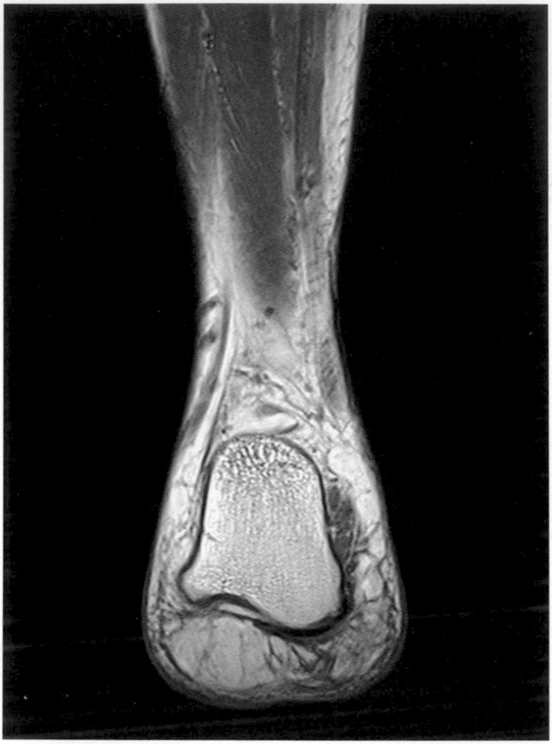

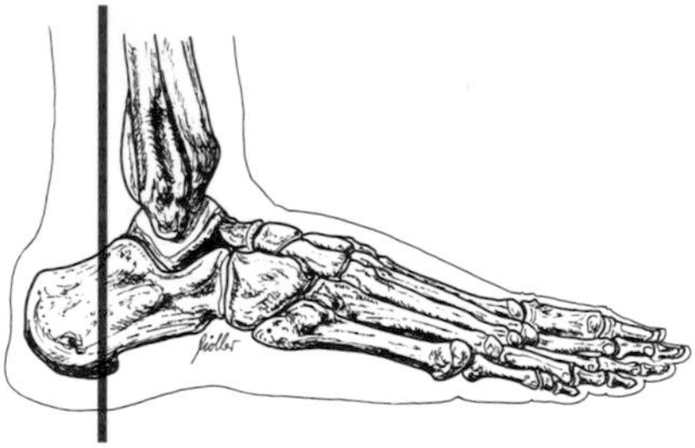

Proximal
Lateral
Medial
Plantar

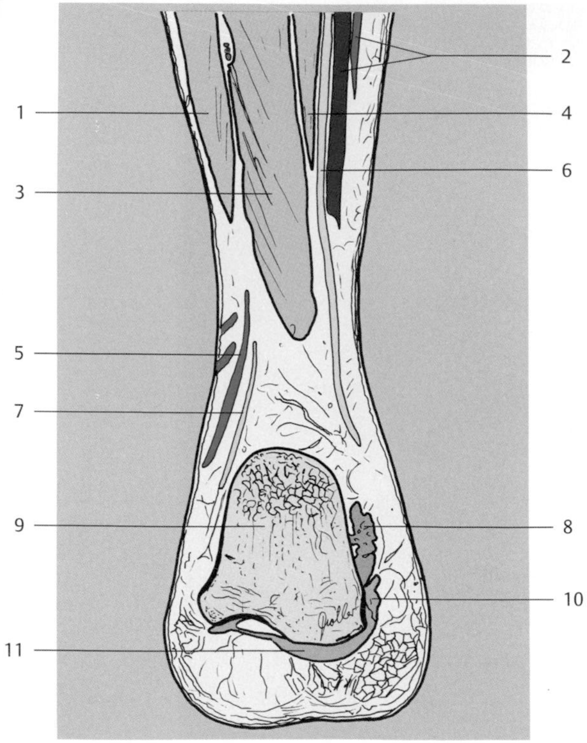

1 Peroneus (fibularis) brevis muscle
2 Posterior tibial artery and vein
3 Flexor hallucis longus muscle
4 Flexor digitorum longus muscle
5 Small saphenous vein
6 Tibial nerve
7 Sural nerve
8 Quadratus plantae muscle
9 Calcaneus
10 Abductor hallucis muscle (tendon)
11 Plantar aponeurosis

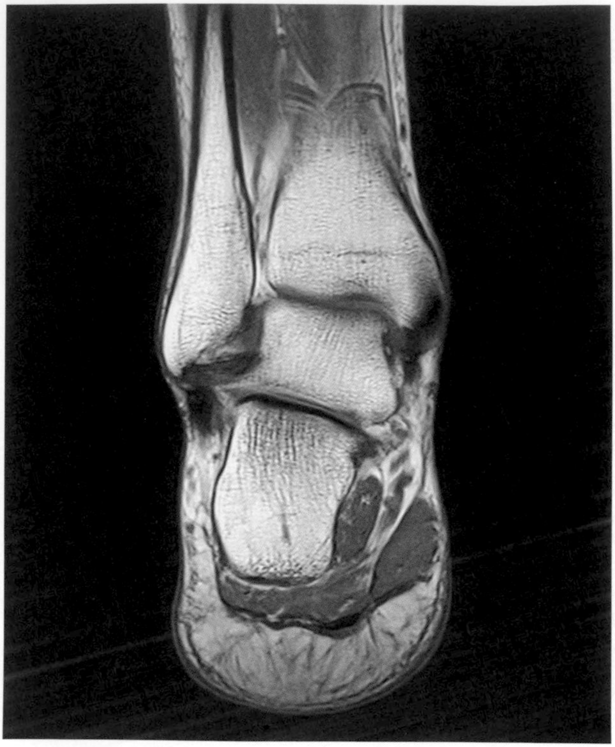

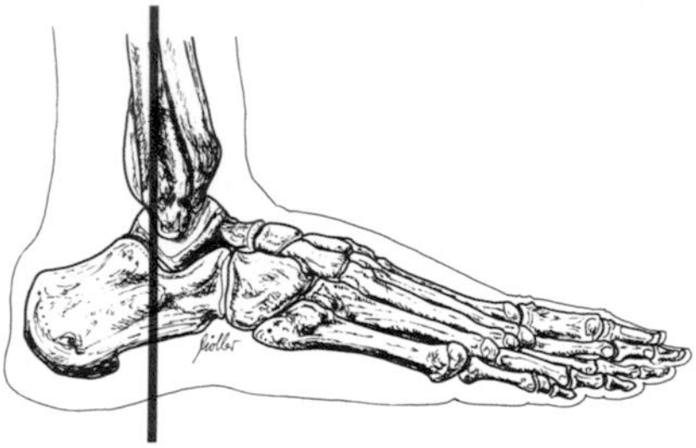

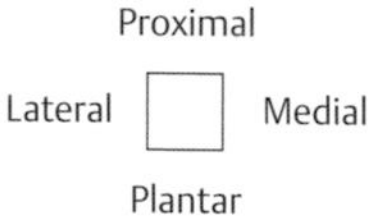
Proximal
Lateral
Medial
Plantar

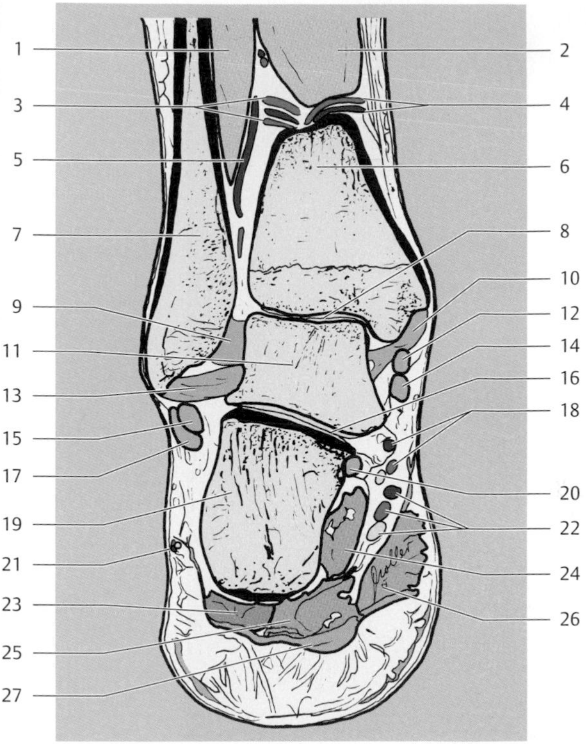

1 Flexor hallucis longus muscle
2 Tibialis posterior muscle
3 Fibular artery and vein (communicating branch)
4 Posterior tibial artery and vein (communicating branch)
5 Fibular artery
6 Tibia
7 Fibula
8 Ankle joint
9 Dorsal capsule
10 Deltoid ligament
11 Talus
12 Tibialis posterior muscle (tendon)
13 Posterior talofibular ligament
14 Flexor digitorum longus muscle (tendon)
15 Peroneus (fibularis) brevis muscle (tendon)
16 Subtalar joint
17 Peroneus (fibularis) longus muscle (tendon)
18 Medial plantar artery, vein, and nerve
19 Calcaneus
20 Flexor hallucis longus muscle (tendon)
21 Sural nerve with accompanying vessels
22 Lateral plantar artery, vein, and nerve
23 Abductor digiti minimi muscle
24 Quadratus plantae muscle
25 Flexor digitorum brevis muscle
26 Abductor hallucis muscle
27 Plantar aponeurosis

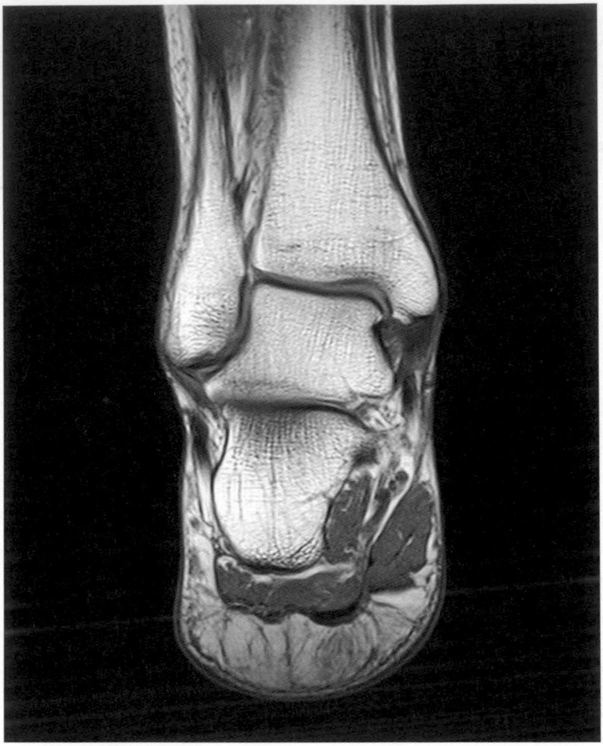

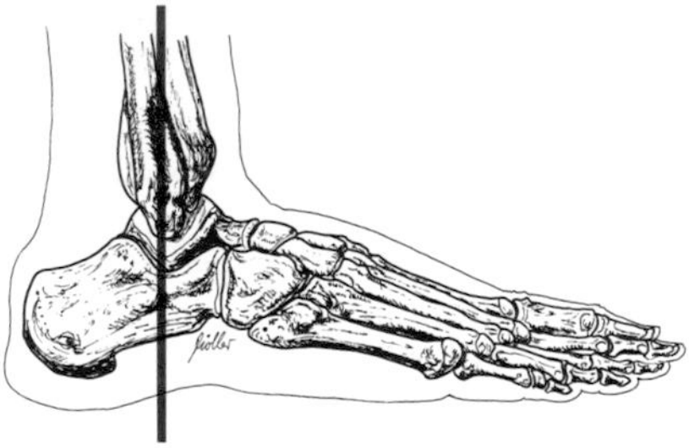

Proximal

Lateral ☐ Medial

Plantar

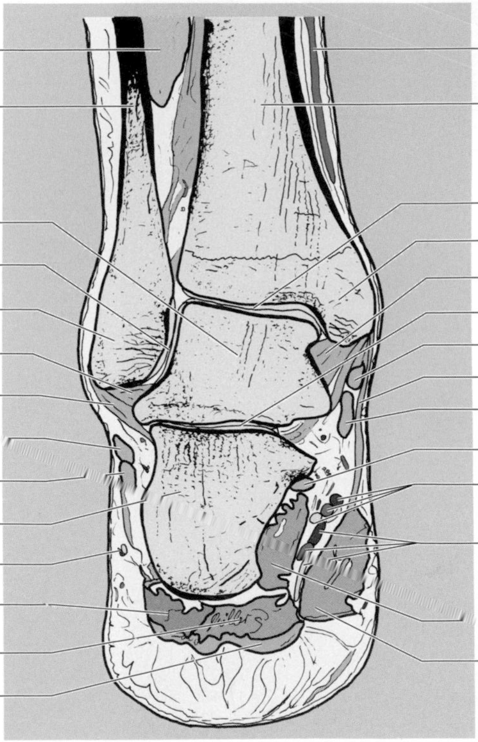

1 Flexor hallucis longus muscle
2 Great saphenous vein
3 Fibula
4 Tibia
5 Talus
6 Ankle joint
7 Talofibular joint
8 Medial malleolus
9 Lateral malleolus
10 Deltoid ligament (posterior tibiotalar part)
11 Posterior talofibular ligament
12 Subtalar joint
13 Calcaneofibular ligament
14 Tibialis posterior muscle (tendon)
15 Peroneus (fibularis) brevis muscle (tendon)
16 Flexor retinaculum
17 Peroneus (fibularis) longus muscle (tendon)
18 Flexor digitorum longus muscle (tendon)
19 Calcaneus
20 Flexor hallucis longus muscle (tendon)
21 Sural nerve with accompanying vessels
22 Medial plantar artery, vein, and nerve
23 Abductor digiti minimi muscle
24 Lateral plantar artery, vein, and nerve
25 Flexor digitorum brevis muscle
26 Quadratus plantae muscle
27 Plantar aponeurosis
28 Abductor hallucis muscle

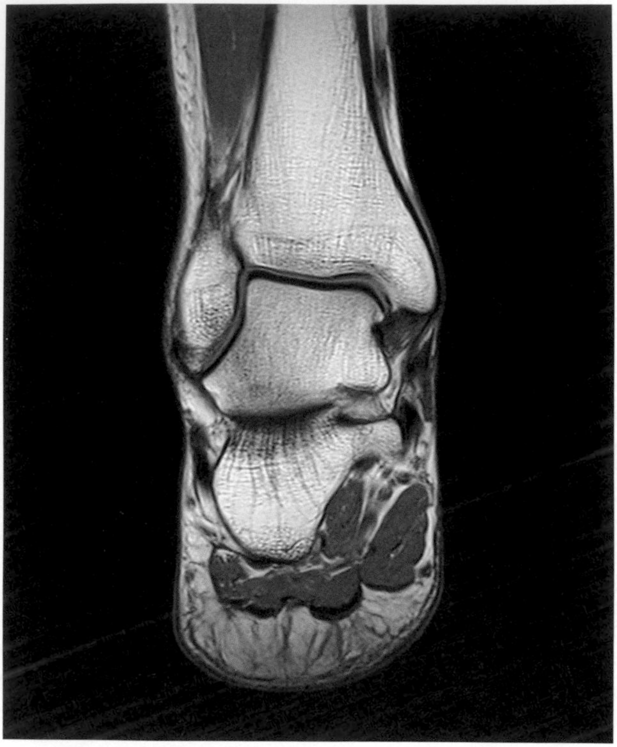

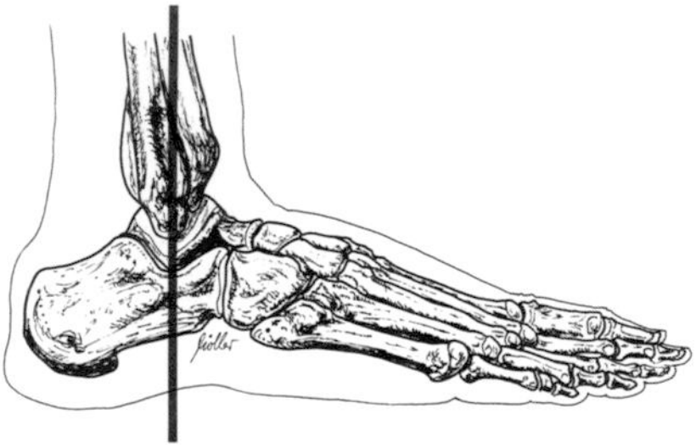
Müller

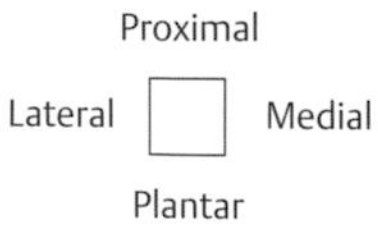
Proximal
Lateral
Medial
Plantar

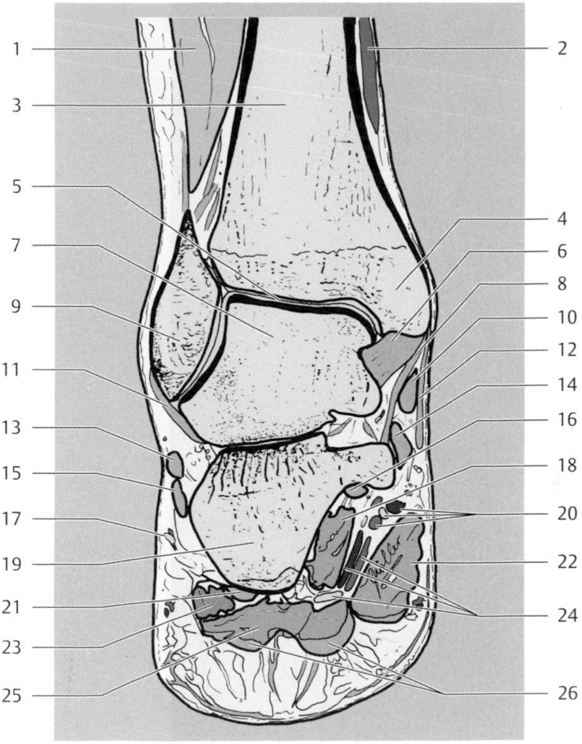

1 Extensor digitorum longus muscle
2 Great saphenous vein
3 Tibia
4 Medial malleolus
5 Ankle joint
6 Deltoid ligament (posterior tibiotalar part)
7 Talus
8 Deltoid ligament (tibiocalcaneal part)
9 Fibula (lateral malleolus)
10 Tibialis posterior muscle (tendon)
11 Calcaneofibular ligament
12 Flexor retinaculum
13 Peroneus (fibularis) brevis muscle (tendon)
14 Flexor digitorum longus muscle (tendon)
15 Peroneus (fibularis) longus muscle (tendon)
16 Flexor hallucis longus muscle (tendon)
17 Sural nerve with accompanying vessels
18 Quadratus plantae muscle
19 Calcaneus
20 Medial plantar artery, vein, and nerve
21 Long plantar ligament
22 Abductor hallucis muscle
23 Abductor digiti minimi muscle
24 Lateral plantar artery, vein, and nerve
25 Flexor digitorum brevis muscle
26 Plantar aponeurosis

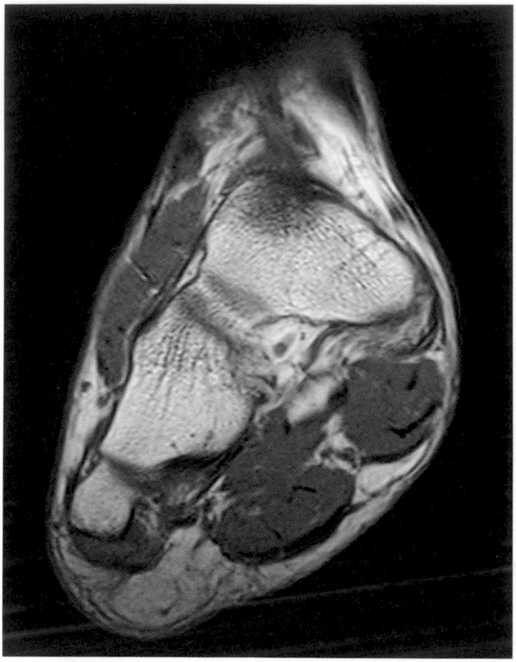

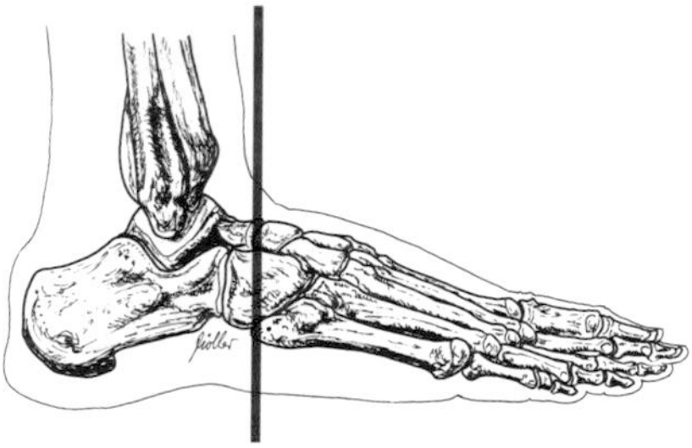

Dorsal

Lateral Medial

Plantar

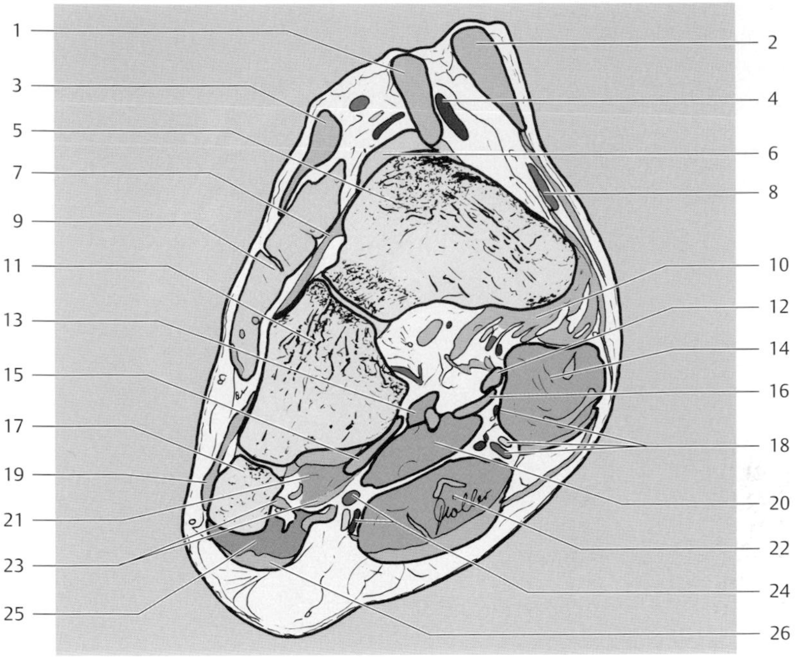

1 Extensor hallucis longus muscle (tendon)
2 Tibialis anterior muscle (tendon)
3 Extensor digitorum longus muscle (tendon)
4 Anterior tibial artery
5 Navicular
6 Extensor hallucis brevis muscle
7 Dorsal tarsal ligaments
8 Great saphenous vein
9 Extensor digitorum brevis muscle
10 Tibialis posterior muscle (tendon)
11 Cuboid
12 Flexor hallucis longus muscle (tendon)
13 Adductor hallucis muscle (oblique head)
14 Abductor hallucis muscle
15 Peroneus (fibularis) longus muscle (tendon)
16 Flexor digitorum longus muscle (tendon)
17 Metatarsal V (base)
18 Medial plantar artery, vein, and nerve
19 Peroneus (fibularis) brevis muscle (tendon)
20 Quadratus plantae muscle
21 Interosseous muscles
22 Flexor digitorum brevis muscle
23 Long plantar ligament
24 Lateral plantar artery, vein, and nerve
25 Abductor digiti minimi muscle
26 Plantar aponeurosis

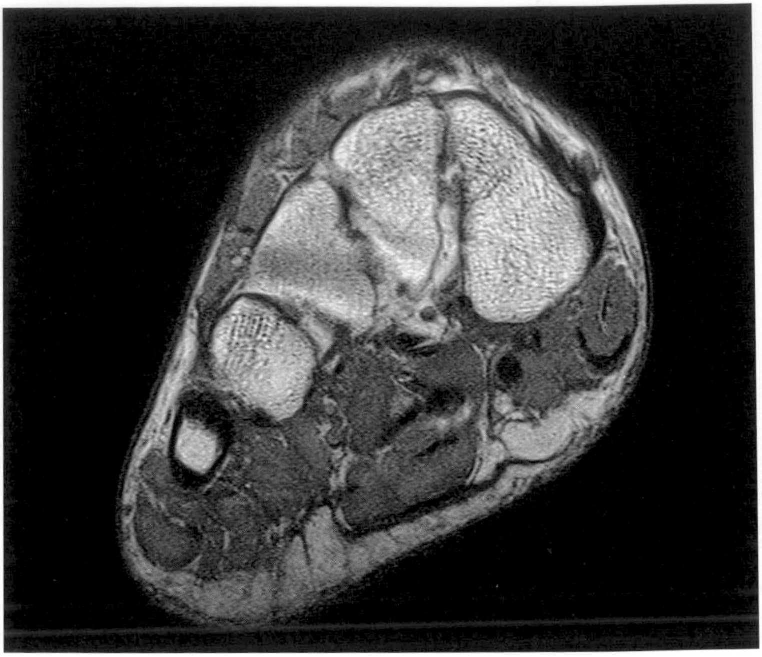

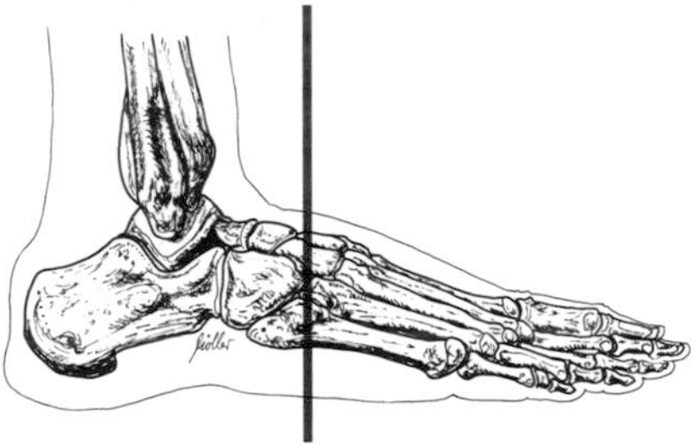

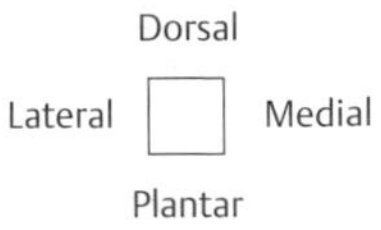

1 Extensor hallucis brevis muscle (tendon)
2 Extensor hallucis longus muscle (tendon)
3 Extensor digitorum brevis muscle
4 Anterior tibial artery
5 Extensor digitorum longus muscle (tendons)

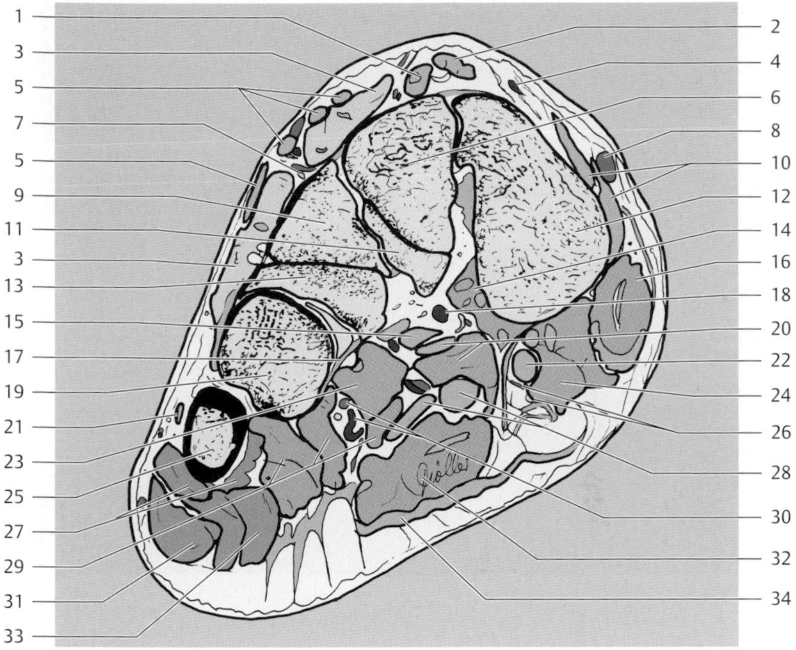

6 Intermediate cuneiform
7 Deep fibular (peroneal) nerve (lateral branch)
8 Great saphenous vein
9 Lateral cuneiform
10 Tibialis anterior muscle (tendon)
11 Metatarsal II (base)
12 Medial cuneiform
13 Metatarsal III (base)
14 Flexor hallucis brevis muscle (lateral head)
15 Peroneus (fibularis) longus muscle (tendon)
16 Abductor hallucis muscle
17 Long plantar ligament
18 Deep plantar arch
19 Metatarsal IV (base)
20 Adductor hallucis muscle (oblique head + tendon)
21 Extensor digiti minimi brevis muscle (tendon)
22 Flexor hallucis longus muscle (tendon)
23 Flexor hallucis brevis muscle (lateral head)
24 Flexor hallucis brevis muscle (medial head)
25 Metatarsal V (base)
26 Medial plantar artery, vein, and nerve (superficial branch)
27 Opponens digiti minimi muscle
28 Flexor digitorum longus muscle (tendon)
29 Interosseous muscles
30 Lateral plantar artery, vein, and nerve
31 Abductor digiti minimi muscle
32 Flexor digitorum brevis muscle
33 Flexor digiti minimi brevis muscle
34 Plantar aponeurosis

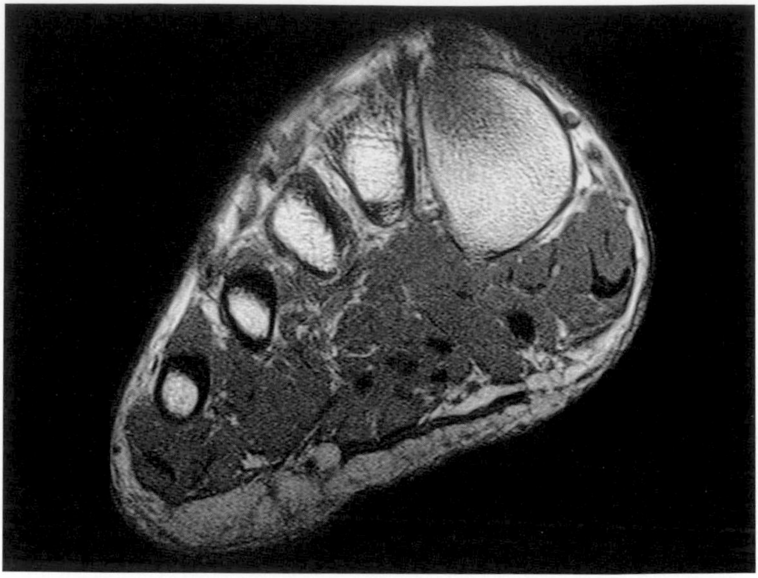

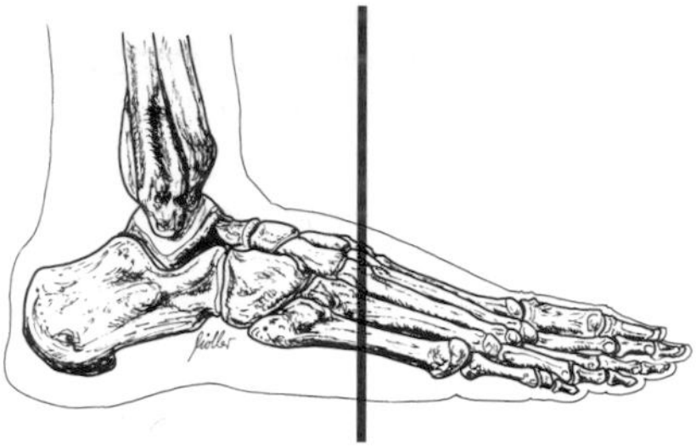

Dorsal

Lateral Medial

Plantar

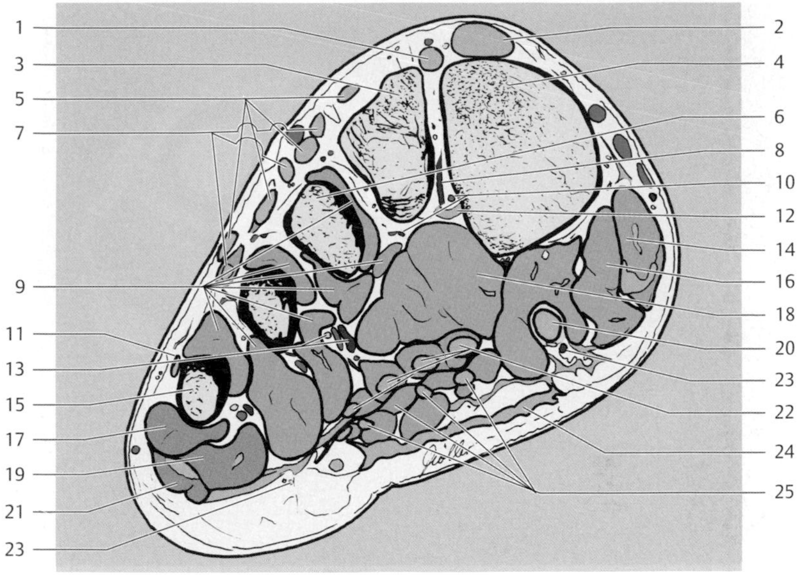

1 Extensor hallucis brevis muscle (tendon)
2 Extensor hallucis longus muscle (tendon)
3 Metatarsal II (base)
4 Metatarsal I (base)
5 Extensor digitorum longus muscle (tendons)
6 Metatarsal III (base)
7 Extensor digitorum brevis muscle (tendon)
8 Plantar metatarsal arteries
9 Interosseous muscles
10 Perforating veins (of first dorsal interosseous muscle)
11 Extensor digiti minimi brevis muscle (tendon)
12 Peroneus (fibularis) longus muscle (attachment)
13 Lateral plantar nerve (deep branch) and plantar metatarsal arteries
14 Abductor hallucis muscle
15 Metatarsal V (base)
16 Flexor hallucis brevis muscle (lateral head)
17 Opponens digiti minimi muscle
18 Adductor hallucis muscle (oblique head)
19 Flexor digiti minimi brevis muscle
20 Flexor hallucis longus muscle (tendon)
21 Abductor digiti minimi muscle
22 Flexor digitorum longus muscle (+ tendon)
23 Proper plantar digital artery
24 Plantar aponeurosis
25 Flexor digitorum brevis muscle (+ tendon)

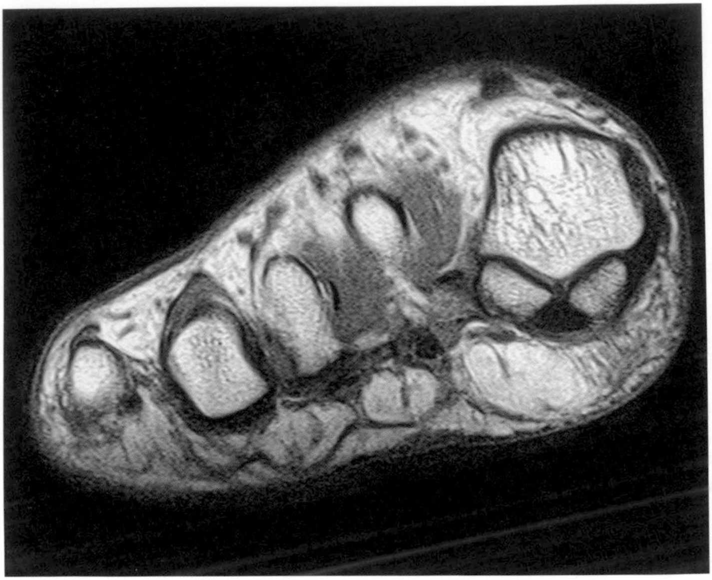

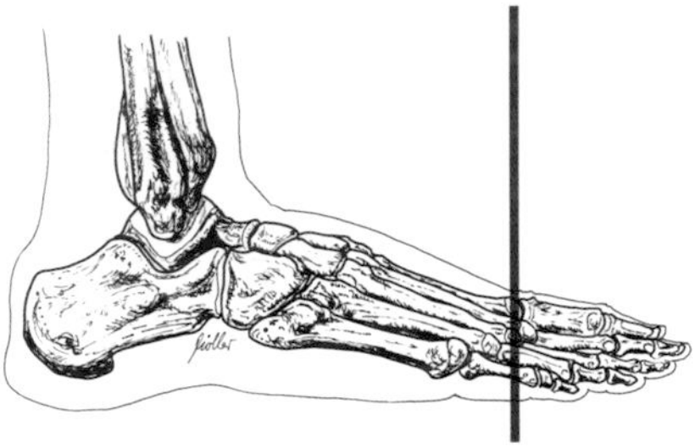

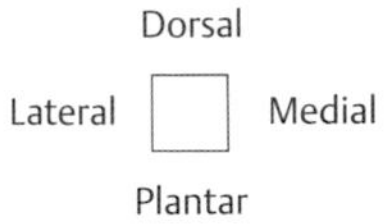
Dorsal
Lateral
Medial
Plantar

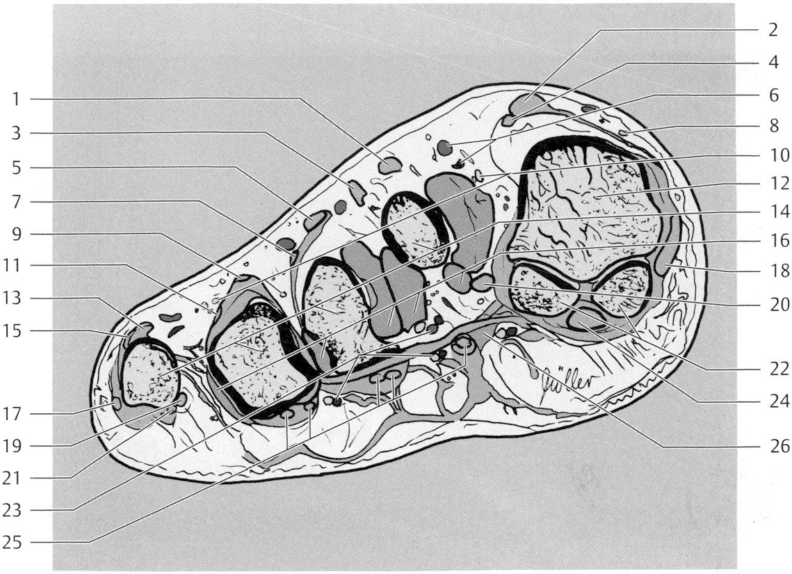

1 Extensor digitorum longus II muscle (tendon)
2 Extensor hallucis longus muscle (tendon)
3 Extensor digitorum brevis II muscle (tendon)
4 Extensor hallucis brevis muscle (tendon)
5 Extensor digitorum longus III muscle (tendon)
6 Dorsal metatarsal arteries and veins
7 Extensor digitorum brevis III muscle (tendon)
8 Medial dorsal cutaneous nerve I
9 Extensor digitorum longus IV muscle (tendon)
10 Dorsal digital nerves of foot
11 Extensor digitorum brevis IV muscle (tendon)
12 Metatarsal I (head)
13 Extensor digiti minimi longus muscle (tendon)
14 Metatarsals II–V
15 Extensor digiti minimi brevis muscle (tendon)
16 Dorsal and plantar interosseous muscles
17 Abductor digiti minimi muscle (tendon attachment)
18 Abductor hallucis muscle (tendon)
19 Flexor digiti minimi longus muscle (tendon)
20 Adductor hallucis muscle (tendon)
21 Flexor digiti minimi brevis muscle (tendon)
22 Sesamoid bones
23 Plantar digital artery and vein proper and proper plantar digital nerve
24 Flexor hallucis longus muscle (tendon)
25 Flexor digitorum longus and brevis muscles (tendons)
26 Adductor hallucis muscle (transverse head)

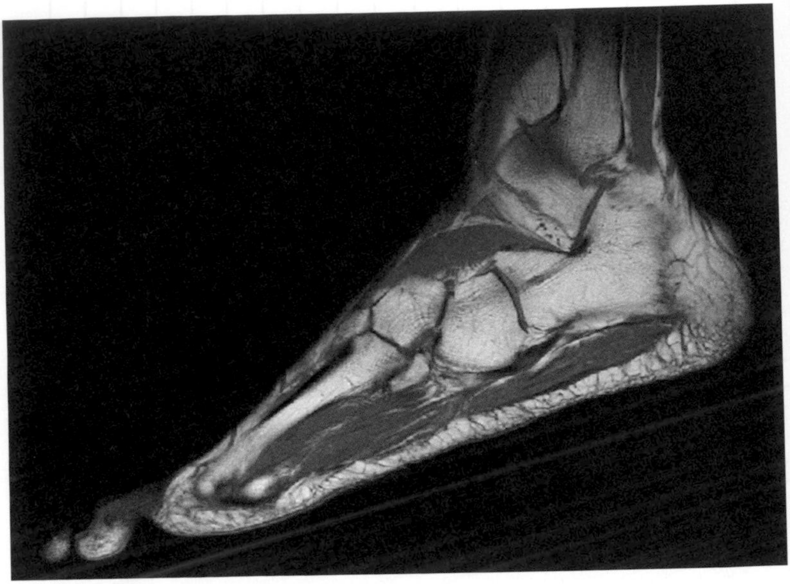

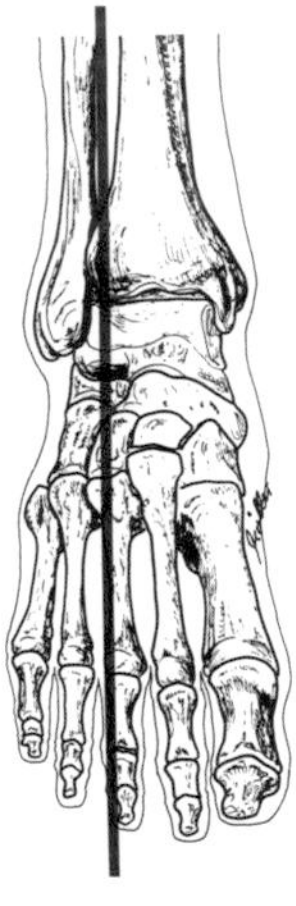

Proximal
Dorsal

Anterior Posterior

Distal
Plantar

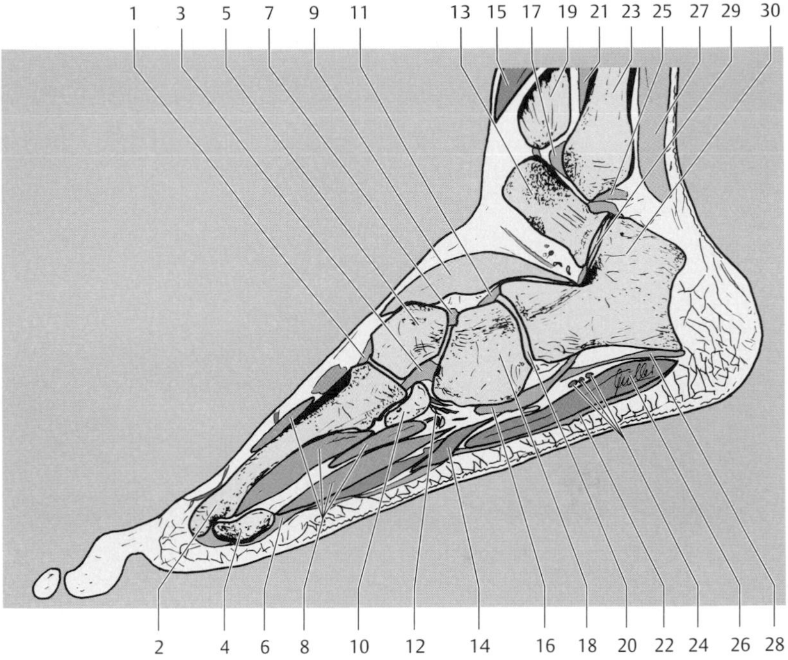

1 Dorsal metatarsal ligaments
2 Metatarsal III
3 Cuneocuboid interosseous ligament
4 Metatarsal IV (head)
5 Lateral cuneiform
6 Flexor digitorum longus muscle (tendon)
7 Dorsal tarsal ligaments
8 Dorsal and plantar interosseous muscles
9 Extensor digitorum brevis muscle
10 Metatarsal IV (base)
11 Bifurcate ligament
12 Deep plantar arch
13 Talus
14 Flexor digiti minimi brevis muscle
15 Extensor digitorum longus muscle
16 Peroneus (fibularis) longus muscle (tendon)
17 Anterior talofibular ligament
18 Cuboid
19 Tibia
20 Calcaneocuboid joint
21 Tibiofibular syndesmosis (anterior tibiofibular ligament)
22 Plantar aponeurosis
23 Fibula
24 Lateral plantar artery, vein, and nerve
25 Posterior talofibular ligament
26 Abductor digiti minimi muscle
27 Peroneus (fibularis) brevis muscle
28 Long plantar ligament
29 Subtalar joint
30 Calcaneus

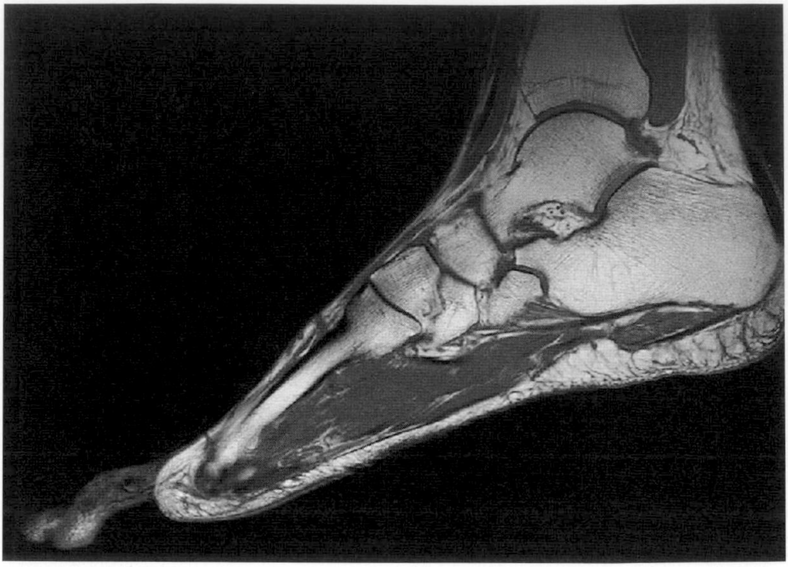

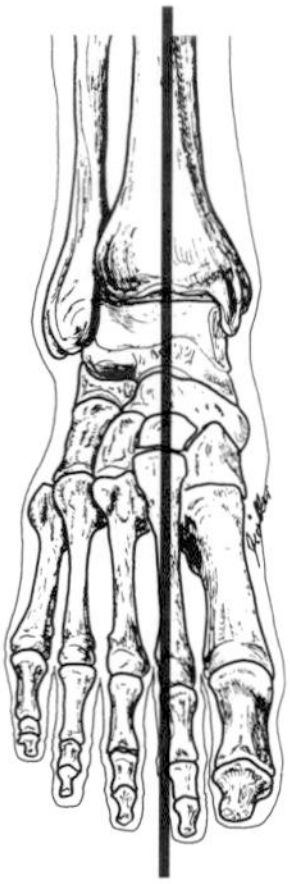

Proximal
Dorsal

Anterior | Posterior

Distal
Plantar

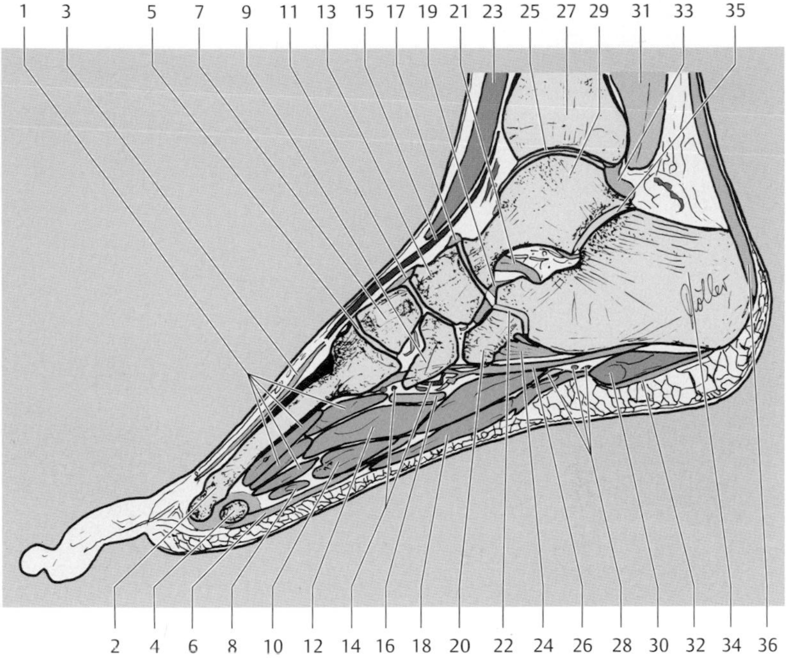

1 Interosseous muscles
2 Metatarsal II
3 Extensor digiti II muscle (tendon)
4 Metatarsal II (head)
5 Tarsometatarsal joint II
6 Flexor digitorum longus muscle (tendon)
7 Intermediate cuneiform
8 Adductor hallucis muscle (transverse head)
9 Lateral cuneiform
10 Lumbrical muscle
11 Dorsal tarsal ligaments
12 Adductor hallucis muscle (oblique head)
13 Navicular
14 Deep plantar arch
15 Dorsalis pedis artery
16 Peroneus (fibularis) longus muscle (tendon)
17 Dorsal talonavicular ligament
18 Flexor digitorum brevis muscle
19 Bifurcate ligament
20 Cuboid
21 Talocalcaneal interosseous ligament
22 Calcaneocuboid joint
23 Extensor digitorum longus muscle
24 Spring ligament (plantar calcaneonavicular ligament)
25 Ankle joint
26 Long plantar ligament
27 Tibia
28 Lateral plantar artery, vein, and nerve
29 Talus
30 Abductor digiti minimi muscle
31 Flexor hallucis longus muscle
32 Plantar aponeurosis
33 Posterior talofibular ligament
34 Calcaneus
35 Subtalar joint
36 Achilles tendon (calcaneal tendon)

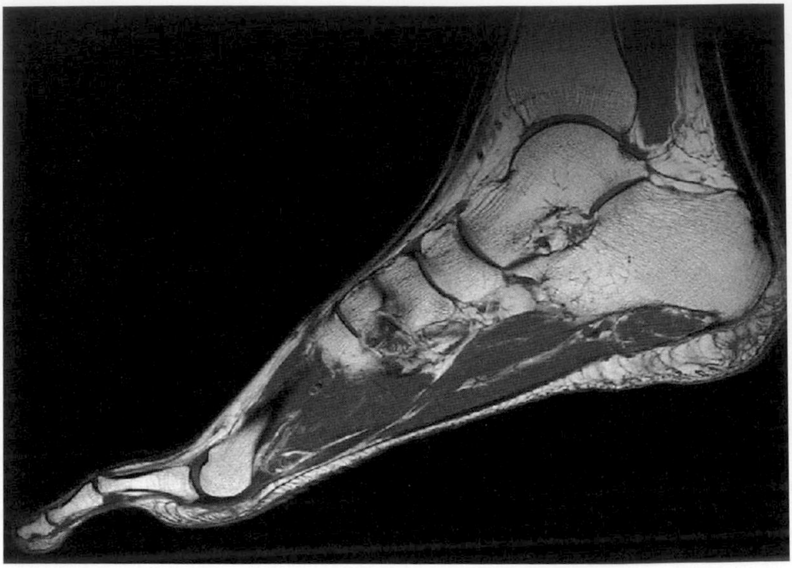

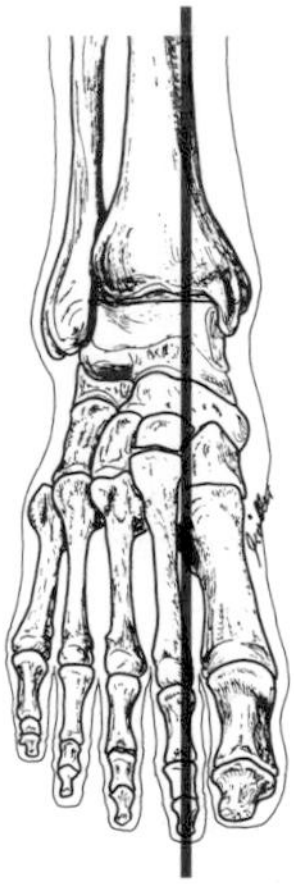

Proximal
Dorsal

Anterior Posterior

Distal
Plantar

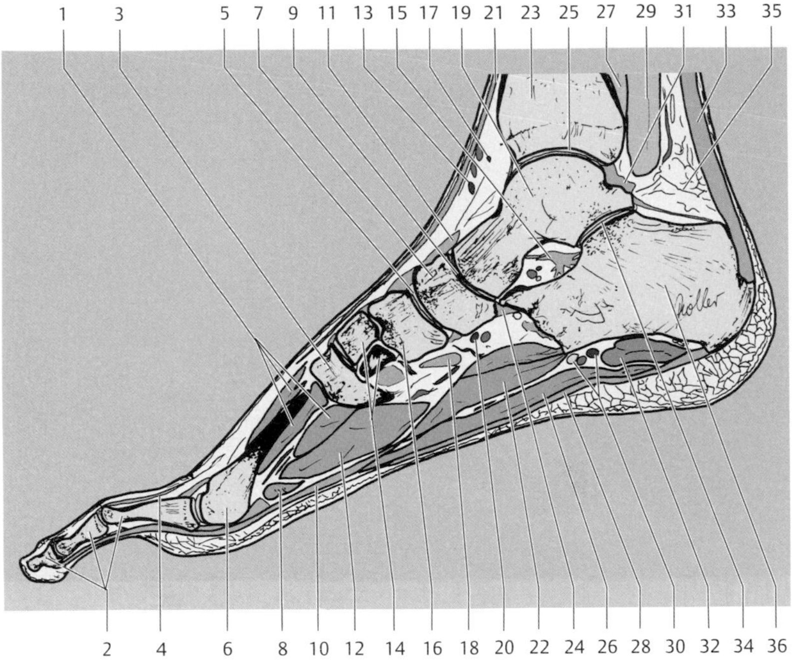

1 Interosseous muscle
2 Proximal, middle, and distal phalanx of second toe
3 Metatarsal I (base)
4 Extensor digitorum muscle (tendon)
5 Cuneonavicular joint
6 Metatarsal II (head)
7 Navicular
8 Adductor hallucis muscle (transverse head)
9 Talonavicular joint
10 Flexor digitorum longus muscle (tendon)
11 Talonavicular ligament
12 Adductor hallucis muscle (oblique head)
13 Medial tarsal artery
14 Medial cuneiform
15 Talocalcaneal interosseous ligament
16 Intermediate cuneiform
17 Anterior medial malleolar artery
18 Peroneus (fibularis) longus muscle (tendon)
19 Talus
20 Deep plantar arch
21 Extensor hallucis longus muscle (tendon)
22 Quadratus plantae muscle
23 Tibia
24 Plantar calcaneonavicular ligament
25 Ankle joint
26 Flexor digitorum brevis muscle
27 Tibialis posterior muscle
28 Plantar aponeurosis
29 Flexor hallucis longus muscle
30 Lateral plantar artery, vein, and nerve
31 Posterior talofibular ligament
32 Abductor digiti minimi muscle
33 Achilles tendon (calcaneal tendon)
34 Subtalar joint
35 Pre-Achilles fat body
36 Calcaneus

- Arteries
- Nerves
- Veins
- Bones
- Fatty tissue
- Cartilage
- Tendon
- Disk, intervertebral cartilage
- Fluid, cerebrospinal fluid
- Lymph nodes
- Esophagus
- Liver, glands
- Air

Erector Spinae Muscles (Lateral Tract):
Iliocostal
Longissimus
Splenius capitis and splenius cervicis
Intertransversarii
Levatores costarum longi and breves

Erector Spinae Muscles (Medial Tract):
Spinal system: interspinous muscles
Spinalis thoracis, cervicis, and capitis
Transversospinal system: rotatores
breves and longi
Multifidus lumborum, thoracis, and cervicis
Semispinalis thoracis, cervicis, and capitis

Peroneus

Short Muscles of Neck and Head Joints:
Rectus capitis posterior major and minor
Obliquus capitis superior and inferior

Prevertebral Cervical Muscles:
Longus capitis and longus colli
Rectus capitis lateralis and anterior

Muscles of Thoracic Cage:
External, internal, and innermost intercostals
Transversus thoracis
Subcostal
Scalenus anterior, medius, minimus, and posterior

Muscles of the Trunk – Shoulder Girdle – Arm:
Rhomboideus major and minor
Sternocleidomastoid
Levator scapulae
Serratus anterior
Pectoralis major and minor
Trapezius
Latissimus dorsi

Muscles of the Trunk – Leg – Abdomen:
Psoas
Quadratus lumborum
Piriformis
Gluteus medius

Muscles of the Face and Ventral Cervical Muscles:
Digastric muscle
Stylohyoid
Sternohyoid

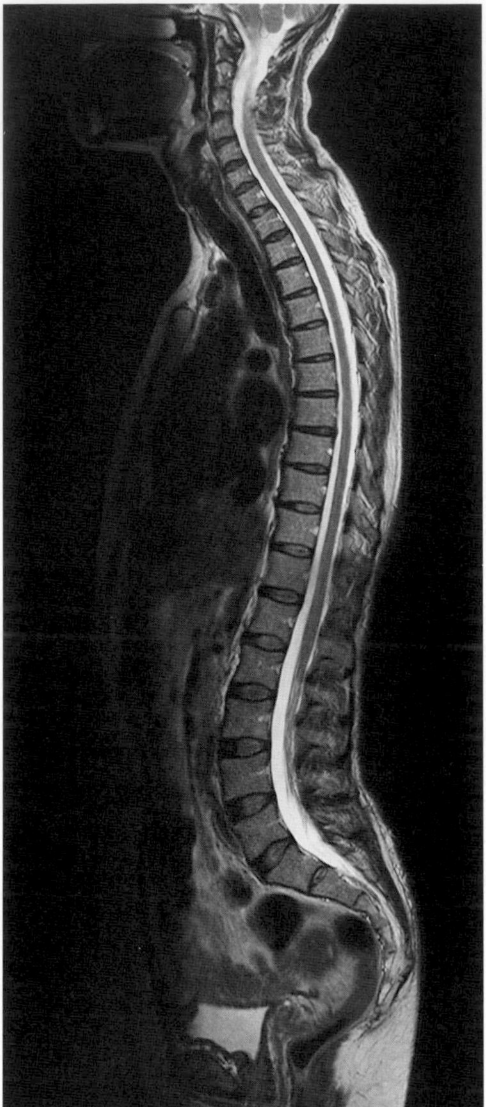

Cranial

Ventral Dorsal

Caudal

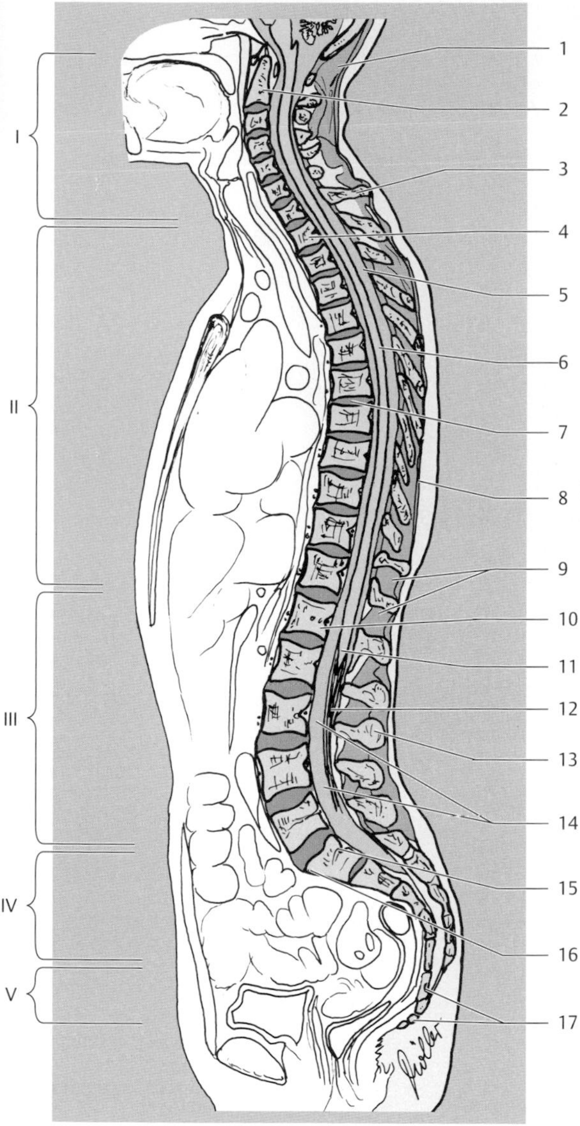

1 Nuchal ligament
2 Dens axis, C2
3 Vertebra prominens, C7
4 Body of thoracic vertebra T1
5 Vertebral canal
6 Thoracic spinal cord
7 Intervertebral disk
8 Supraspinous ligament
9 Interspinous ligaments
10 Body of lumbar vertebra L1
11 Conus medullaris
12 Cauda equina
13 Spinous process
14 Thecal sac
15 Sacrum (S1)
16 Promontory of sacrum
17 Coccyx

I Cervical vertebrae C1–C7
II Thoracic vertebrae T1–T12
III Lumbar vertebrae L1–L5
IV Sacrum (sacral vertebrae S1–S5)
V Coccyx (coccygeal vertebrae Co1–Co3 or Co1–Co4)

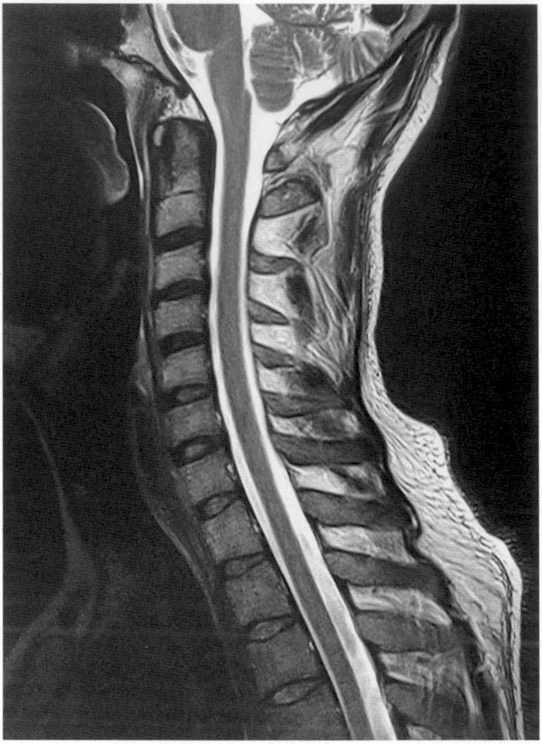

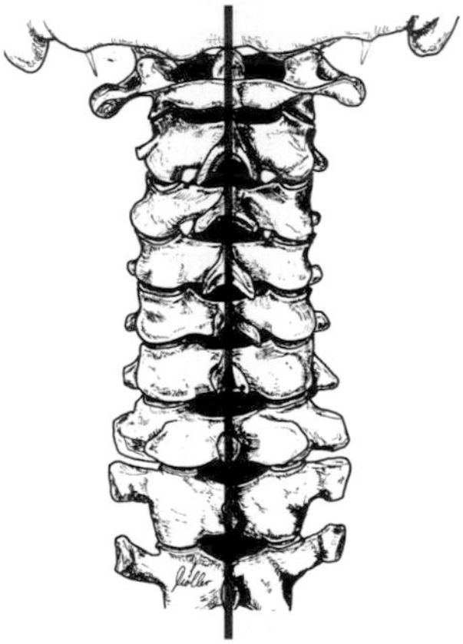

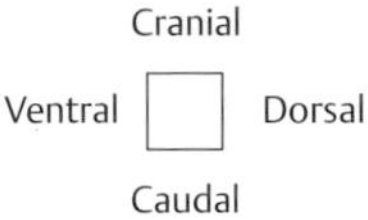

1 Foramen magnum
2 Trapezius muscle (descending part)
3 Tectorial membrane
4 Occipital bone (internal occipital protuberance)
5 Anterior atlanto-occipital membrane
6 Semispinalis capitis muscle

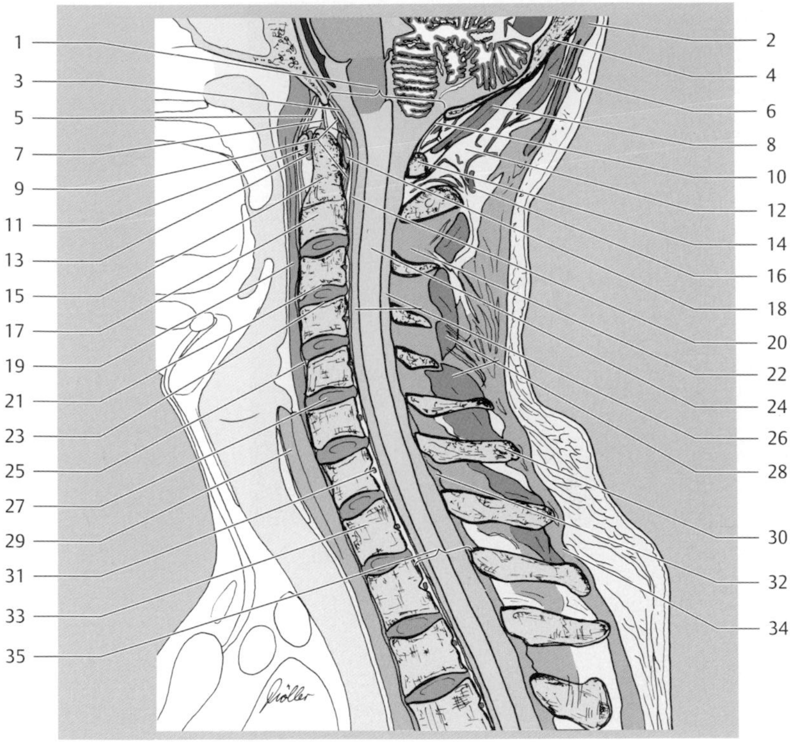

7 Apical ligament of dens
8 Rectus capitis posterior minor muscle
9 Longitudinal fasciculi
10 Posterior atlanto-occipital membrane
11 Atlas (anterior arch)
12 Suboccipital fatty tissue
13 Median atlanto-axial joint
14 Atlas (posterior arch)
15 Axis (dens)
16 Deep cervical veins
17 Axis (vertebral body)
18 Transverse ligament of atlas
19 Longus capitis muscle
20 Posterior longitudinal ligament
21 Inferior vertebral end plate C3
22 Interspinous ligament
23 Superior vertebral end plate C4
24 Cervical spinal cord
25 Anterior longitudinal ligament
26 Premedullary and postmedullary subarachnoid space
27 Intervertebral disk
28 Interspinales muscles
29 Esophagus
30 Spinous process C7
31 Basivertebral veins
32 Ligamentum flavum
33 Thoracic vertebral body T1
34 Supraspinous ligament
35 Bony vertebral canal

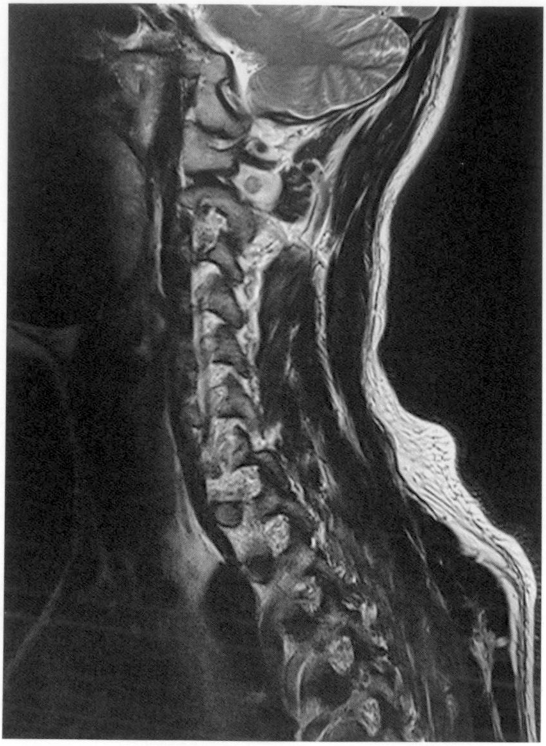

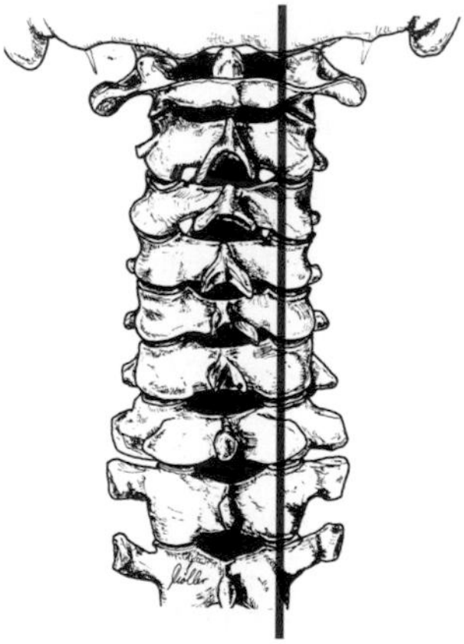

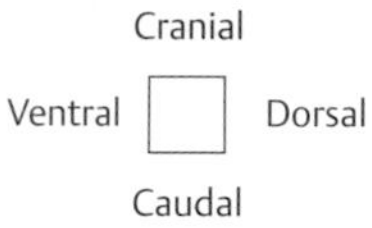

1 Vertebral artery
2 Occipital bone
3 Occipital condyle
4 Semispinalis capitis muscle
5 Atlanto-occipital joint
6 Rectus capitis posterior minor muscle
7 Atlas (lateral mass)

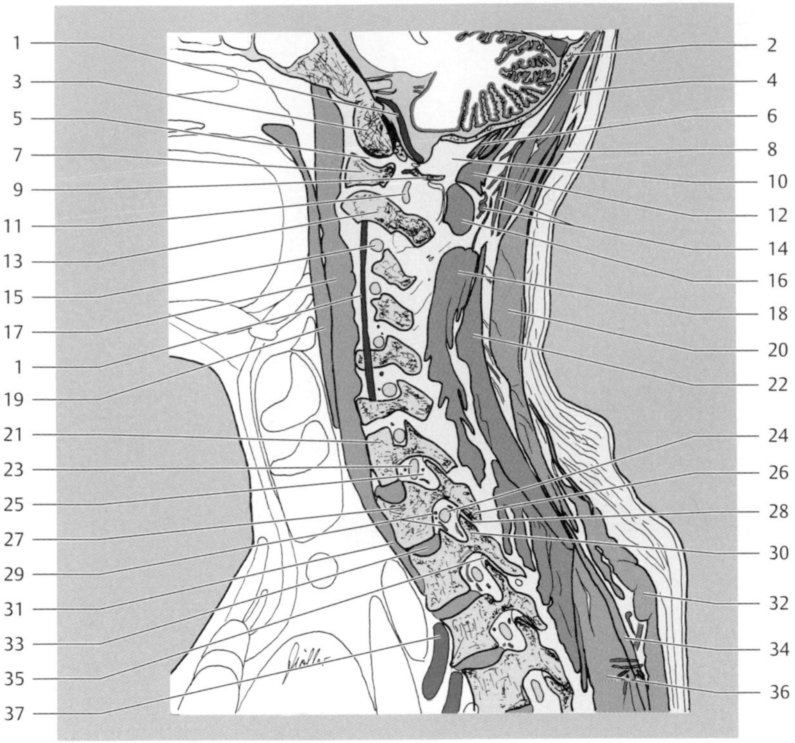

8 Trapezius muscle (descending part)
9 Atlas (posterior arch)
10 Suboccipital fatty tissue
11 Spinal nerve C2
12 Rectus capitis posterior major muscle
13 Axis (body)
14 Deep cervical veins
15 Spinal ganglion C3
16 Obliquus capitis inferior muscle
17 Longus capitis muscle
18 Spinalis cervicis and multifidus muscles
19 Palatopharyngeus muscle
20 Splenius capitis muscle
21 Body of cervical vertebra C7
22 Semispinalis cervicis muscle
23 Spinal ganglion C8
24 Spinal ganglion T1
25 Intervertebral foramen
26 Inferior articular process
27 First thoracic vertebral body
28 Zygapophysial joint
29 Posterior intercostal artery (spinal and radicular branches of dorsal branch)
30 Superior articular process
31 Longus colli muscle
32 Trapezius muscle (transverse part)
33 Intervertebral disk
34 Rhomboid muscle
35 Ligamentum flavum
36 Splenius cervicis muscle
37 Posterior intercostal vein

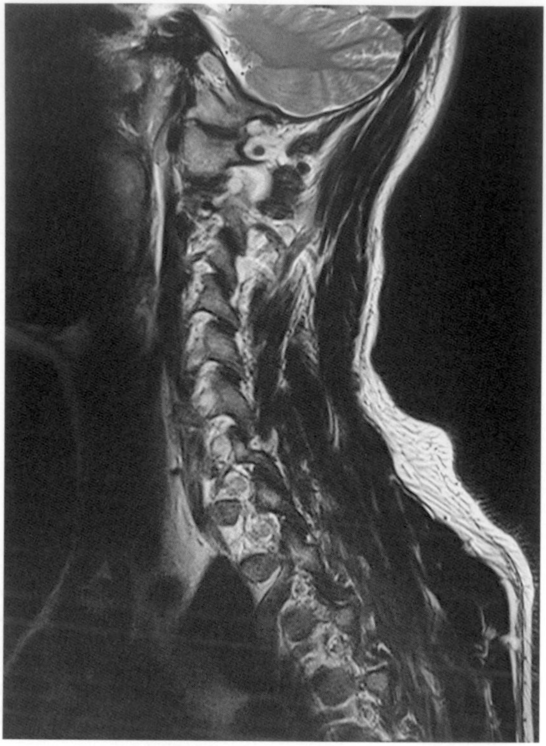

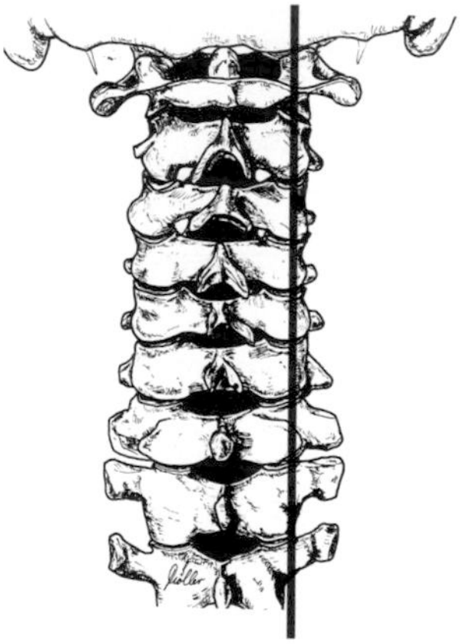

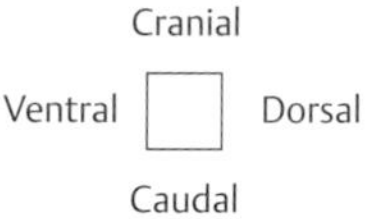
Cranial
Ventral
Dorsal
Caudal

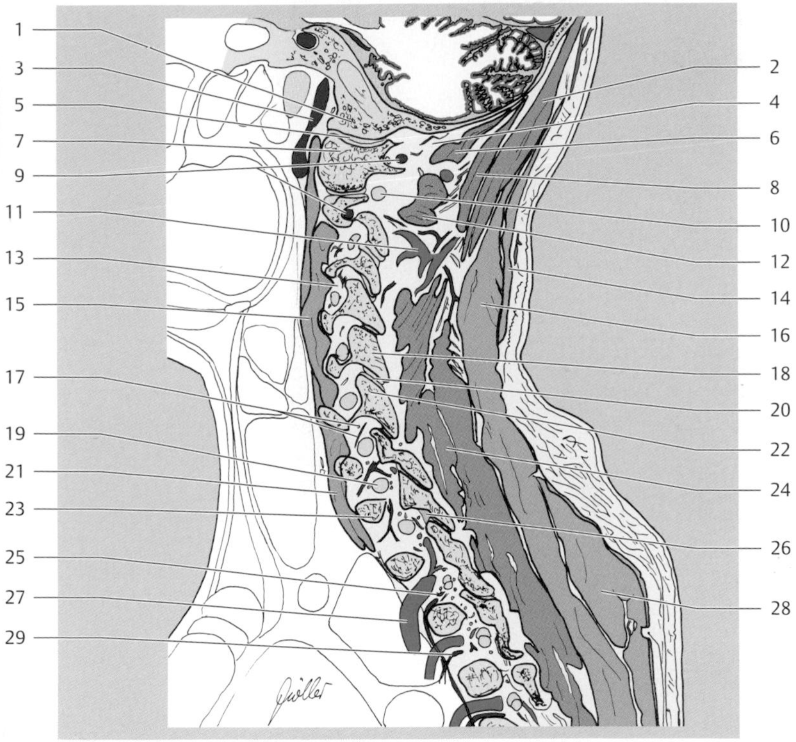

1 Occipital condyle
2 Semispinalis capitis muscle
3 Internal carotid artery
4 Suboccipital fatty tissue
5 Atlanto-occipital joint
6 Rectus capitis posterior minor muscle
7 Atlas (lateral mass)
8 Rectus capitis posterior major muscle
9 Vertebral artery
10 Spinal nerve C2
11 Deep cervical veins
12 Obliquus capitis inferior muscle
13 Intervertebral foramen
14 Trapezius muscle (descending part)
15 Longus capitis muscle
16 Splenius capitis muscle
17 Vertebral artery (spinal and radicular branches)
18 Inferior articular process
19 Spinal ganglion C8
20 Zygapophysial joint
21 Longus colli muscle
22 Superior articular process
23 First thoracic vertebral body
24 Spinalis cervicis and multifidus muscles
25 Posterior intercostal artery (spinal and radicular branches of dorsal branch)
26 Ligamentum flavum
27 Posterior intercostal vein
28 Trapezius muscle (transverse part)
29 Posterior intercostal artery (dorsal branch)

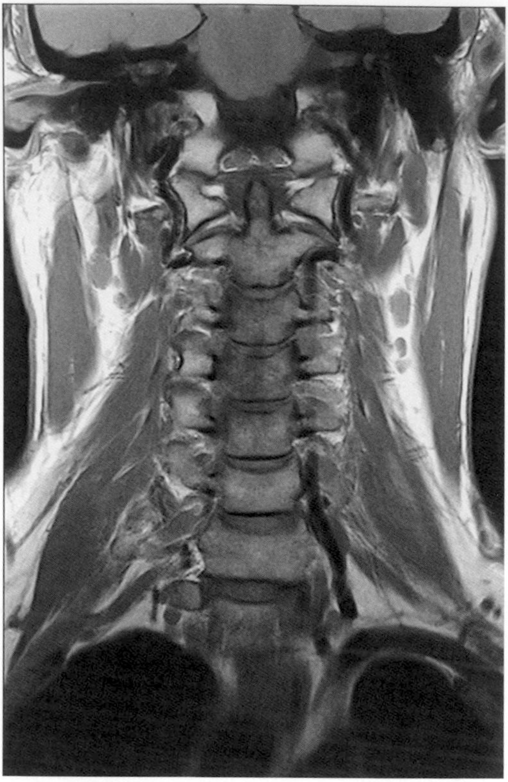

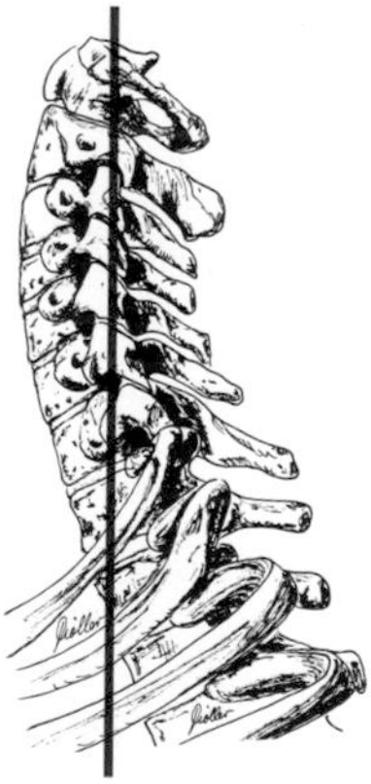

Cranial

Right ☐ Left

Caudal

1 External auditory canal
2 Stylomastoid foramen
3 Vertebral vein
4 Internal jugular vein
5 Occipital condyle
6 Mastoid process
7 Parotid gland

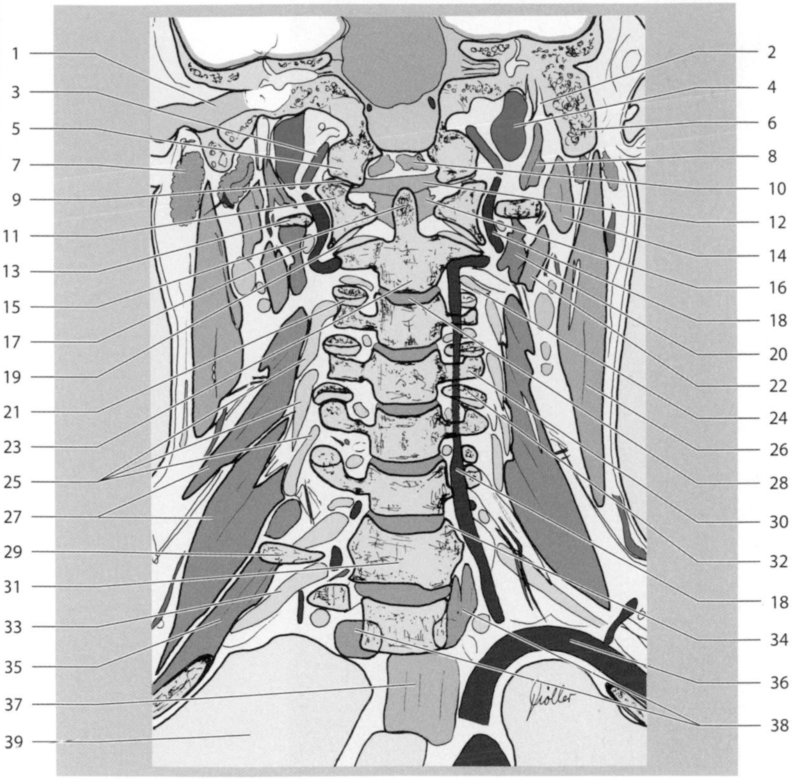

8 Rectus capitis lateralis muscle
9 Atlanto-occipital joint
10 Tectorial membrane
11 Atlas (lateral mass)
12 Transverse ligament
13 Atlas (transverse process)
14 Digastric muscle (posterior belly)
15 Axis (dens)
16 Alar ligaments
17 Spinal nerve C2
18 Vertebral artery
19 Lateral atlantoaxial joint
20 Obliquus capitis inferior muscle
21 Zygapophysial joint
22 Levator scapulae muscle
23 Axis (vertebral body)
24 Spinal ganglion C3
25 Cervical plexus
26 Sternocleidomastoid muscle
27 Scalenus medius muscle
28 Intervertebral disk (C2/C3)
29 Transverse process C7
30 Superior articular process C4
31 Cervical vertebral body C7
32 Inferior articular process
33 Spinal nerve C8
34 Uncinate process C7
35 Scalenus posterior muscle
36 Subclavian artery
37 Esophagus
38 Longus colli muscle
39 Lung

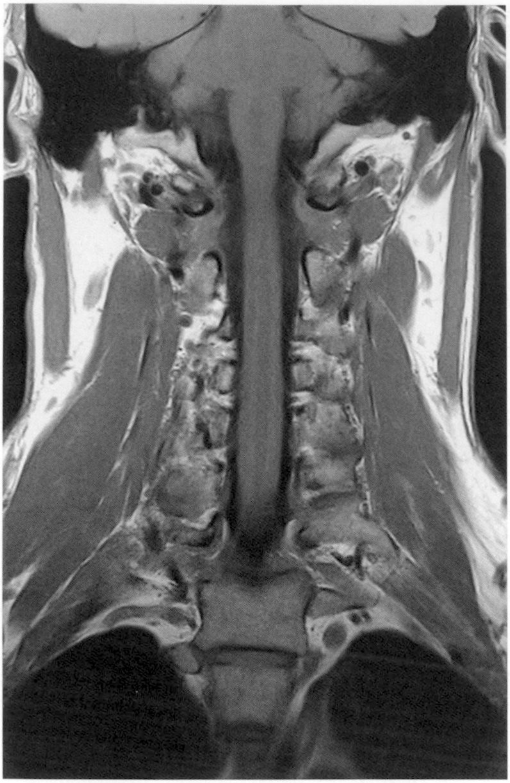

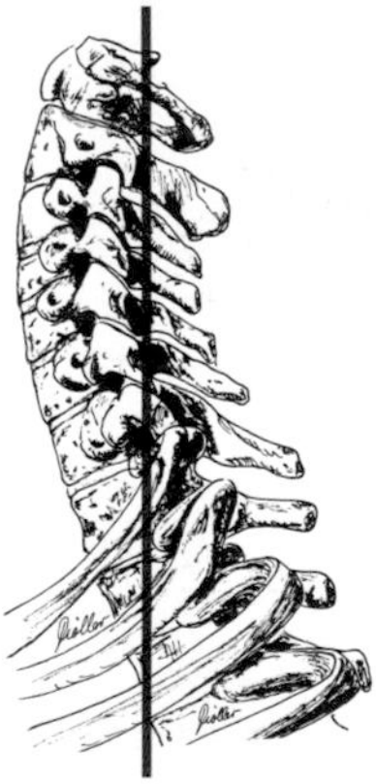

Cranial

Right ☐ Left

Caudal

1 Medulla oblongata
2 Sigmoid sinus
3 Mastoid process
4 Foramen magnum
5 Vertebral artery
6 Splenius capitis muscle

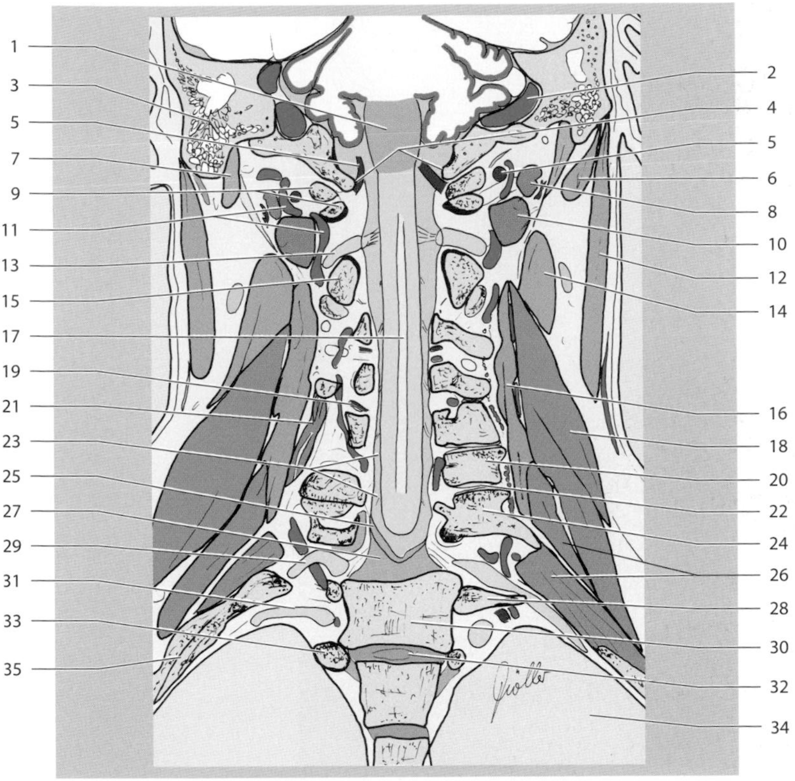

7 Digastric muscle (posterior belly)
8 Obliquus capitis superior muscle
9 Atlas (posterior arch)
10 Obliquus capitis inferior muscle
11 Vertebral artery
12 Sternocleidomastoid muscle
13 Spinal ganglion C2
14 Levator scapulae muscle
15 Axis (vertebral arch)
16 Splenius cervicis muscle
17 Spinal cord (cervical pulp with central canal)
18 Scalenus medius muscle
19 Posterior intercostal artery (spinal and radicular branches of dorsal branch)
20 Inferior articulate process C6
21 Semispinalis cervicis muscle
22 Zygapophysial joint
23 Cerebrospinal fluid in spinal canal
24 Superior articular process C7
25 Spinal dura mater
26 Scalenus posterior muscle
27 Posterior longitudinal ligament
28 First rib (neck)
29 Spinal nerve C8
30 Thoracic vertebral body T1
31 Spinal nerve T1
32 Intervertebral disk
33 Second rib (head)
34 Left lung
35 First rib (body)

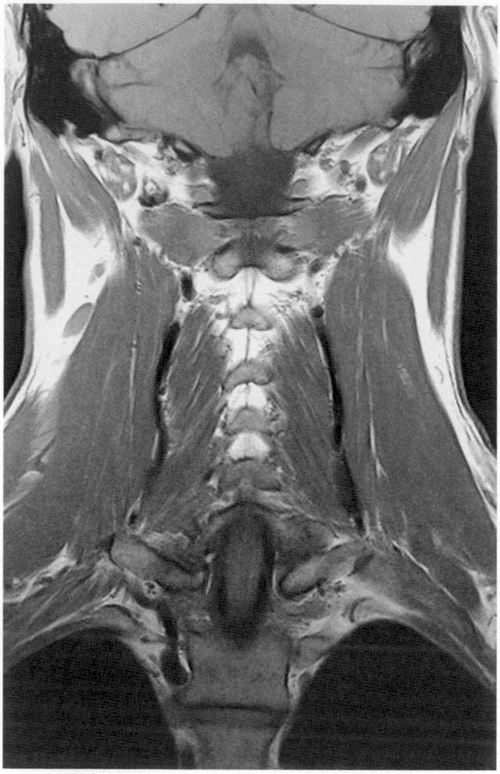

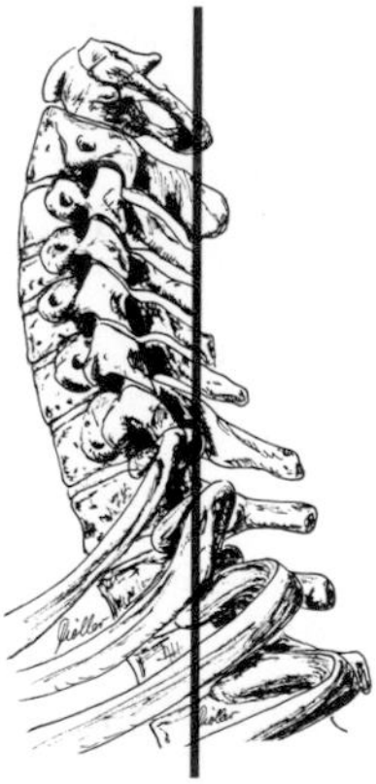

Cranial

Right ☐ Left

Caudal

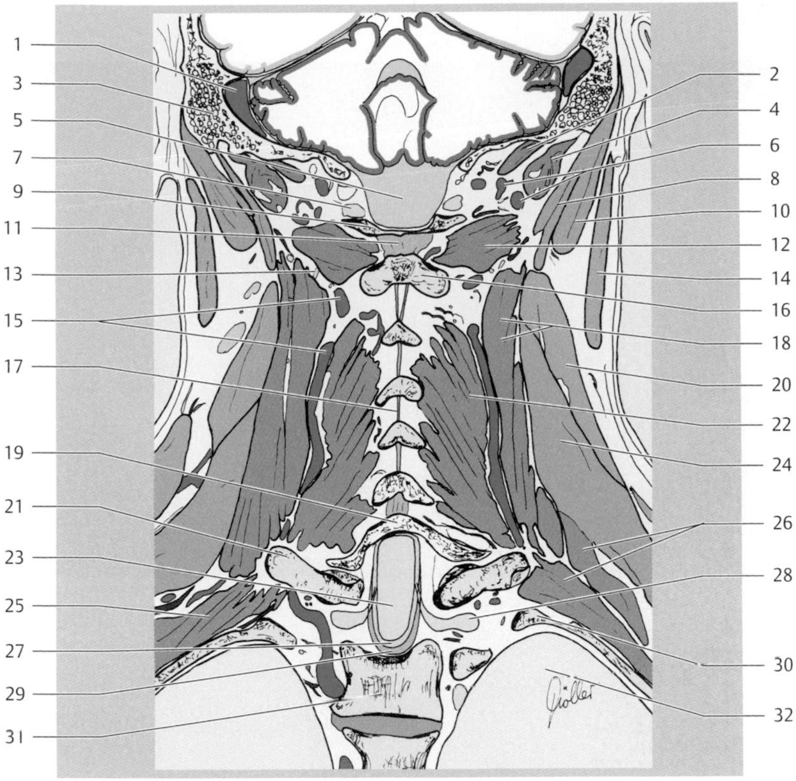

1 Sigmoid sinus
2 Rectus capitis posterior major muscle
3 Mastoid process
4 Obliquus capitis superior muscle
5 Cisterna magna
6 Suboccipital venous plexus
7 Suboccipital nerve
8 Longissimus capitis muscle
9 Atlas (posterior arch)
10 Splenius capitis muscle
11 Nuchal ligament
12 Obliquus capitis inferior muscle
13 Major occipital nerve
14 Sternocleidomastoid muscle
15 Deep cervical vein
16 Spinous process C2
17 Interspinous ligament
18 Semispinalis cervicis muscle
19 Vertebral arch C7
20 Levator scapulae muscle
21 First rib (neck and tubercle)
22 Spinalis cervicis and multifidus muscles
23 Thoracic spinal cord
24 Splenius cervicis muscle
25 Intercostal muscles
26 Scalenus posterior muscle
27 Cerebrospinal fluid in vertebral canal
28 Spinal ganglion T1
29 Spinal dura mater and posterior longitudinal ligament
30 Second rib
31 Second thoracic vertebral body
32 Left lung

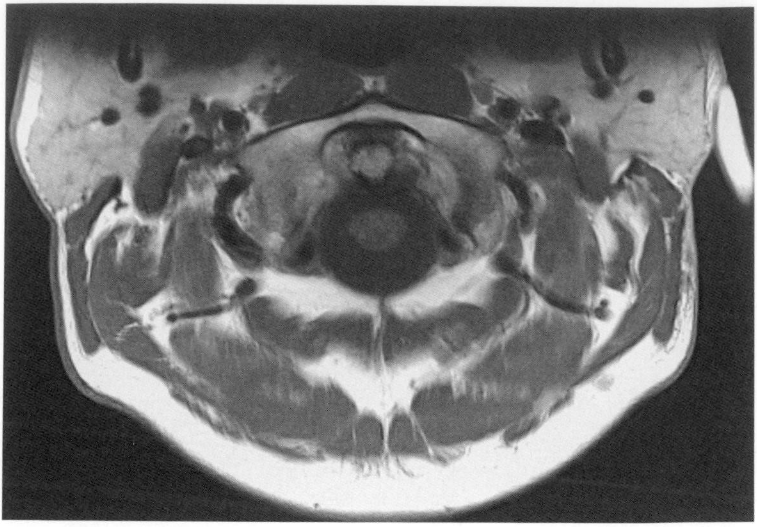

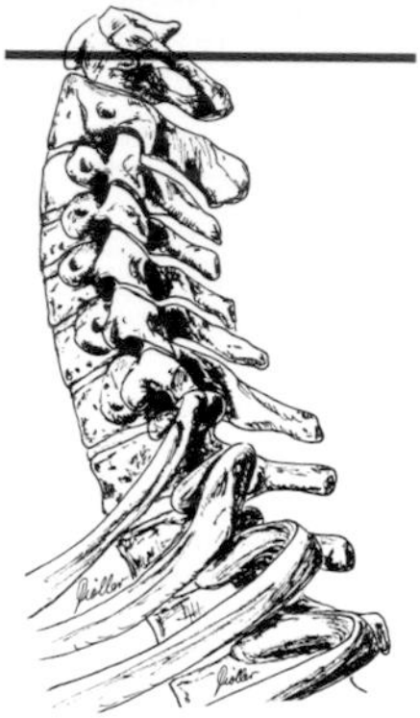

Ventral

Right Left

Dorsal

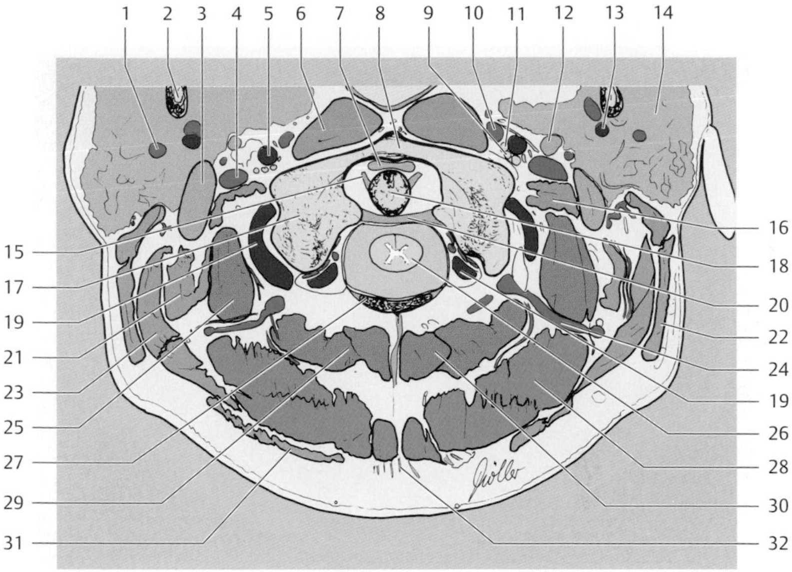

1 Retromandibular vein
2 Mandible
3 Digastric muscle (posterior belly)
4 Internal jugular vein
5 Internal carotid artery
6 Longus capitis muscle
7 Median atlantoaxial joint
8 Atlas (anterior arch)
9 Hypoglossal nerve (XII)
10 Pterygoid venous plexus
11 Vagus nerve (X)
12 Stylohyoid muscle
13 Maxillary artery (mandibular part)
14 Parotid gland
15 Alar ligaments
16 Rectus capitis lateralis muscle
17 Atlas (lateral mass)
18 Dens of axis
19 Vertebral artery
20 Cruciate ligament of atlas (longitudinal bands [= central part] and transverse ligament of atlas [= lateral parts])
21 Longissimus capitis muscle
22 Sternocleidomastoid muscle
23 Splenius capitis muscle
24 Deep cervical vein
25 Obliquus capitis superior muscle
26 Spinal cord
27 Atlas (posterior arch)
28 Semispinalis capitis muscle
29 Rectus capitis posterior major muscle
30 Rectus capitis posterior minor muscle
31 Trapezius muscle
32 Nuchal ligament

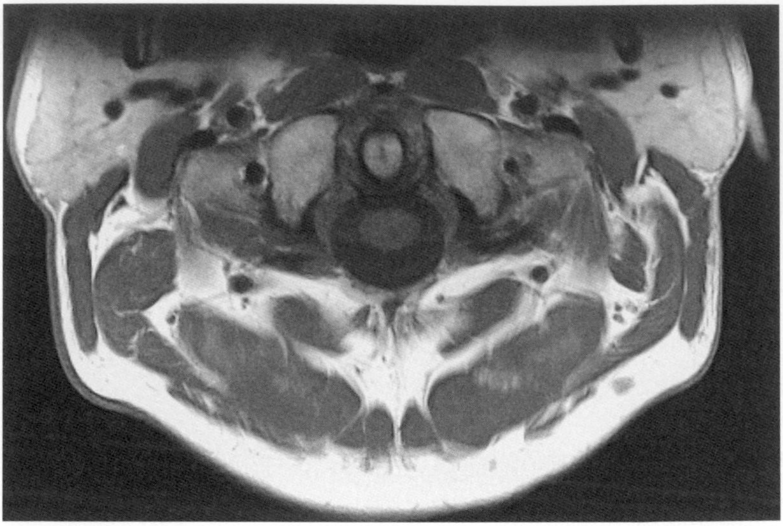

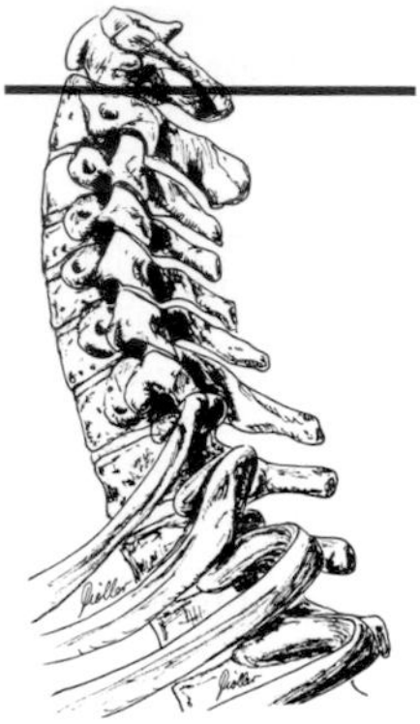

Ventral

Right Left

Dorsal

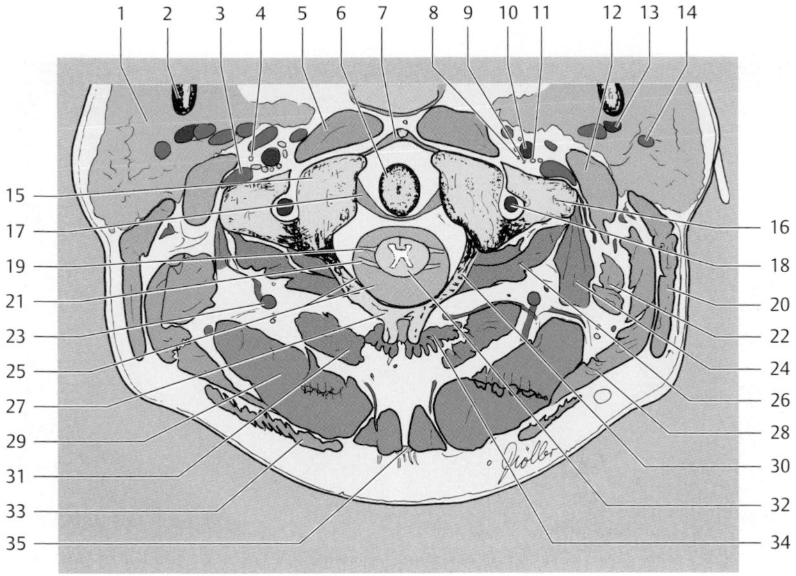

1 Parotid gland
2 Mandible (ramus)
3 Internal jugular vein
4 Glossopharyngeal nerve (IX)
5 Longus capitis muscle
6 Dens of axis
7 Anterior longitudinal ligament
8 Vagus nerve (X)
9 Hypoglossal nerve (XII)
10 Internal carotid artery
11 Accessory nerve (XI)
12 Digastric muscle (posterior belly)
13 Maxillary artery (mandibular part)
14 Retromandibular vein
15 Atlas (lateral mass)
16 Atlas (transverse process)
17 Transverse ligament of atlas
18 Vertebral artery
19 Ventral root
20 Sternocleidomastoid muscle
21 Dorsal root
22 Longissimus capitis muscle
23 Deep cervical vein
24 Obliquus capitis superior muscle
25 Dura mater and cerebrospinal fluid (subarachnoid space)
26 Obliquus capitis inferior muscle
27 Spinous process
28 Splenius capitis muscle
29 Semispinalis capitis muscle
30 Axis (posterior arch)
31 Rectus capitis posterior major muscle
32 Spinal cord
33 Trapezius muscle
34 Rectus capitis posterior minor muscle
35 Nuchal ligament

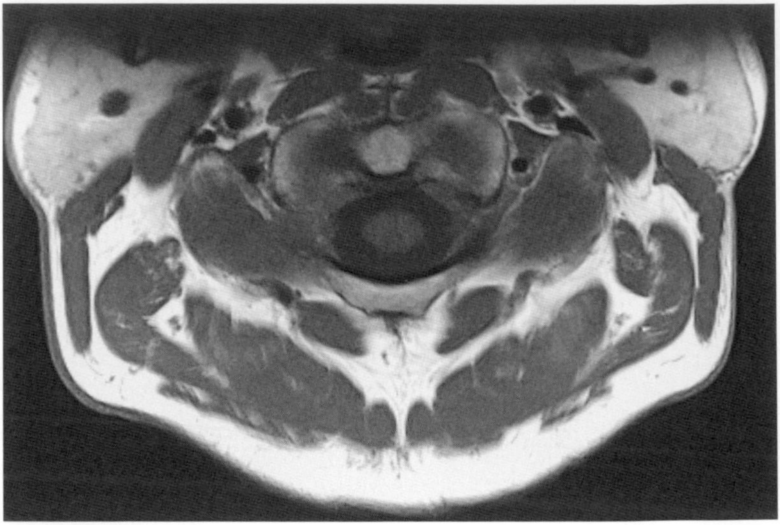

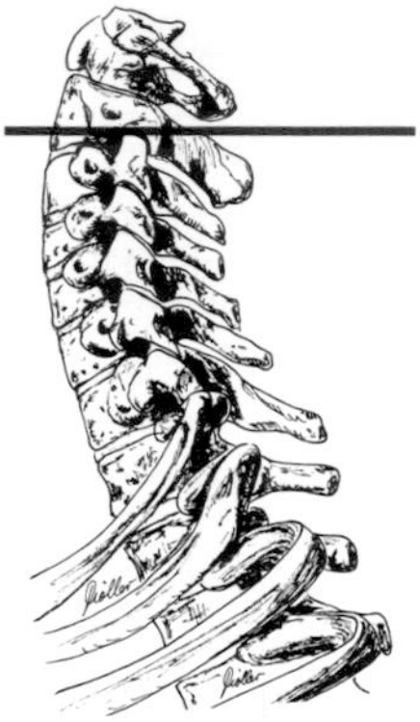

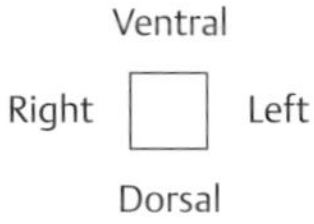
Ventral
Right
Left
Dorsal

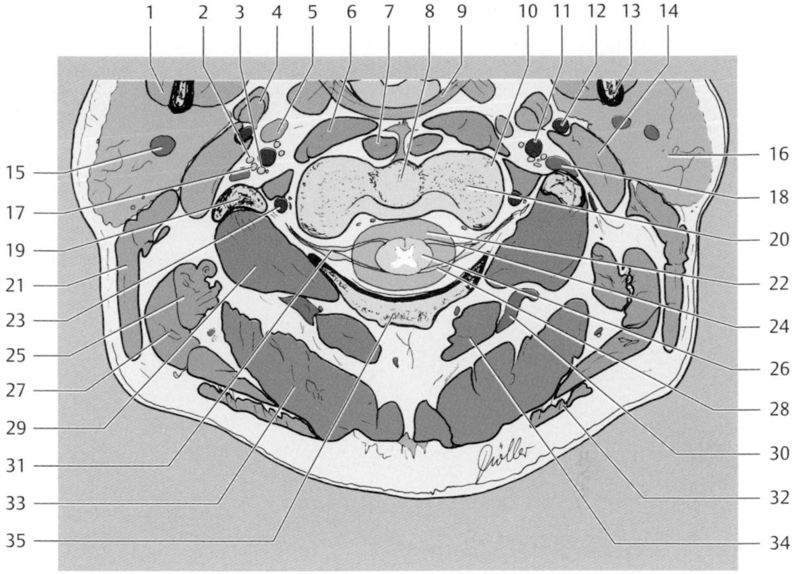

1 Medial pterygoid muscle
2 Vagus nerve (X)
3 Accessory nerve (XI)
4 Styloglossus muscle
5 Stylopharyngeus muscle
6 Longus capitis muscle
7 Longus colli muscle
8 Axis (body)
9 Superior constrictor muscle of pharynx
10 Atlas (articular process)
11 Internal carotid artery
12 External carotid artery
13 Mandible (ramus)
14 Digastric muscle (posterior belly)
15 Retromandibular vein
16 Parotid gland
17 Hypoglossal nerve (XII)
18 Internal jugular vein
19 Atlas (transverse process)
20 Axis (body)
21 Sternocleidomastoid muscle
22 Premedullary subarachnoid space
23 Vertebral artery
24 Ventral root of spinal nerve C2
25 Longissimus capitis muscle
26 Spinal cord
27 Splenius capitis muscle
28 Dorsal root of spinal nerve C2
29 Obliquus capitis inferior muscle
30 Deep cervical vein
31 Spinal ganglion (nerve root)
32 Trapezius muscle
33 Semispinalis capitis muscle
34 Rectus capitis posterior major muscle
35 Axis (posterior arch)

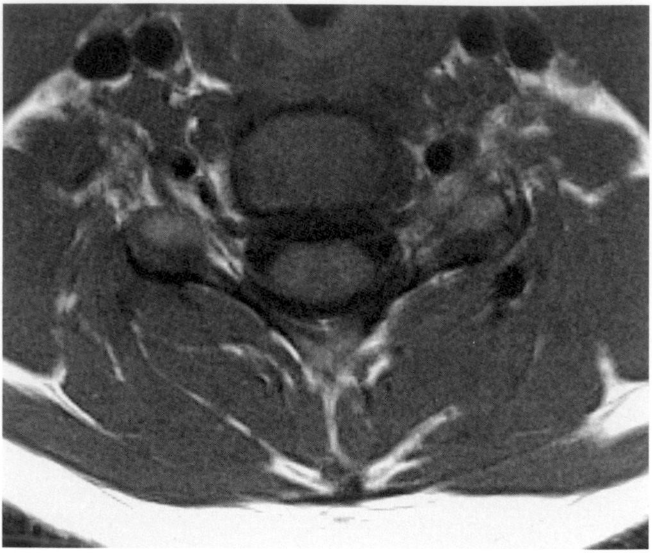

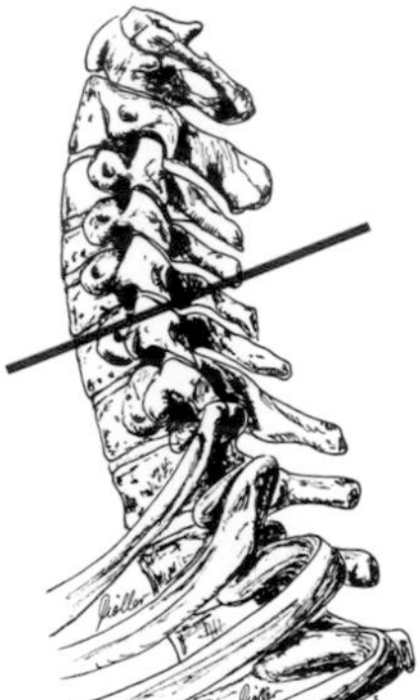

Ventral

Right ☐ Left

Dorsal

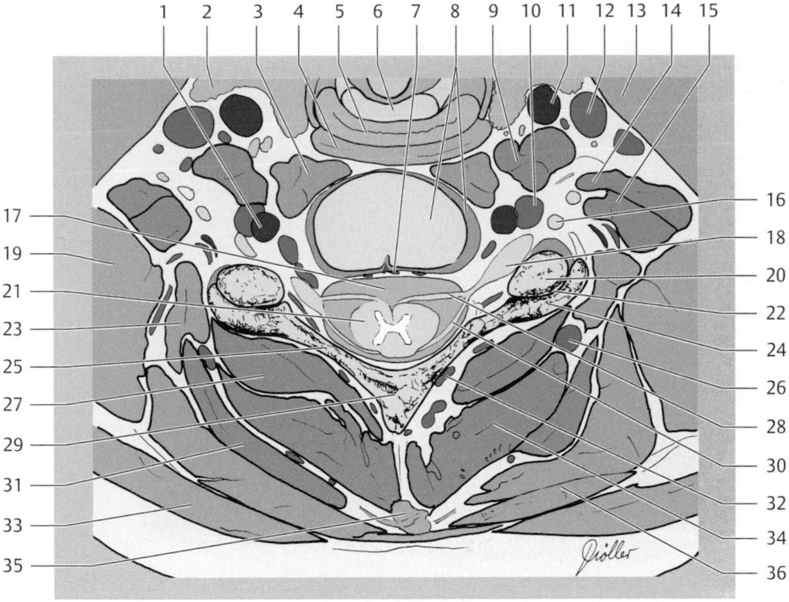

1 Vertebral artery
2 Thyroid gland
3 Longus colli muscle
4 Superior constrictor muscle of pharynx
5 Esophagus
6 Cricoid cartilage
7 Basivertebral veins
8 Cervical vertebral body C5 and intervertebral space C5/C6
9 Scalenus anterior muscle
10 Vertebral vein
11 Common carotid artery
12 Internal jugular vein
13 Sternocleidomastoid muscle
14 Scalenus medius muscle
15 Scalenus posterior muscle
16 Spinal nerve C5
17 Premedullary subarachnoid space
18 Spinal ganglion (nerve root)
19 Levator scapulae muscle
20 Superior articular process
21 Spinal cord
22 Zygapophysial joint
23 Longissimus cervicis muscle
24 Inferior articular process
25 Posterior vertebral arch C5 (lamina)
26 Deep cervical vein
27 Spinalis cervicis and multifidus muscles
28 Ventral root C6
29 Spinous process
30 Dorsal root C6
31 Semispinalis capitis muscle
32 Posterior external vertebral venous plexus
33 Trapezius muscle
34 Semispinalis cervicis muscle
35 Nuchal ligament
36 Splenius capitis muscle

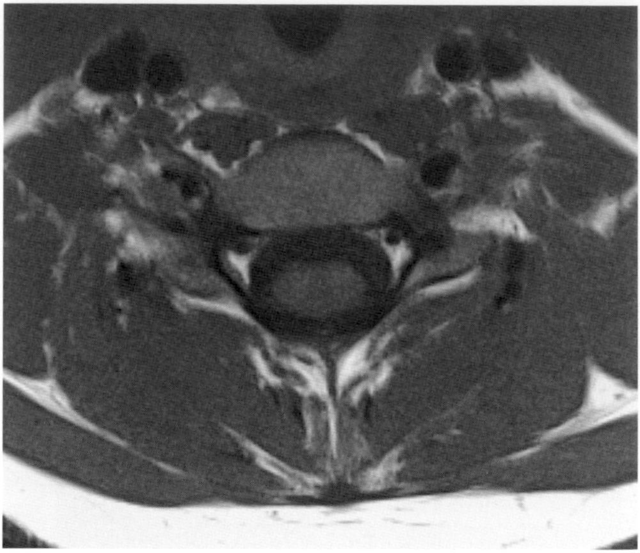

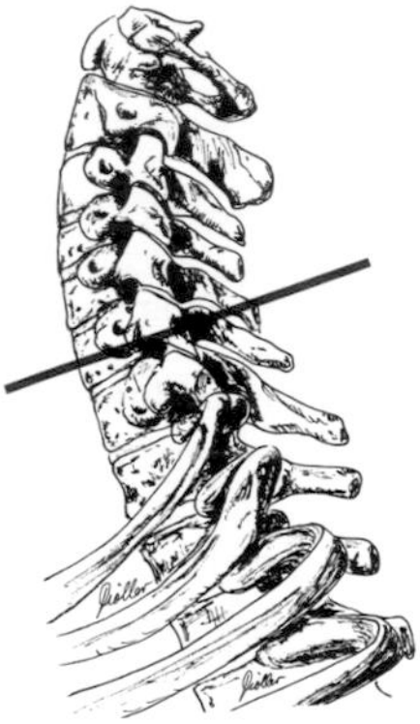

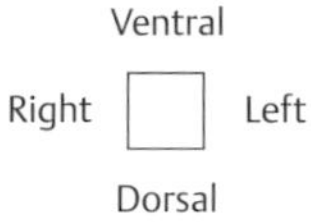
Ventral
Right
Left
Dorsal

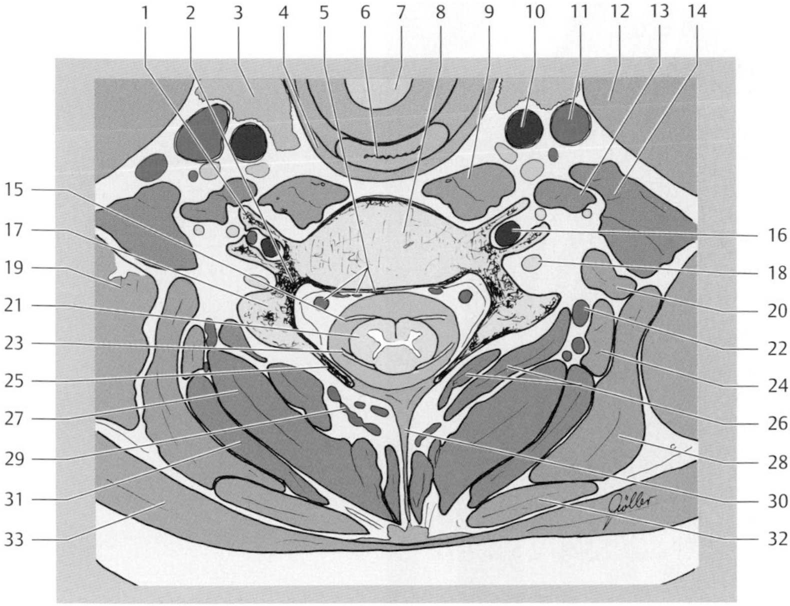

1 Transverse process
2 Pedicle of vertebral arch
3 Thyroid gland
4 Superior constrictor muscle of pharynx
5 Anterior internal vertebral venous plexus
6 Esophagus
7 Larynx
8 Cervical vertebral body C6
9 Longus colli muscle
10 Common carotid artery
11 Internal jugular vein
12 Sternocleidomastoid muscle
13 Scalenus anterior muscle
14 Scalenus medius muscle
15 Ventral root C7
16 Vertebral artery
17 Articular process
18 Spinal nerve C6
19 Levator scapulae muscle
20 Longissimus capitis muscle
21 Spinal cord
22 Deep cervical vein
23 Dorsal root C7
24 Longissimus cervicis muscle
25 Posterior vertebral arch C6 (lamina)
26 Spinalis cervicis and multifidus muscles
27 Semispinalis cervicis muscle
28 Splenius cervicis muscle
29 Posterior external vertebral venous plexus
30 Nuchal ligament
31 Splenius capitis muscle
32 Rhomboid minor muscle
33 Trapezius muscle

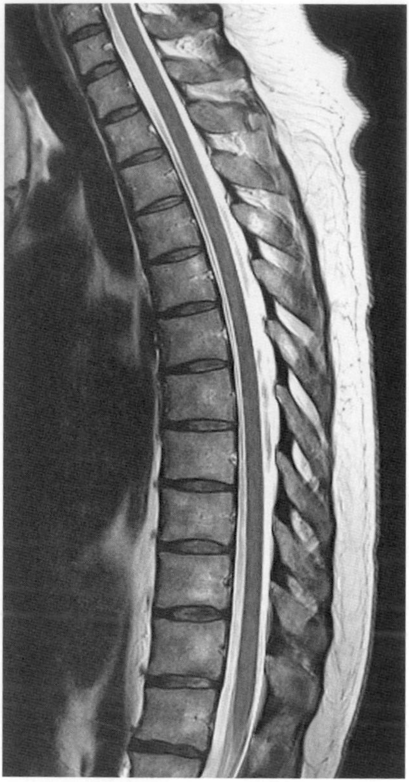

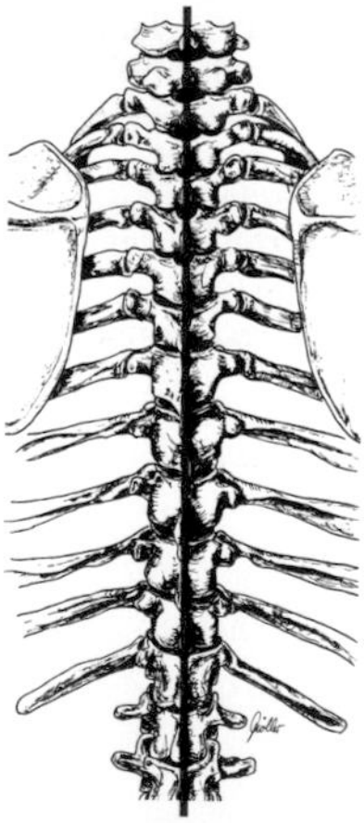

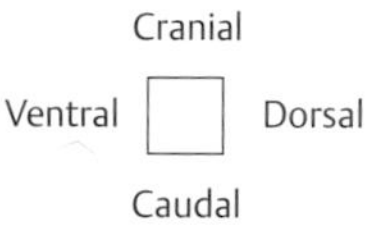
Cranial
Ventral
Dorsal
Caudal

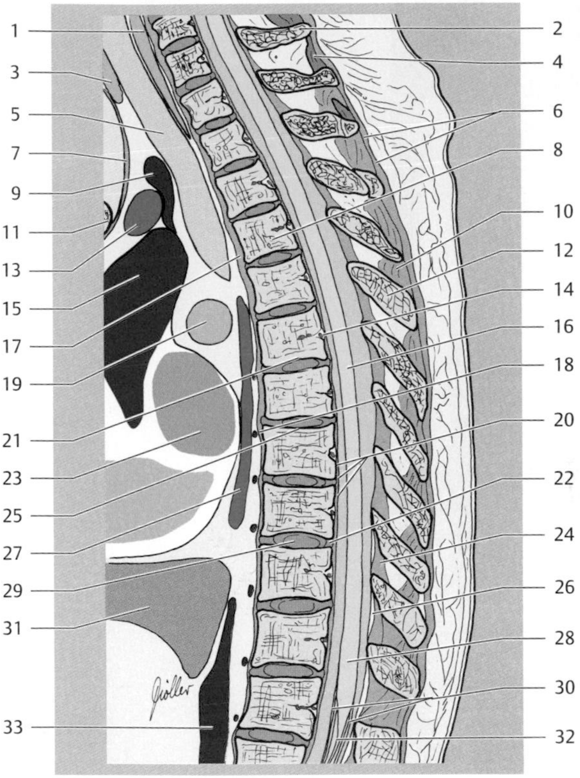

1 Esophagus
2 Vertebra prominens C7
3 Thyroid gland
4 Interspinalis cervicis muscle
5 Trachea
6 Supraspinous ligament
7 Sternohyoid muscle
8 Thoracic vertebral body T4
9 Brachiocephalic trunk
10 Interspinous ligament
11 Sternum (manubrium)
12 Spinous process
13 Left brachiocephalic vein
14 Basivertebral vein
15 Ascending aorta
16 Thoracic spinal cord
17 Anterior longitudinal ligament
18 Posterior intercostal artery
19 Pulmonary artery
20 Posterior longitudinal ligament
21 Inferior vertebral end plate T6
22 Intervertebral disk T9–10 (anulus fibrosus)
23 Left atrium
24 Ligamentum flavum
25 Superior vertebral end plate T7
26 Epidural fatty tissue (retrospinal fat)
27 Azygos vein
28 Conus medullaris
29 Intervertebral disk T9–10 (nucleus pulposus)
30 Cauda equina
31 Liver
32 Filum terminale
33 Descending aorta

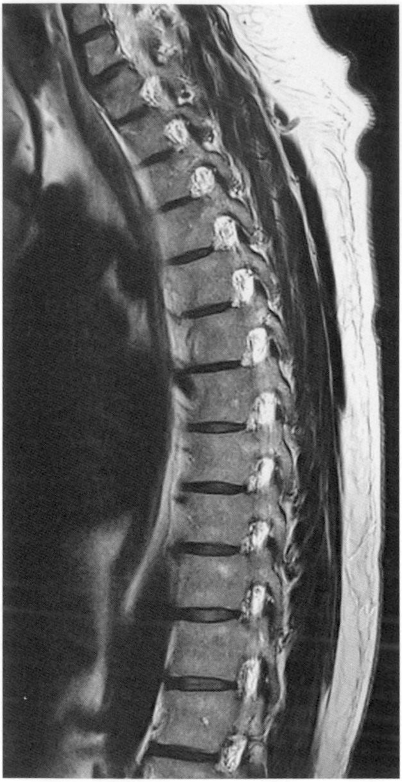

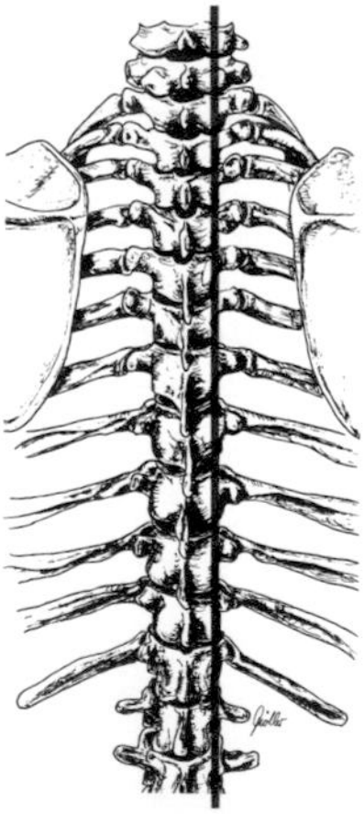

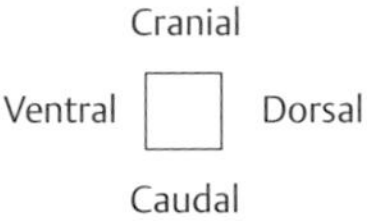

1 Trachea
2 Splenius cervicis muscle
3 Thyroid gland
4 Semispinalis capitis muscle
5 Sternohyoid muscle
6 Serratus posterior superior muscle
7 Esophagus
8 Rhomboid major muscle

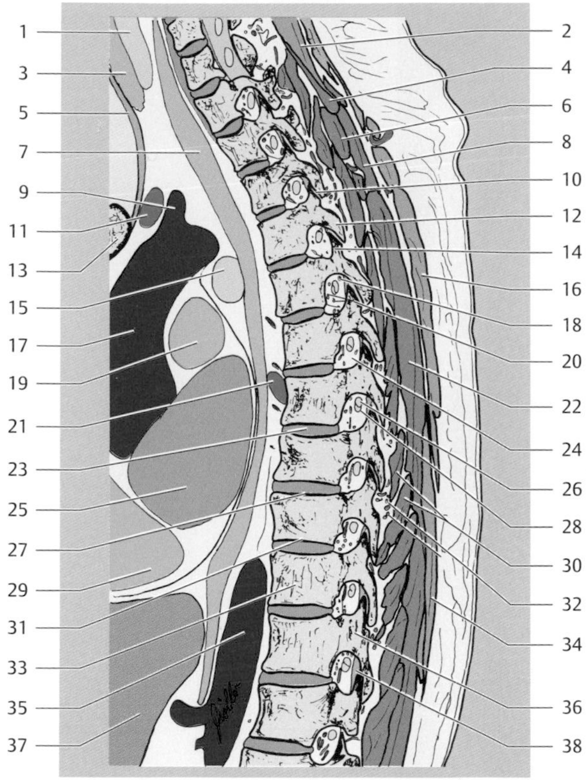

9 Brachiocephalic trunk
10 Zygapophysial joint T3–4
11 Left brachiocephalic vein
12 Inferior articular process T4
13 Sternum (manubrium)
14 Superior articular process T5
15 Left main bronchus
16 Trapezius muscle
17 Ascending aorta
18 Posterior intercostal artery (spinal branch)
19 Pulmonary artery
20 Intervertebral vein
21 Hemi-azygos vein
22 Erector spinae muscle
23 Intervertebral disk T7–8
24 Intervertebral foramen
25 Left atrium
26 Spinal ganglion (dorsal root)
27 Superior vertebral end plate T9
28 Spinal ganglion (ventral root)
29 Right atrium
30 Multifidus and semispinalis thoracis muscles
31 Inferior vertebral end plate T9
32 Posterior external vertebral venous plexus
33 Thoracic vertebral body T10
34 Latissimus dorsi muscle
35 Descending aorta
36 Pedicle of vertebral arch (interarticular portion)
37 Liver
38 Ligamentum flavum

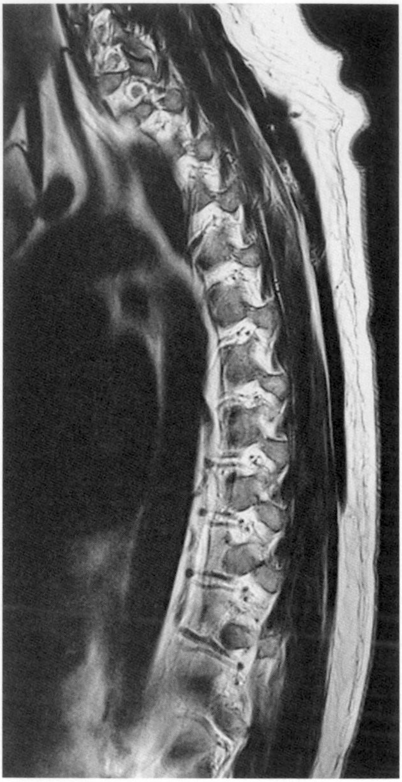

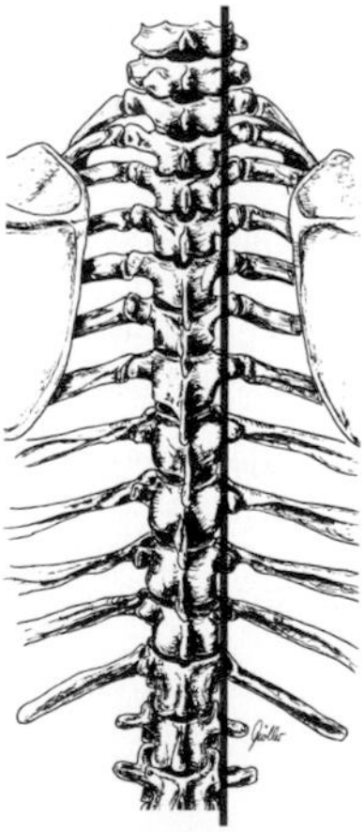

Cranial

Ventral Dorsal

Caudal

1 Thyroid gland
2 Splenius cervicis muscle
3 Longus capitis muscle
4 Spinalis cervicis muscle and multifidus muscle

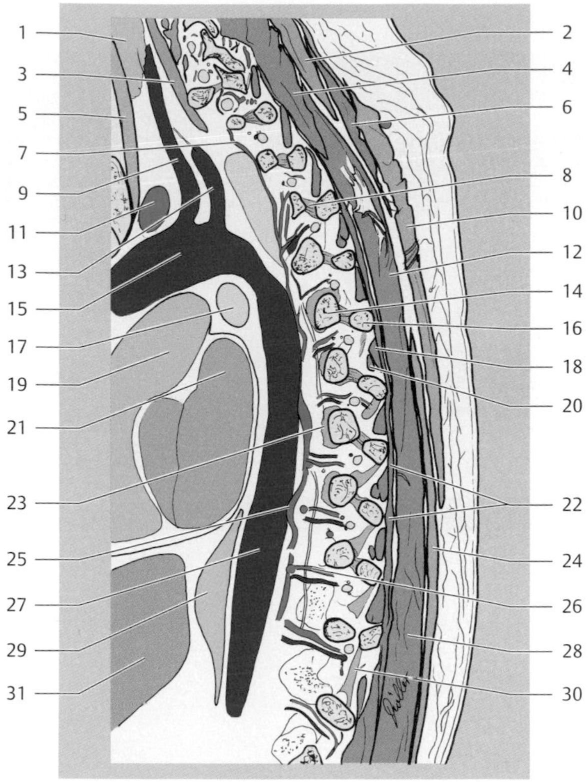

5 Sternohyoid muscle
6 Rhomboid major muscle
7 Accessory hemi-azygos vein
8 Costotransverse ligament
9 Common carotid artery
10 Trapezius muscle
11 Left brachiocephalic vein
12 Spinalis thoracis muscle
13 Subclavian artery
14 Sixth rib (head)
15 Aortic arch
16 Transverse process T6
17 Left main bronchus
18 Intertransversarius muscle
19 Pulmonary trunk
20 Rotatores muscles
21 Left atrium
22 Multifidus muscle
23 Radiate ligament of head of rib T8
24 Latissimus dorsi muscle
25 Hemi-azygos vein
26 Posterior intercostal artery and vein (dorsal branch)
27 Descending aorta
28 Erector spinae muscle
29 Esophagus
30 Superior costotransverse ligament
31 Liver

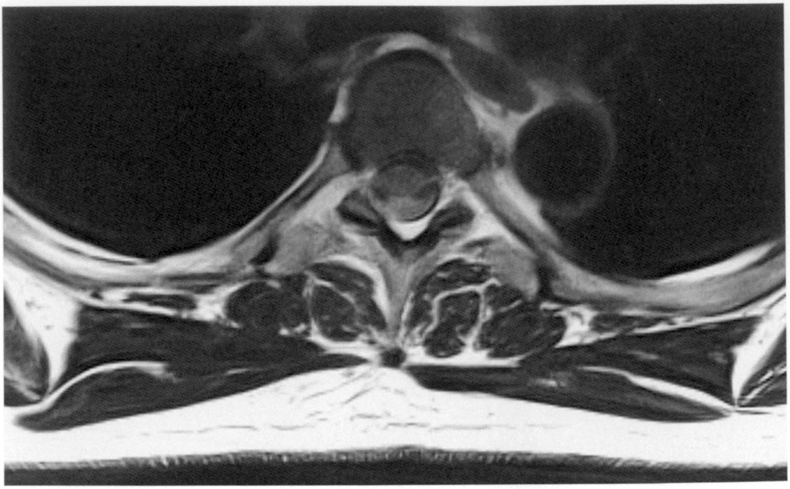

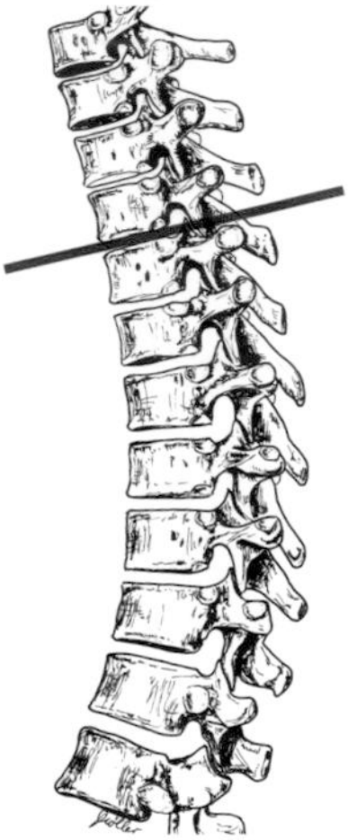

Ventral

Right Left

Dorsal

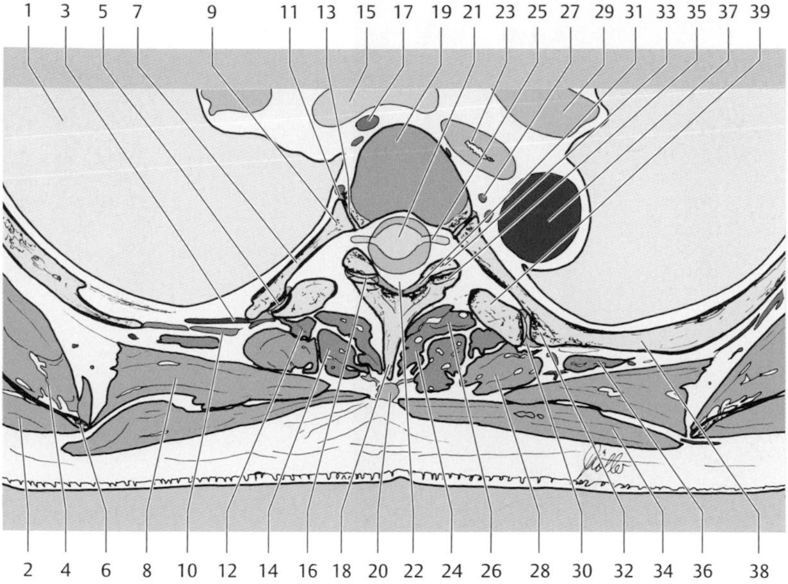

1 Right lung
2 Infraspinatus muscle
3 Intercostal artery
4 Subscapularis muscle
5 Costotransverse joint
6 Scapula
7 Rib (neck)
8 Rhomboid major muscle
9 Fifth rib (head)
10 Intercostal muscles
11 Radiate ligament of head of rib
12 Rotatores thoracis muscles
13 Joint of head of rib
14 Semispinalis thoracis muscle
15 Trachea (bifurcation)
16 Zygapophysial joint T4–5
17 Azygos vein
18 Spinous process
19 Intervertebral disk T4–5
20 Supraspinous ligament
21 Thoracic spinal cord
22 Retrospinal fatty triangle (epidural fat)
23 Esophagus
24 Spinalis thoracis muscle
25 Spinal ganglion
26 Multifidus muscle
27 Accessory hemi-azygos vein
28 Longissimus thoracis muscle
29 Left pulmonary artery
30 Costotransverse ligament (lateral)
31 Ligamentum flavum
32 Fifth rib (tubercle)
33 Superior articular process T5
34 Trapezius muscle
35 Inferior articular process T4
36 Iliocostalis thoracis muscle
37 Descending aorta
38 Fifth rib (body)
39 Transverse process T5

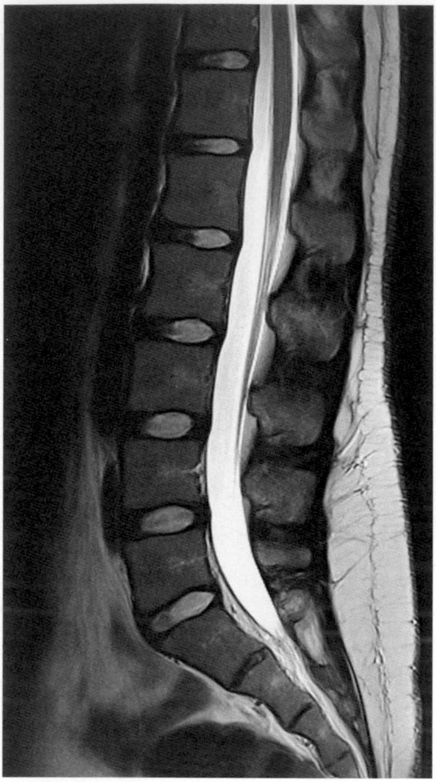

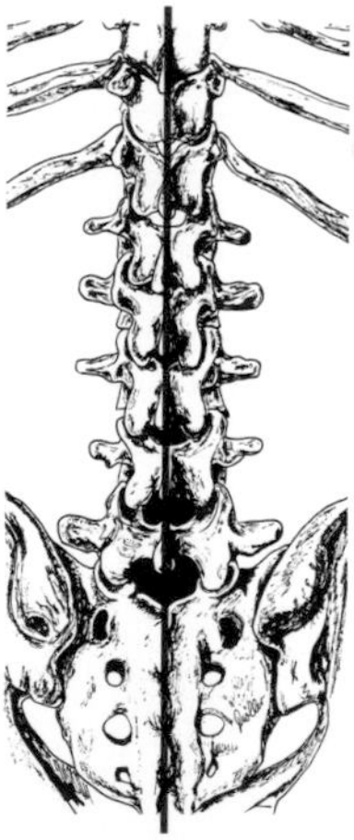

Cranial

Ventral Dorsal

Caudal

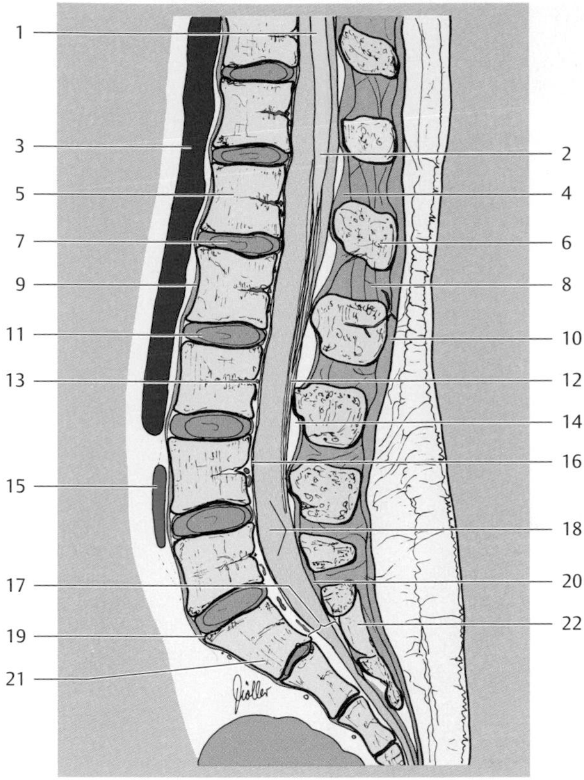

1 Spinal cord
2 Conus medullaris
3 Abdominal aorta
4 Ligamentum flavum
5 Lumbar vertebral body L1
6 Spinous process L1
7 Intervertebral disk L1–2 (nucleus pulposus)
8 Interspinous ligament
9 Anterior longitudinal ligament
10 Supraspinous ligament
11 Intervertebral disk L2–3 (anulus fibrosus)
12 Cauda equina
13 Basivertebral vein
14 Epidural fatty tissue
15 Left common iliac vein
16 Posterior longitudinal ligament
17 Sacral canal
18 Thecal sac (lumbar cistern)
19 Promontory of sacrum
20 Dura mater
21 Sacrum (S1)
22 Median sacral crest

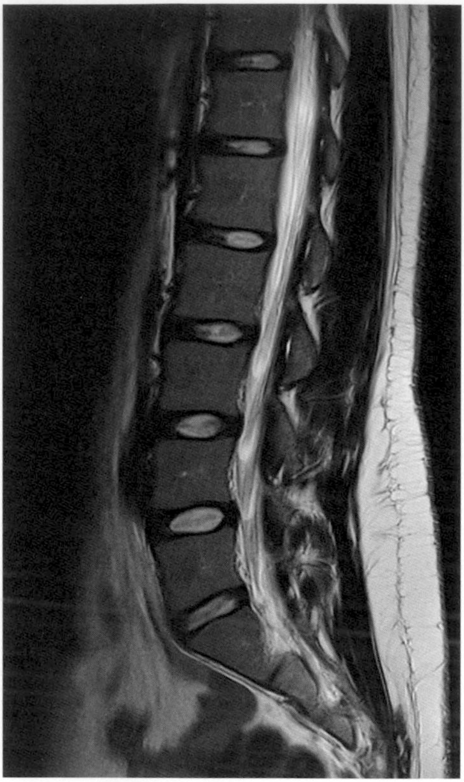

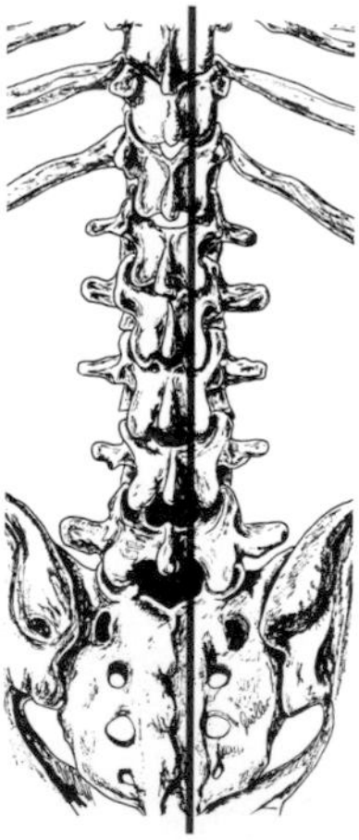

Cranial

Ventral Dorsal

Caudal

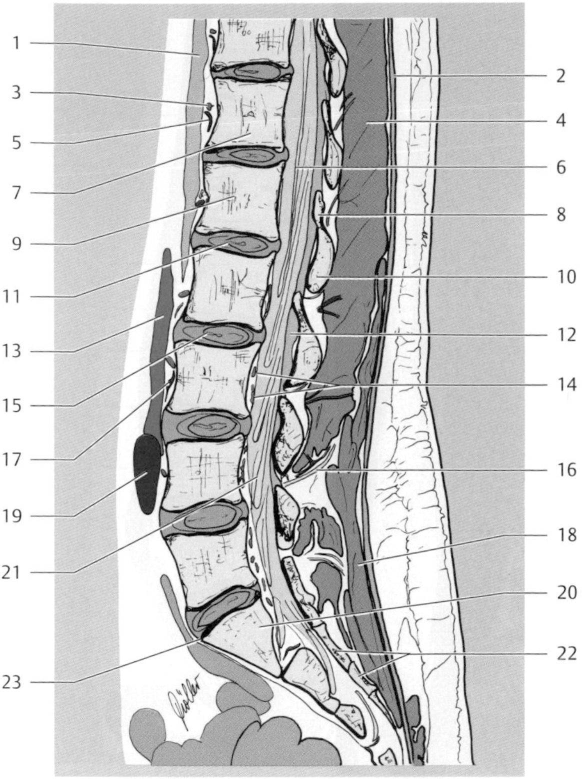

1 Diaphragm (lumbar part)
2 Thoracolumbar fascia
3 Anterior external vertebral venous plexus
4 Erector spinae muscle (spinalis muscle)
5 Posterior intercostal artery
6 Nerve filaments
7 Thoracic vertebral body T12
8 Superior articular process
9 Lumbar vertebral body L1
10 Posterior vertebral arch (lamina)
11 Intervertebral disk L1–2 (nucleus pulposus)
12 Ligamentum flavum
13 Inferior vena cava
14 Anterior internal vertebral venous plexus
15 Intervertebral disk L2–3 (anulus fibrosus)
16 Lumbar artery and nerve (medial cutaneous branch of dorsal branch)
17 Lumbar artery
18 Multifidus muscle
19 Common iliac artery
20 Sacrum (S1)
21 Spinal ganglion
22 Median sacral crest
23 Promontory of sacrum

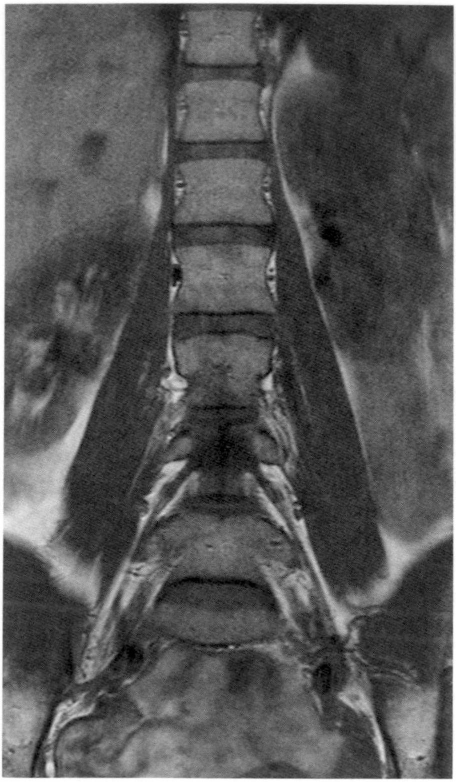

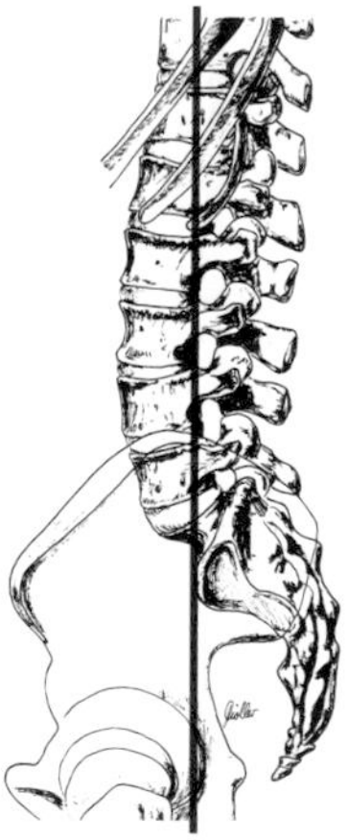

Cranial

Right Left

Caudal

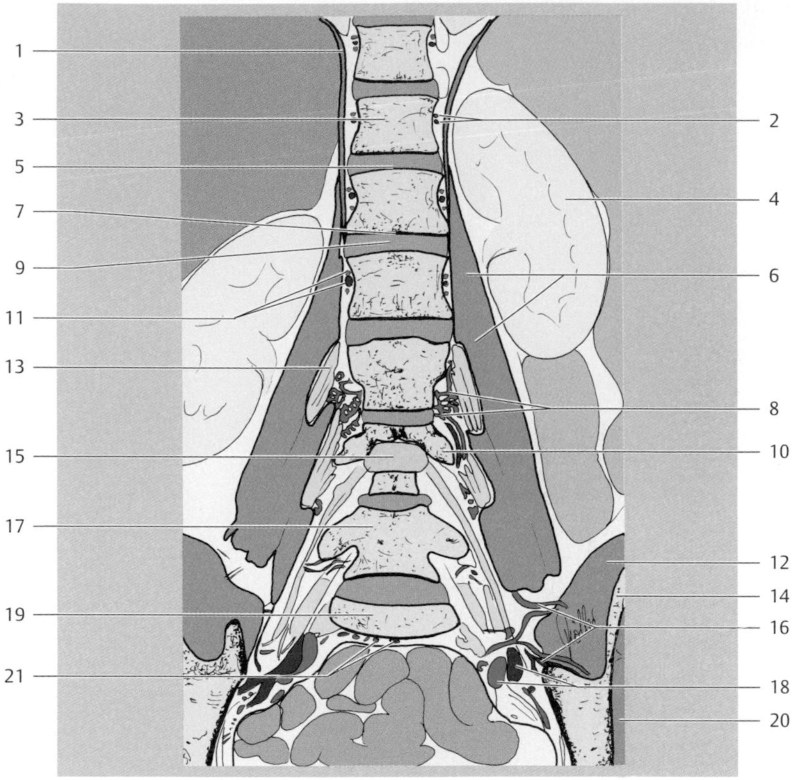

1 Diaphragm (lumbar part)
2 Posterior intercostal artery and vein
3 Thoracic vertebral body T12
4 Left kidney
5 Superior vertebral end plate L1
6 Psoas major muscle
7 Inferior vertebral end plate L1
8 Anterior external vertebral venous plexus
9 Intervertebral disk L1–2 (anulus fibrosus)
10 Transverse process L4
11 Lumbar artery and vein
12 Iliacus muscle
13 Lumbar plexus
14 Ilium
15 Thecal sac (lumbar cistern)
16 Iliolumbar artery and vein
17 Lumbar vertebral body L5
18 Internal iliac artery and vein
19 Promontory of sacrum
20 Gluteus medius muscle
21 Median sacral artery and vein

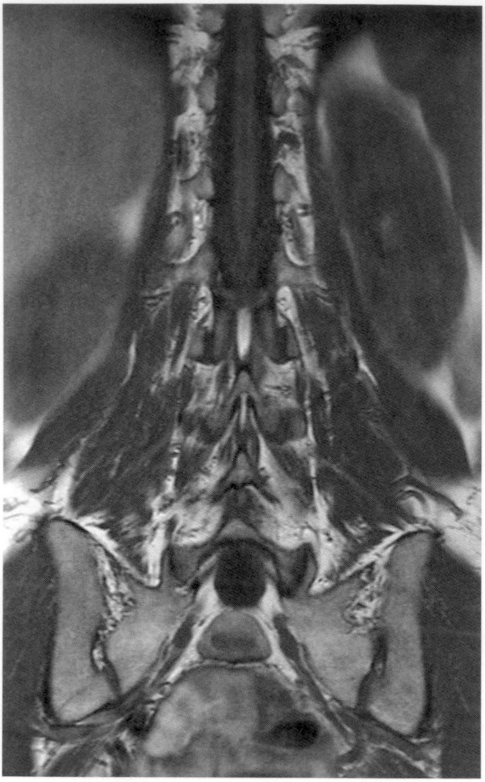

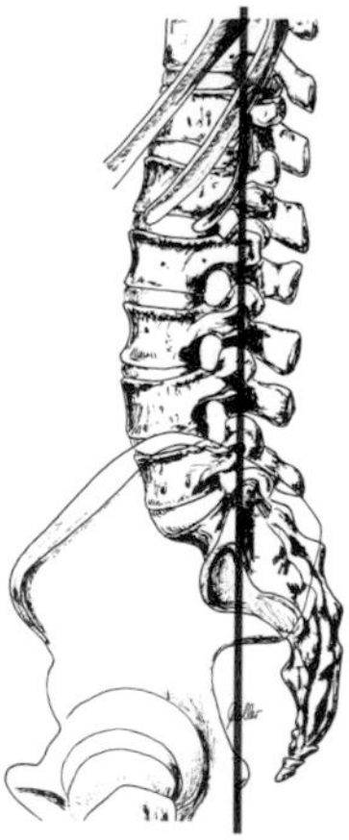

Cranial

Right Left

Caudal

1 Right lung
2 Cerebrospinal fluid in thecal sac (lumbar cistern)
3 Pedicle of vertebral arch T12
4 Psoas major muscle
5 Twelfth rib (head)
6 Conus medullaris

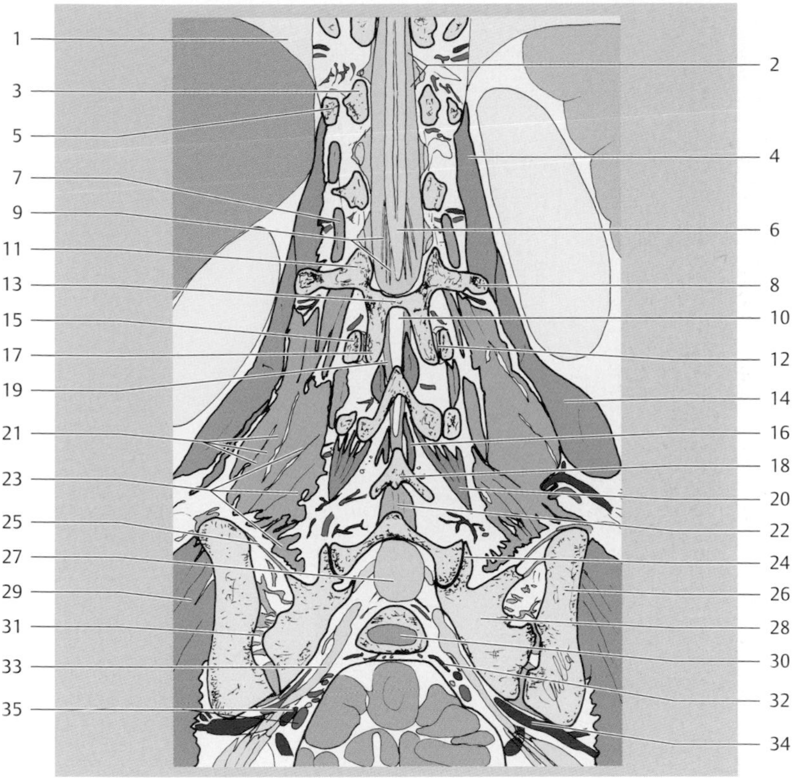

7 Intertransversarius muscle
8 Transverse process L2
9 Cauda equina
10 Posterior epidural fat (retrospinal fat, dorsal fat)
11 Posterior vertebral arch L2 (lamina)
12 Zygapophysial joint
13 Pedicle of vertebral arch L2
14 Quadratus lumborum muscle
15 Superior articular process L3
16 Interspinalis muscle
17 Inferior articular process L2
18 Spinous process L4
19 Ligamentum flavum
20 Multifidus muscle
21 Iliocostalis lumborum muscle
22 Interspinous ligament
23 Longissimus muscle
24 Lumbosacral Zygapophysial joint L5–S1
25 Sacro-iliac ligaments
26 Ilium
27 Thecal sac (lumbar cistern)
28 Sacrum (lateral mass)
29 Gluteus medius muscle
30 Intervertebral space S1–2
31 Sacro-iliac joint
32 Lateral sacral artery and vein
33 Sacral plexus
34 Superior gluteal artery
35 Internal iliac artery and vein

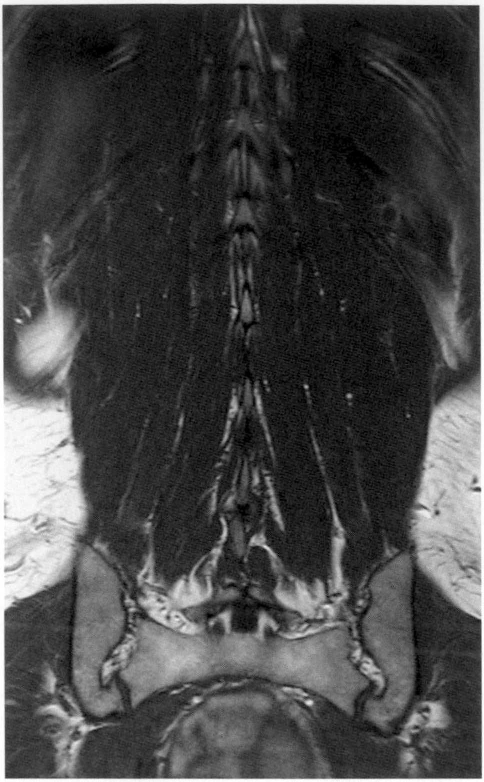

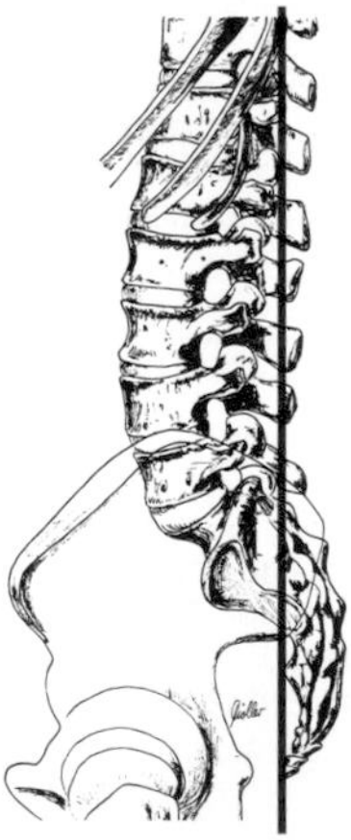

Cranial

Right Left

Caudal

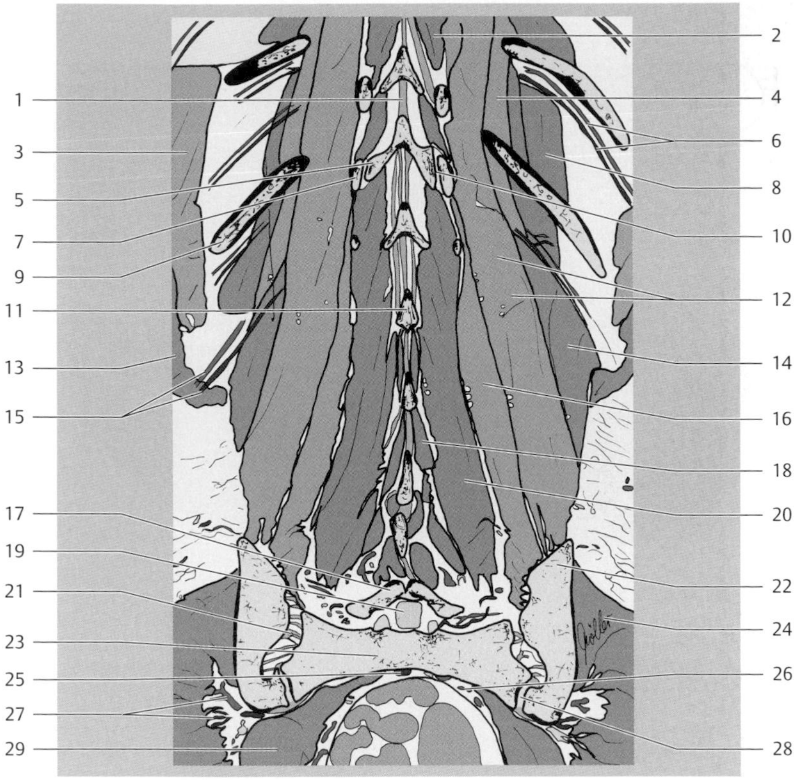

1 Interspinous ligament
2 Spinalis thoracis muscle and rotatores thoracis muscles
3 Serratus anterior muscle
4 Levatores costarum muscles
5 Inferior articular process T12
6 Posterior intercostal artery and vein
7 Superior articular process L1
8 Intercostal muscles
9 Eleventh rib
10 Zygapophysial joint
11 Spinous process L2
12 Iliocostalis lumborum muscle
13 Latissimus dorsi muscle
14 Quadratus lumborum muscle
15 Lumbar artery and vein
16 Longissimus muscle
17 Posterior vertebral arch S1 (lamina)
18 Interspinales lumborum muscles
19 Cerebrospinal fluid in thecal sac (lumbar cistern)
20 Multifidus muscle
21 Sacro-iliac ligaments
22 Ilium
23 Sacrum
24 Gluteus medius muscle
25 Median sacral artery and vein
26 Lateral sacral artery and vein
27 Superior gluteal artery and vein
28 Sacro-iliac joint
29 Piriformis muscle

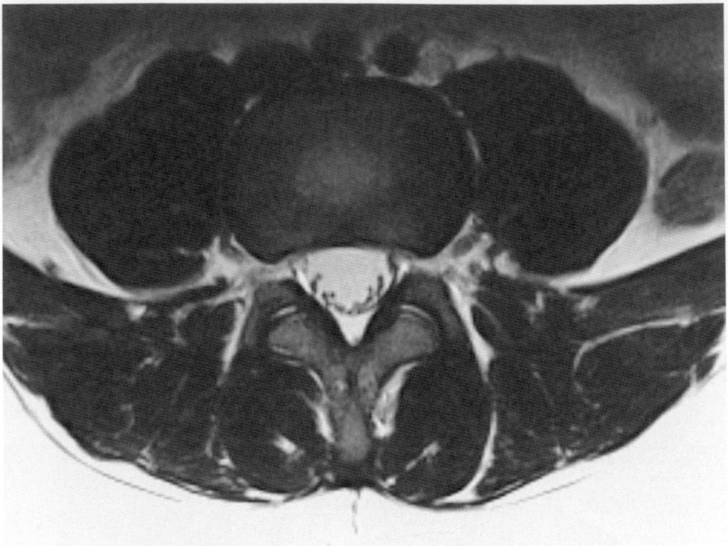

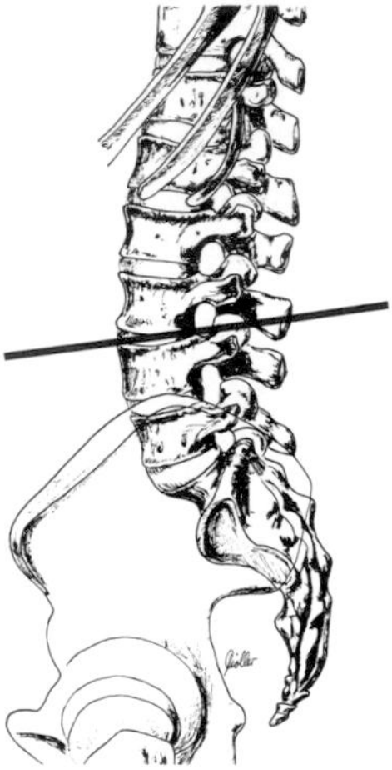

Ventral

Right ☐ Left

Dorsal

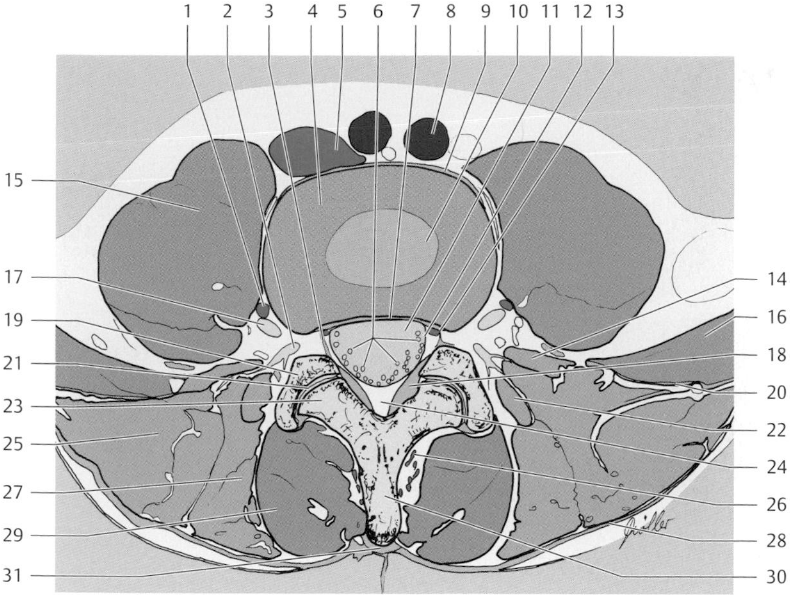

1 Lumbar vein
2 Spinal nerve (dorsal ramus)
3 Neuroforaminal ligament
4 Intervertebral disk L3–4 (anulus fibrosus)
5 Inferior vena cava (confluence)
6 Nerve filaments
7 Posterior longitudinal ligament
8 Left common iliac artery
9 Anterior longitudinal ligament
10 Intervertebral disk L3–4 (nucleus pulposus)
11 Thecal sac (lumbar cistern)
12 Spinal dura mater
13 Internal vertebral venous plexus
14 Erector spinae muscle (lateral tract: intertransversarii laterales muscles)
15 Psoas major muscle
16 Quadratus lumborum muscle
17 Spinal ganglion L3
18 Ligamentum flavum
19 Inferior articular process
20 Thoracolumbar fascia (anterior layer)
21 Zygapophysial joint
22 Erector spinae muscle (lateral tract: intertransversarii mediales muscles)
23 Superior articular process
24 Epidural fatty tissue (retrospinal/dorsal fatty triangle)
25 Erector spinae muscle (lateral tract: iliocostalis lumborum muscle)
26 Posterior external vertebral venous plexus
27 Erector spinae muscle (lateral tract: longissimus muscle)
28 Thoracolumbar fascia (posterior layer)
29 Erector spinae muscle (medial tract: multifidus muscle)
30 Spinous process
31 Supraspinous ligament

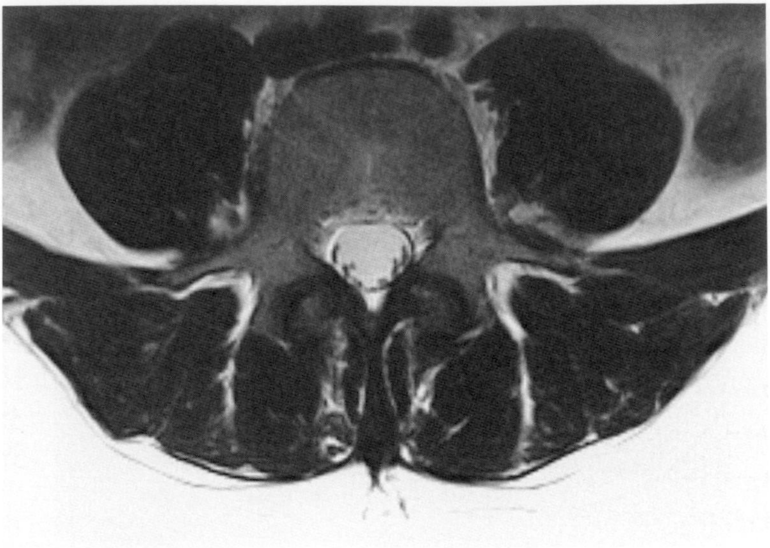

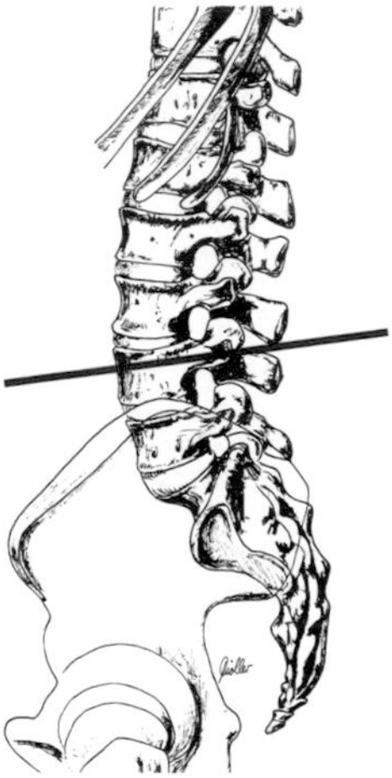

Ventral

Right Left

Dorsal

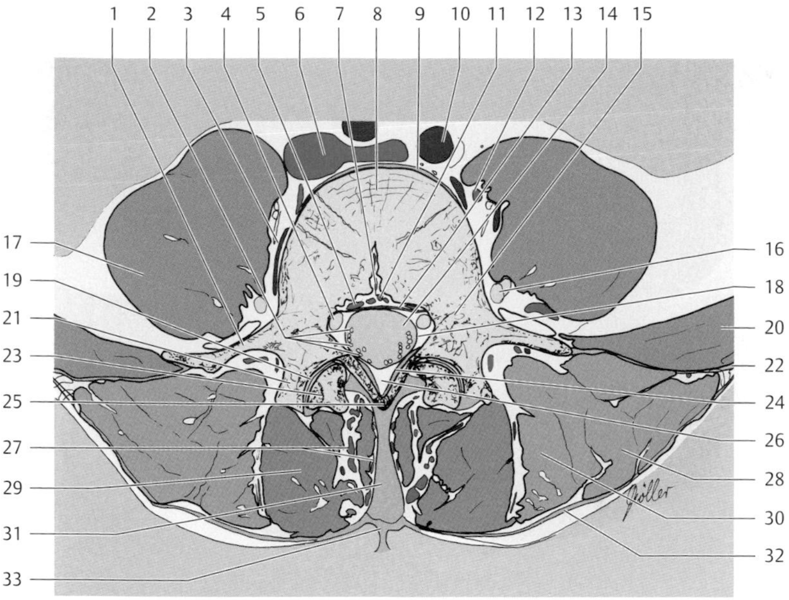

1 Costal process
2 Nerve filaments
3 Lumbar artery
4 Spinal ganglion in lateral recess L4
5 Anterior internal vertebral venous plexus
6 Inferior vena cava (confluence)
7 Nutrient foramen
8 Lumbar vertebral body L4
9 Anterior longitudinal ligament
10 Left common iliac artery
11 Basivertebral vein
12 Ascending lumbar vein
13 Posterior longitudinal ligament
14 Thecal sac (lumbar cistern)
15 Interarticular portion L4
16 Spinal ganglion L3
17 Psoas major muscle
18 Spinal dura mater
19 Zygapophysial joint
20 Quadratus lumborum muscle
21 Superior articular process
22 Thoracolumbar fascia (anterior layer)
23 Inferior articular process
24 Ligamentum flavum
25 Posterior vertebral arch (lamina)
26 Epidural fatty tissue (retrospinal/dorsal fatty triangle)
27 Posterior external vertebral venous plexus
28 Erector spinae muscle (lateral tract: iliocostalis lumborum muscle)
29 Erector spinae muscle (medial tract: multifidus muscle)
30 Erector spinae muscle (lateral tract: longissimus muscle)
31 Interspinous ligament
32 Thoracolumbar fascia (posterior layer)
33 Supraspinous ligament

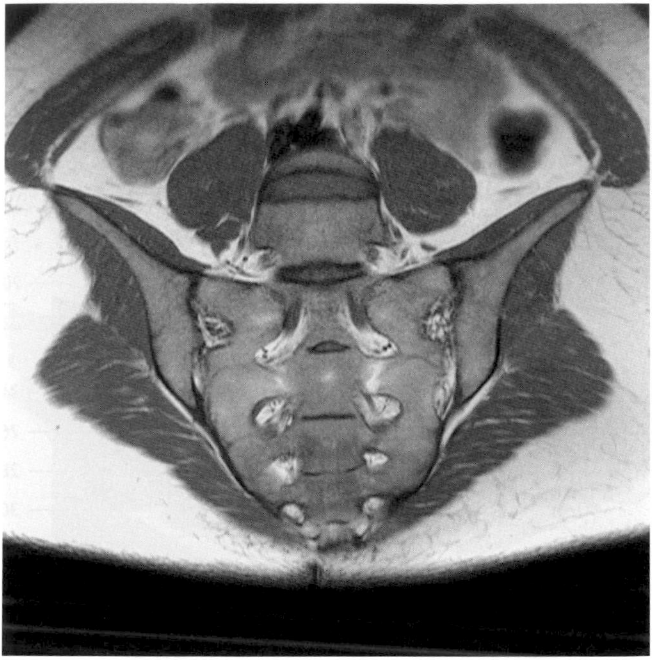

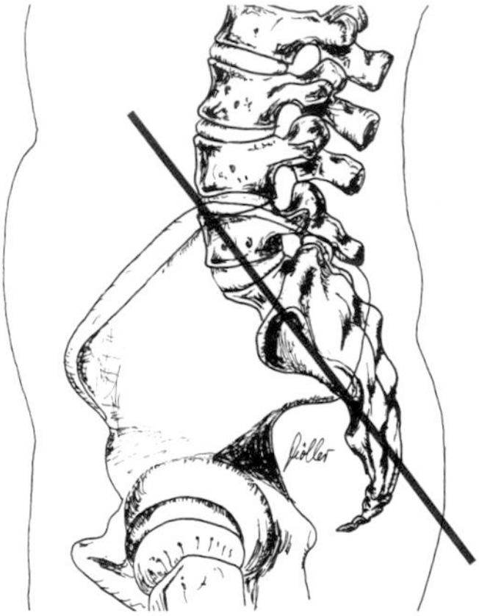

Cranial
Ventral

Right Lateral

Left Lateral

Caudal
Dorsal

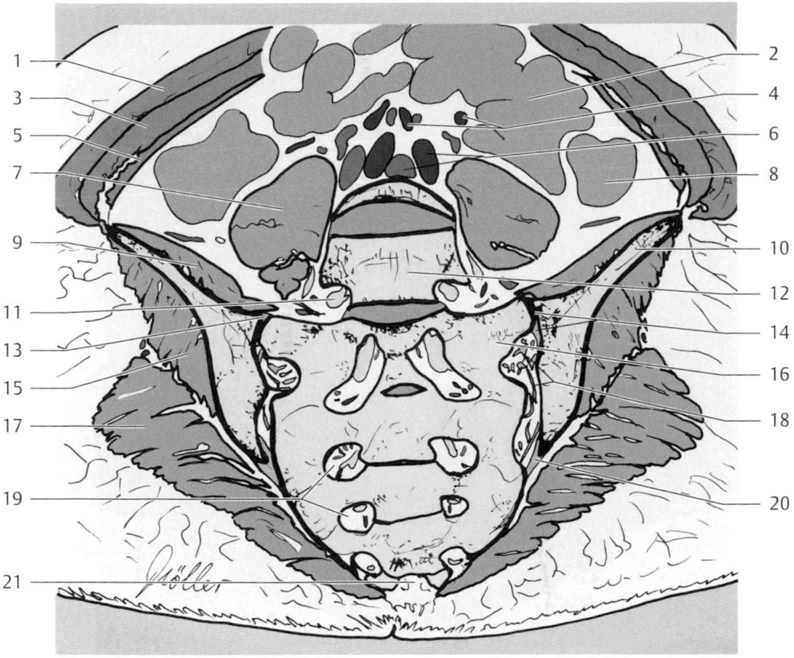

1 External oblique (abdominal) muscle
2 Ileum
3 Internal oblique (abdominal) muscle
4 Iliac arteries
5 Transversus abdominis muscle
6 Common iliac artery and vein (left)
7 Psoas major muscle
8 Descending colon
9 Iliacus muscle
10 Ilium (wing)
11 Fifth lumbar nerve root
12 Fifth lumbar vertebra (body)
13 Anterior sacro-iliac ligaments
14 Sacro-iliac joint
15 Gluteus medius muscle
16 Sacrum (lateral mass)
17 Gluteus maximus muscle
18 Interosseous sacro-iliac ligaments
19 Anterior sacral foramina
20 Posterior sacro-iliac ligaments
21 Sacral canal

Index

B

U

V

W

Z